EXERCISE AND SPORTS CARDIOLOGY

Volume 1: Cardiac Adaptations and Environmental Stress During Exercise

Sports Medicine for the Orthopedic Resident
edited by Julie A Neumann, Donald T Kirkendall and Claude T Moorman, III
ISBN: 978-981-4324-65-6
http://www.worldscientific.com/worldscibooks/10.1142/7936

Sports medicine including care of the athlete can be an exciting and unique aspect of ortho-
paedic residency training and beyond. Many of us develop a lifelong passion for helping
athletes get back to competition, but, at times, the challenge of mastering sports medicine
can be daunting. This book is written by health care providers specifically to help residents
prepare to effectively manage conditions seen in athletes both on the field and in clinical
situations.

Sports Innovation, Technology and Research
edited by Dominic F L Southgate, Peter R N Childs and Anthony M J Bull
ISBN: 978-1-78634-041-2
http://www.worldscientific.com/worldscibooks/10.1142/Q0012

Sports Innovation, Technology and Research gives an insight into recent research and
design projects at Imperial College London. It presents the on-going development of a
diverse range of areas from elite rowing performance to impact protection to sporting
amenities in communities.

Also included are descriptions of some of the latest innovations that have been
developed as part of the Rio Tinto Sports Innovation Challenge, an initiative that tasked
engineering students to design, build and implement Paralympic and other sporting equipment. It offers a glimpse at the breadth of creativity that can be achieved when human
centred design is applied to an area such as disabled sport. It also shows the potential that
design and engineering have to contribute to healthy lifestyles and the generation of whole
new sporting domains.

This book will be valuable for anyone with an interest in sports technology, including those
in industry, academia, sports organisations and athletes themselves.

EXERCISE AND SPORTS CARDIOLOGY

Volume 1: Cardiac Adaptations and Environmental Stress During Exercise

Editors

Paul D Thompson, MD
Antonio B Fernandez, MD

Hartford Hospital, USA & University of Connecticut, USA

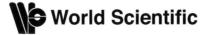

World Scientific

NEW JERSEY · LONDON · SINGAPORE · BEIJING · SHANGHAI · HONG KONG · TAIPEI · CHENNAI · TOKYO

Published by

World Scientific Publishing Europe Ltd.

57 Shelton Street, Covent Garden, London WC2H 9HE

Head office: 5 Toh Tuck Link, Singapore 596224

USA office: 27 Warren Street, Suite 401-402, Hackensack, NJ 07601

Library of Congress Cataloging-in-Publication Data

Names: Thompson, Paul D. (Cardiologist), editor. | Fernandez, Antonio B., editor.
Title: Exercise and sports cardiology / edited by Paul D Thompson (Hartford Hospital, USA &
    University of Connecticut, USA), Antonio B Fernandez (Hartford Hospital, USA &
    University of Connecticut, USA).
Other titles: Exercise and sports cardiology (World Scientific) | Based on (work):
    Exercise and sports cardiology. 2001.
Description: New Jersey : World Scientific, 2017. | Based on Exercise and sports cardiology /
    editor, Paul D. Thompson. New York : McGraw-Hill, Medical Pub. Div., c2001. |
    Includes bibliographical references.
Identifiers: LCCN 2016055370| ISBN 9781786341556 (hc-set : alk. paper) |
    ISBN 9781786342560 (hc : v. 1 : alk. paper) | ISBN 9781786342584 (hc : v. 2 : alk. paper) |
    ISBN 9781786342607 (hc : v. 3 : alk. paper)
Subjects: | MESH: Cardiovascular Diseases--prevention & control | Sports--physiology |
    Adaptation, Physiological | Cardiovascular Physiological Phenomena |
    Exercise--physiology | Risk Assessment | Sports Medicine--methods
Classification: LCC RC1236.H43 | NLM WG 141 | DDC 612.1/7088796--dc23
LC record available at https://lccn.loc.gov/2016055370

British Library Cataloguing-in-Publication Data
A catalogue record for this book is available from the British Library.

For any available supplementary material, please visit
http://www.worldscientific.com/worldscibooks/10.1142/Q0045#t=suppl

Desk Editors: Dr. Sree Meenakshi Sajani/Mary Simpson

Typeset by Stallion Press
Email: enquiries@stallionpress.com

Printed in Singapore

Foreword

The first edition of Paul Thompson's textbook of *Exercise and Sports Cardiology*, published 15 years ago, was paradigm shifting. Written with the cardiologist in mind, it pulled together for the first time, the clinical science required to understand how to take care of athletes with heart disease, and implement exercise-based interventions in both patients and healthy individuals. Indeed, this book could be said to have formed the core knowledge base for the nascent field of Sports Cardiology; the European Society of Cardiology established the first special interest group in sports cardiology in 2005 and the American College of Cardiology followed suit in 2011. This second edition of the Sports Cardiologist's "bible" reflects the tremendous growth in the specialty itself. It now includes 3 separate volumes divided into the physiology (cardiac adaptations to exercise and environmental stress) and pathophysiology (specific diseases in athletes) of exercise, as well as some of the controversial aspects of the field (exercise risks, cardiac arrhythmias, and unusual problems in athletes). The list of authors represents both the established and rising leaders in the field of sports cardiology, and each chapter has been meticulously edited by Dr. Thompson, widely recognized as the "father" of sports cardiology. This trilogy should be on the book shelves (and at the fingertips) of every cardiologist who sees athletes, whether or not they consider themselves members of the sports cardiology community.

Benjamin D. Levine

Department of Internal Medicine
University of Texas Southwestern Medical Center
Dallas, TX, USA

Preface

This preface to *Exercise and Sports Cardiology* must start with a story. The story is about Paul's correspondence with John Naughton, MD, the originator of the Naughton stress test protocol, when he was a 3rd year medical student and trying to run fast enough to qualify for the 1972 US Olympic Marathon Trials. He had decided that he wanted to be an exercise cardiologist, whatever that was, so wrote to Dr. Naughton to inquire how he could create such a career. Dr. Naughton's reply was essentially to "work hard to be the best medical student, the best internal medical resident, and the best cardiology fellow that you can be. Then become an exercise cardiologist because if you are not a solid clinician first, you will never be respected especially as an exercise cardiologist."

Exercise and Sports Cardiology is written to provide the general clinical knowledge that Dr. Naughton knew one would need and also to provide the specific clinical expertise required by the increasing number of cardiologists who have developed, or are developing, careers in sports and exercise cardiology.

The book is divided into 3 volumes. The first volume of this trilogy describes the development of sports cardiology as a field, reviews normal exercise physiology, and examines the cardiac response to different exercises and environmental stress. This first volume includes chapters on altitude and heat stress as well as on diving medicine. The second volume addresses how to manage exercise and sports participation in individuals with specific cardiac conditions. This includes chapters on hypertension, atherosclerosis, coronary anomalies, heart failure, and valvular heart disease. The third volume is dedicated to the risks of exercise, cardiac arrhythmias, and unusual problems with exercise and in athletes. This volume reviews arrhythmias, the issue of myocardial fibrosis in athletes, thromboembolism, and genetic diseases. It also includes a chapter on preparing for cardiac emergencies in various sporting venues.

We hope that you find this textbook as educational to read as we did in preparing it. Its breadth should make it useful to the many practitioners of sports medicine, but especially to those cardiologists specializing in sports cardiology. Sports cardiology has emerged as a subspecialty of cardiology, something we would not have predicted a decade ago. We hope that this book will serve as a resource for those clinicians practicing in this field.

We will like to thank the contributing authors for their efforts and their tolerance of our editing, our families for allowing us to focus on this work, and to Jennifer Brough, Koe Shi Ying, Jane Sayers, and the staff of World Scientific Publishing for their editorial assistance and for publishing this text.

Paul D. Thompson
Antonio B. Fernandez

Contents

Summary

Cardiac problems in athletic individuals are rare, but when they occur can be devastating. This volume, the first of the *Exercise and Sports Cardiology* trilogy, looks at the athlete's capabilities to adapt to different exercises and environmental stress. It provides a definitive review of the development of sports cardiology, followed by studies of an athlete's coronary, electrophysiological, and cardiac structural adaptations to exercise and sustained training. It concludes with a look at the increased stress on the heart as a result of high altitude training, swimming and diving, and higher temperatures.

Based on their earlier work *Exercise and Sports Cardiology* (2001), editors Paul Thompson and Antonio Fernandez have provided an updated, improved text for cardiologists, physicians, coaches, trainers and medical students, and researchers with a comprehensive go-to reference for modern day concerns in the expanding field of sports cardiology research and treatment.

Chapter 1

Growth and Development of Sports and Exercise Cardiology in the US

Christine E. Lawless

Sports Cardiology Consultants LLC
Chicago, IL, USA

History of Sports Cardiology

Long-standing beliefs in the health benefits of exercise

Sports Cardiology is considered a new and rapidly evolving subspecialty in medicine[1,2]; but its roots can be traced back to the 5th century BC. Ancient Greek physicians were among the first to recognize and promote the health benefits of exercise. Herodicus (5th century BC), often referred to as "The Father of Sports Medicine," had a unique background as both a sports teacher and a physician, which allowed him to combine both disciplines for the benefit of his patients.[3] Considering bad health to be the result of imbalance between nutrition and physical activity, Herodicus recommended a strict diet and regular athletic training to his patients. In fact, he routinely prescribed that his patients walk from Athens to Megara, a distance of over 20 mi. Herodicus taught, and in turn, influenced Hippocrates (460–370 BC), the "Father of Western Medicine." Hippocrates, too, often promoted athletic training, and included a chapter on it in his book "Regimens in Health."[4] Hippocratic medicine, including the promotion of exercise for its health benefits, influenced medical school curriculums through the late 1700s. Contemporary epidemiologic research has since confirmed this long-held belief that regular exercise confers health benefits and longevity.[5]

Cardiovascular risks of exercise

Similarly, exercise-related sudden cardiac events can also be traced back to antiquity. Legend has it that in 490 BC, the Athenian courier Pheidippides (530–490 BC) collapsed and died after running 24 mi from Marathon to Athens to announce a Greek victory over Persia.[6] Historians note that he probably ran a total of 150 mi (or more) over the days preceding his collapse.[6] Widely felt to represent the first recorded episode of exercise-related sudden cardiac death (SCD), at least one author questions whether Pheidippides actually did die that day, and suggests there may be some confusion between the Pheidippides story and that of Eucles, a courier who, some 50 years later, ran a similar distance and did die.[7] Nonetheless, these collapses were among the first to suggest that exercise could serve as a trigger for a sudden cardiac event.

The contemporary risk of exercise began to be quantified in the late '70s and early '80s. Reports from Opie,[8] Maron,[9] and Thompson[10] described the clinical profiles of small numbers of athletes who died suddenly during sporting activity. Later, Thompson reported SCD was seven times more likely during jogging than at rest and estimated an annual SCD incidence of 1:15,240 among healthy joggers.[11] Siscovick (in 1984) reported a risk of SCD/sudden cardiac arrest (SCA) of 1:18,000 for previously healthy men, with the greatest risk for the habitually least active subjects.[12] In 1993, Mittleman[13] and Willich[14] showed that vigorous exercise increases the risk of acute myocardial infarction, and that the risk was greatest for the physically least active. Studies of cross-country skiers and endurance cyclists have shown that while SCD risk is increased DURING events, long-term risk of SCD is actually decreased compared to the general population.[15–17] Collectively, these data imply that while exercise serves as a short-term trigger for cardiac events, long-term athletic participation actually protects against such events. Younger athletes were studied in 1995. Using data compiled by the National Center for Catastrophic Sports Injury Research, Van Camp estimated the risk of SCD among high school and college athletes as 1:133,000 in males, and 1:770,000 in females.[18] Contemporary epidemiologic studies have challenged these findings, and suggest that the risk of SCD in young athletes is highly variable, dependent upon age, sex, ethnicity, level of play, and sport.[19–23] Other risks of long-term participation in sports include atrial fibrillation,[24] acute myocardial stunning after endurance events,[25] and adverse right ventricular remodeling.[26]

Athletic adaptation (athlete's heart)

The concept that regular exercise could lead to cardiac enlargement surfaced in the late 19th century. In 1892, Sir William Osler wrote: "In the process of training, the getting wind as it is called, is largely a gradual increase in the capability of the heart.... The large heart of athletes may be due to the prolonged use of their muscles, but no man becomes a great runner or oarsman who has not naturally a capable if not a large heart."[27] Autopsy studies in animals at that time showed differences in heart size between wild animals compared to domesticated controls.[28] In 1899, the Swedish physician Henschen first introduced the term "athlete's heart" in the literature.[29] Using only cardiac percussion to estimate heart size in cross-country skiers, Henschen proposed that cardiac enlargement was due to both dilation and hypertrophy, and that the dilation was symmetrical (both left and right). As radiographs became available, it was demonstrated that cardiothoracic ratios ≥0.50 were more common in athletes.[30] Not being able to distinguish between cardiomegaly due to pathology and that from athletic adaptation, concern surfaced that chronic training and competition actually resulted in pathology, and could potentially shorten athletes' lifespans. As modern methods of defining athletic adaptation came into practice, this concern gradually dissipated, but has not been eliminated.

Morganroth (in 1975), first described the echocardiographic features of athletic adaptation.[31] In 1982, when Italian law mandated all competitive athletes undergo preparticipation screening with ECG, researchers seized the opportunity to accumulate significant amounts of data in athletic populations. Pelliccia and colleagues demonstrated that athletic adaptation varied according to gender, size, age, and type of sport.[32] Black athletes, underrepresented in early studies of athletic adaptation, have now been studied early in the 21st century, and their unique athletic adaptations described.[33–36]

As technology and research have progressed, further details of the athlete's heart have been described. These include the limits of athletic right ventricular (RV) enlargement,[26] and use of advanced echocardiographic indices, such as strain and tissue Doppler, to differentiate adaptation from pathology.[37–39] Beyond chamber size and thickness, electrophysiologic gray zones have been identified[2]; and athlete ECG interpretation criteria have been proposed and refined.[40–42] Cardiac MRI has shown unexpected myocardial scarring in some athletes, but its significance remains uncertain.[43]

Era of ECG screening

In 1971, Italy enacted legislation requiring National-caliber Italian athletes to undergo preparticipation physical examination (PPE) consisting of family and personal history, physical examination, resting 12-lead ECG, and limited exercise testing (Montoye step test). Additional tests, such as echocardiography, 24-hour ambulatory Holter monitoring, or submaximal exercise testing, were performed on subjects who had positive findings at the initial evaluation. This approach was deemed responsible for an 89% reduction in athlete SCD over a 25-year period,[44] prompting the European Society of Cardiology (ESC), the International Olympic Committee (IOC), and the Fédération Internationale de Football Association (FIFA, soccer's governing body) to recommend that ECG screening be performed prior to sports participation in all athletes.[40,45,46] These powerful endorsements have served to drive the adoption of ECG screening practices in many countries throughout the world.

In the US, adoption of ECG-based screening has been selective, and somewhat polarizing. Notwithstanding European enthusiasm, major US cardiology organizations have not supported the mandatory ECG movement. In 2014, the American Heart Association (AHA) and American College of Cardiology (ACC) concluded that "mandatory and universal mass screening with 12-lead ECGs in large general populations of young healthy people 12–25 years of age (including on a national basis in the US) to identify genetic/congenital and other cardiovascular abnormalities is not recommended for athletes and non-athletes alike (Class III, no evidence of benefit; Level of Evidence C)."[47] Despite this strong statement, ECG-based screening is occurring in the US at some levels. US professional sports governing bodies such as the National Basketball Association (NBA), National Football League (NFL), and Major League Soccer (MLS) embrace the practice,[48] while up to 47% of NCAA member schools have adopted some degree of ECG screening.[49] At the US high school level, screening ECG is not generally performed as part of the preparticipation physical examination (PPE), but, some local screening organizations do offer ECG screening on either a volunteer basis, or for a fee.[50]

Aside from driving the global growth of ECG-based screening, and igniting a worldwide debate as to the "value-added" by ECG, the Italian screening experience has greatly advanced what we know about athletic adaptations, and early identification of cardiomyopathies. This adds yet another layer to what was already known about the "athlete's heart," while unearthing a whole new set of diagnostic conundrums. High prevalence of training-related changes that mimic features of inherited diseases, accompanied by what is likely low disease prevalence in athletes, can place athletes into a unique category known as the "gray zone." Classically applied to LV cavity and wall thickness,[51] the gray zone can also apply to the RV, QT interval, repolarization, and cardiac rhythms.[1,2] Training-related enlargement of the right ventricle must be distinguished from ARVC. The corrected QT interval, longer in athletes compared with non-athletes, requires differentiation from long QT syndromes. Early repolarization patterns prevalent in athletic populations should not be confused with Brugada patterns or other potentially lethal conditions. Benign T-waves, especially in black athletes, need to be differentiated from those associated with ARVC or HCM.[34,52] Benign ventricular beats and rhythms may be seen in athletes, but need to be distinguished from pathologic conditions.[53]

What Competencies are Necessary to Practice Sports Cardiology?

The ACC continues its work on core competencies. However, the ESC proposed a core curriculum (or, set of competencies) in 2012[1] (Figure 4). These can be divided into several broad categories.

Basic exercise physiology

Sports Cardiology begins with an understanding of the basics of exercise physiology. Athletic adaptation occurs in response to training, while certain physiologic reflexes or responses may be triggered by the sports environment.

CV screening

Regardless of which side of the ECG screening debate one ascribes to, cardiologists providing CV care to athletes are advised to be well-versed in the process of preparticipation evaluation, and athlete ECG and echocardiogram interpretation.

Choice of cardiac testing

Choice of testing must be tailored to the athlete. Athletes frequently require ambulatory monitoring; but, difficulty with lead adherence during physical activity, or contact with an opponent, can impede monitoring. During athletic activity, wearable patches, cellular phone applications, wireless heart rate monitors, special water-resistant external devices, implantable loop recorders, or smart shirts may be superior to conventional ambulatory monitoring.[2,56–59] Bruce protocol stress testing, intended to diagnose coronary artery disease (CAD) may be insufficient to reproduce athlete symptoms. Clinicians are advised to either monitor during the sporting activity, or to recreate exercise loads and conditions in the exercise laboratory.[2,55] Upright tilt table testing is considered unreliable in athletes, perhaps related to the interaction of high vagal tone with neurocardiogenic responses.[60]

Interpretation of CV testing: Differentiating normal athletic adaptation from inherited diseases

Training-related adaptations mimic the phenotypic appearance of inherited diseases (the gray-zone). The clinician has access to a variety of specialized tools (cardiopulmonary exercise testing, advanced echocardiography, cardiac MRI, supervised detraining, pharmacologic infusion, genetic testing) to differentiate between normal and true pathology.[51,61] But, to successfully navigate this minefield, cardiologists must have a clear understanding of both the "normal" limits to cardiac athletic adaptations, and the cardinal features of the inherited diseases that cause athlete SCA/SCD. Clinicians should be aware that disease, if present, is likely occurring in its early stages in athletic individuals.

Tailored management of CV conditions

When making treatment recommendations, cardiologists must tailor therapies to the needs of the athlete. Some CV pharmacologic agents may be on the World Anti-Doping Agency (WADA) prohibited list and, thus, not suitable for certain athletes. Beta-blockade may not be the best choice due to negative effects on cardiac performance.[62] Need for anticoagulant therapy may influence choice of valve replacement vs. repair in those wishing to resume contact sports after surgery. Ablation may be recommended earlier for athletes with reentrant arrhythmias or accessory pathways.[63] In athletes with pacemakers, upper rate limit behaviors can negatively impact athletic performance. In these cases, custom-made devices or custom programming can be helpful.[64]

Determine if CV cause of symptoms

This is one of the more common reasons a cardiologist may be asked to see an athlete. While it has been shown that prodromal symptoms are common in those who succumb to SCA/SCD,[65–67] the predictive value of exertional and non-exertional chest pain, syncope, fatigue, palpitations, and shortness of breath in athletes is not known with certainty. Clearly, more research is necessary to define the predictive value of symptoms in this patient group.

Participation recommendation in those with known or suspected CV disease

In the US, the 36th Bethesda Conference has been the gold standard for participation recommendation in athletes with established heart disease.[68] This document has been criticized for being too restrictive and lacking an evidence base.[69] Preliminary data in athletes and exercising individuals with implanted defibrillators (ICDs),[70] and long QT,[71] suggest that the risk of exercise and/or sports may be acceptably low in certain individuals with these conditions. Further studies are planned, but outcome data like this will provide the Bethesda (participation recommendation) writers with information they need to allow the guidelines to evolve. Updated sports participation recommendations have recently been published.[72]

How to Practice Sports Cardiology: A Practical Approach to the Sports-Specific CV Care of any Athlete

When working with athletes, one of the greatest challenges is sifting through large amounts of published data, and organizing it in some fashion that allows comfortable navigation through the sports' culture, assessment of sports-specific CV risk, and accurate interpretation of CV testing in any individual athlete. In the US, athletes can be grouped as high school, collegiate, professional, and older or master athletes (over age 35 years). Beyond that, athletes can be grouped according to sport, gender, size, ethnicity, and type of training. Since CV risk, cardiac adaptations, and appearance of cardiac tests will all vary considerably based upon individual demographic characteristics, I recommend a systematic, sports-specific, 5-step approach to the CV care of any athlete. This approach lends itself particularly well to professional and endurance athletes, where the most published data are available.

5-Step Approach to the Cardiovascular Care of an Athlete

Step 1. *Understand the sport, how it is governed, and the role of the team doctor and cardiologist*

If one is going to be serving as team cardiologist or team physician, it is essential to develop a basic knowledge of the sport, how it is governed, and your specific role. Most physicians serving as team or event medical staff have actively participated in that sport; but this is not always the case. As a figure skater, I knew nothing about the sport of soccer when asked to serve as the Major League Soccer (MLS) cardiologist in 2007. However, I was not one to miss an opportunity, so I quickly learned.

Step 2. *Define CV demands of the sport*

Classification of sport (from the AHA/ACC Eligibility and Disqualification Recommendations for Competitive Athletes With Cardiovascular Abnormalities), is based on components achieved during competition.[68,72] Increasing dynamic component is defined as percent maximal oxygen uptake (VO_2 max) attained, from A (lowest) to C (highest); increasing static component is defined as percent maximal voluntary contraction (MVC), from I (lowest) to III (highest). Using this scheme, examples of lowest demand sports are golf, curling, and riflery (IA sports), and highest demand sports are cycling, rowing, and triathlon (IIIC). In soccer (1C sport), VO_2 max values range from 55–68 mL/kg/min.[73] In contrast, in American football (2B sport), mean VO_2 max is somewhat lower, at 53.1 mL/kg/min,[74] and probably higher in running backs than linemen. Lower than the expected VO_2 max on cardiopulmonary testing might tip the scales towards a diagnosis of pathology when evaluating "gray-zone" athletes. For example, a black soccer player with deep infero-lateral T-waves on ECG, left ventricular wall thickness of 1.5 cm on echocardiogram, and a VO_2 max of 38.2 mL/kg/min is more likely to have hypertrophic cardiomyopathy than normal athletic adaptation. Aside from assisting in the diagnosis, matching the VO_2 max of a sport with what the athlete-patient is able to achieve can assist clinicians in prescribing safe levels of exercise in those with cardiac disease.

Step 3. *Consider the internal and external sports environment*

Aside from the CV demands, the sports cardiologist needs an understanding of the environmental demands posed by that sport. For instance, during a 90-min soccer match, catecholamines and cortisol levels increase significantly compared to resting values.[75,76] Like marathoners, troponin-I is elevated in 43% of soccer players after a match,[77] and may remain elevated for up to 48 h.[78] Core temperature increases during play, starting at 20 min, and often reaching 39°C at the end of a match.[79] In contrast, troponin release has not been reported in American football, but much like soccer, core temperature increases during play, greater in linemen compared to backs, and can approach 39°C at the end of a game.[80] The environmental influences may add to risk, especially when players are deconditioned early in the season.

Step 4. *Identify range of normal CV adaptations for this sport*

To successfully interpret ECGs, echocardiograms, and other imaging, the sports cardiologist must know the published "normal" for that sport. In soccer, studied at the 2006 FIFA World Cup, 4.8% of athletes can be expected to have a potentially "pathologic" ECG, most commonly due to T-wave inversion.[81] 30% demonstrate left ventricular end-diastolic dimension >5.5 cm, 10% show right ventricular end-diastolic dimension >3.0 cm (ref), and 3% demonstrate left ventricular wall thickness >1.3 cm.[81] Studies at the NFL combine have produced three sets of normative data for American football players.[36,82,83] Unlike soccer, 11% of American football players demonstrate left ventricular wall thickness greater than 1.3 cm. Dimensions vary according to size, player position, and ethnicity.[36] This type of detail is extremely helpful to cardiologists when determining whether an athlete's heart is "normal," "gray-zone," or pathologic.

Step 5. *Evaluate CV risk, including that from performance enhancing agents in this sport*

Risk of SCD appears to vary by gender, ethnicity, and type and level of sport,[19–23] with highest relative risk occurring in black collegiate basketball players.[21] Adding to CV risk is the use of performance enhancing agents (PEAs), primarily anabolic steroids, and stimulants (ephedrine, amphetamines, and cocaine). In 2011, WADA recorded 117 anti-doping rule violations among FIFA-registered athletes, which was the highest number of positive tests in any of the professional sports committed to WADA regulations. Each year, 2–3% of professional American football players will be suspended for anti-doping violations, generally caused by steroids, and marijuana.

Summary

This 5-step approach to the CV care of an athlete may seem over-simplistic, but that is the intention. It can be adapted to fit any athlete, in any sport. Adolescent athletes demonstrate distinct training responses,[84] echocardiographic adaptations,[85] and CV risk,[86] while older athletes are well represented in endurance athlete literature.[87] An individual approach to interpretation of cardiac testing in athletes is advised.

Conclusions

Sports cardiology can be said to have had its beginnings in the 5th century BC with the ancient Greeks, but it was not until the end of the 19th century that clinicians made the connection between exercise and cardiac enlargement (athlete heart). Later, cardiac testing and imaging allowed for further refinement and characterization of athletic adaptations. In the last part of the 20th century and early 21st century, observations by Italian researchers, combined with strong endorsements from global sports governing bodies, have inspired wide-spread use of ECG-based screening throughout the world, especially at the elite athlete level. This has led to further growth of sports cardiology, accompanied by an emergence of a unique set of competencies.

While I am pleased to have played a very small part in the development of sports cardiology in the US, we are still at a very early stage of this journey. In the absence of formal competencies in the US, clinicians are advised to develop a working knowledge of the basics of sports cardiology, and to practice a systematic approach to the cardiovascular care of any athlete. Remaining challenges include traversing the pro-ECG/anti-ECG divide, defining sports cardiology core competencies for US providers, and determining ways to work collaboratively with sports medicine physicians. If these challenges can be overcome, this specialty has a very bright future in the US.

Personal Perspective on Sports Cardiology

Much like Herodicus, my own interest in sports cardiology grew from my background as both a sports teacher and physician. As a national competitor in the sport of figure skating, skating instructor, and physician, I was invited to be a team physician for the US Figure Skating World Team in 2002. But, as an academic heart failure/transplant cardiologist for 25 years, I felt my background was insufficient to provide comprehensive care to elite skating athletes. So, I completed a 2-year fellowship in primary care sports medicine, leading to American Board of Internal Medicine (ABIM) board certification in Sports Medicine in 2004, and American College of Sports Medicine (ACSM) fellowship in 2007. The combination of cardiology and sports medicine training would serve as a personal inspiration to organize and further the sports cardiology movement in the US.

I reached out to a small group of cardiologists with an interest in sports cardiology, and we began to meet informally in 2007. Gradually, we grew from 5 individuals to a group of 150, including many of the 36th Bethesda Conference Guideline writers. In 2009, a medical education company assisted me in conducting a sports cardiology needs assessment among five different types of medical practitioners, including cardiologists (Figures 1 and 2).[54] We discovered that while a significant number of cardiologists cleared ≥50 athlete-patients annually (Figure 1(A)), several important knowledge gaps existed. Only 11% consistently used the 36th Bethesda Guidelines, while 46% were either unaware of, or did not use, the guidelines (Figure 1(B)). The majority of cardiologists felt ECG should be added to preparticipation screening (Figure 1(C)); but, almost 50% tended to over-read the athlete ECG (Figure 1(D)). The greatest educational needs identified included: athletic adaptations, *commotio cordis*, Marfan's and aortic diseases, channellopathies, cardiac MRI, and the use of genetic testing (Figure 2). In 2011, this information was used to support a

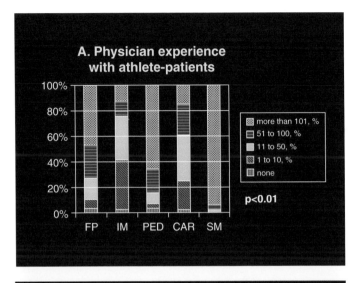

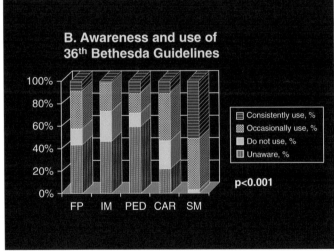

Figure 1.   Sports cardiology assessment conducted in 2009 indicated 39% of cardiologists cleared ≥50 athlete-patients annually (A). Only 11% consistently used the 36th Bethesda Guidelines, while 46% were either unaware of, or did not use, the guidelines (B). Around 93% of cardiologists felt ECG should be added to preparticipation screening (C); but, 49% would not allow play for left ventricular hypertrophy by voltage only (over-reading or false positives) (D). (FP = Family Practice; IM = Internal Medicine; PED = Pediatrics; CAR = Cardiologists; SM = Primary Care Sports Medicine Specialists).

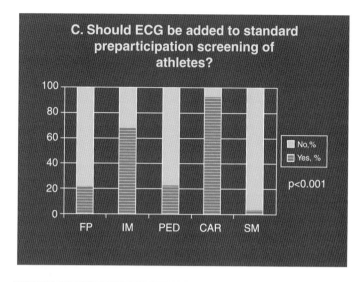

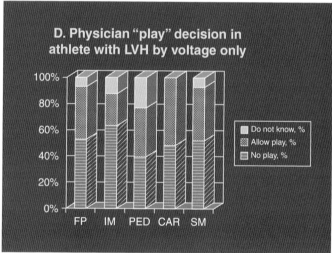

Figure 1.   (*Continued*)

petition to the American College of Cardiology (ACC) to create the Sports and Exercise Cardiology Council and Section.

The ACC Sports and Exercise Cardiology Council and Section can only be described as an unqualified and overnight success. We started with 150 members from the original petition, but rapidly grew to over 4,000 members by 2013. The 14 member Leadership Council provided a sounding board for sports cardiology issues to be discussed and vetted within the ACC. Early Council activities included

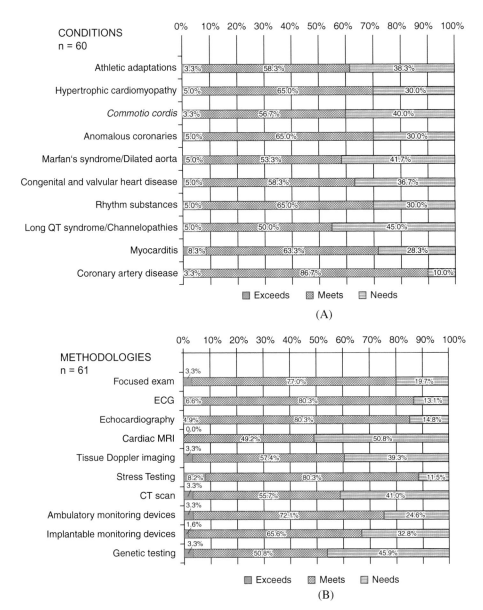

Figure 2. Cardiologists felt their greatest educational needs were athletic adaptations, *commotio cordis*, Marfan's and aortic diseases, channelopathies, cardiac MRI, and use of genetic testing.

a "Sports Cardiology in The United States" white paper,[2] and a 2012 Think Tank on "Protecting the Heart of the American Athlete."[55] The latter brought together a multidisciplinary group of 40 major stakeholder organizations with an interest in athlete CV care. The Council designed and implemented a stand-alone continuing medical educational (CME) program entitled the Annual ACC Sports Cardiology Summit, which provided a basic curriculum in sports and exercise cardiology. Held annually for 3 years (2012–2014), this 1.5 day course has attracted over 200 attendees each year.

Despite our successes, the ACC Sports and Exercise Cardiology Council and Section has had its share of challenges, as would be expected from any new endeavor. Three main areas of conflict were traversing the pro-ECG/anti-ECG divide, defining sports cardiology core competencies, and working collaboratively with sports medicine physicians.

The global ECG debate served to polarize the Council and Section into pro-ECG and anti-ECG factions. Consensus papers were painful to write, and took longer than usual, because of passionate feelings on both sides. Going forward, I would encourage Council leadership to make every attempt to stay neutral, and allow science and truth to prevail.

Similar to the story of the blind men and the elephant, every cardiologist had their own view of what sports cardiology should be. Cardiologists who care directly for athletes felt there were competencies unique to sports cardiology, such as basic exercise physiology, interpretation of cardiac symptoms in athletes, and athletic adaptations. Cardiac disease experts viewed sports cardiology from the aspect of how exercise adds risk to their disease states, such as exercise triggering SCD in Long QT 1 or hypertrophic cardiomyopathy. Defining sports cardiology competencies in the US proved more challenging than one might think. ACC educational policies insist that competencies fall into one of the existing Learning Pathways (Figure 3(A)). Lacking formal competencies, and faced with defining the relationship between sports cardiology and Learning Pathways, the first ACC Sports Council came to the preliminary conclusion there were competencies unique to sports cardiology, that there exists an overlap with virtually every current Learning Pathway, and that exercise has an effect on each disease state or condition within the Learning Pathway[2] (Figure 3(A)). Not surprisingly, this diagram looks very similar to the Maron "gray zone" diagram[51] (Figure 3(B)).

One of my original hopes upon forming the Council and Section was to allow mixing of cardiologists with sports medicine physicians into one major sports cardiology interest group, based within the ACC. Although we appealed to ACC leadership to allow sports medicine physician, non-members to participate in the activities of the ACC Sports and Exercise Cardiology Council and Section, ACC policies would not allow it. It's my belief that sports cardiologists and sports medicine physicians could learn a lot from one another; I remain optimistic that this goal can be accomplished in the future, if not within the ACC, then perhaps as a result of collaboration between medical societies.

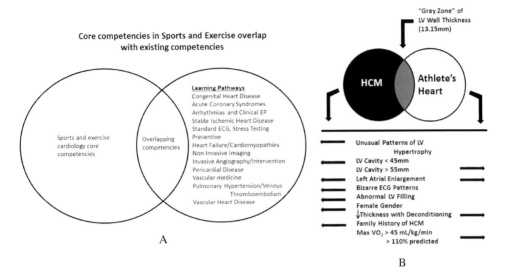

Figure 3.   (A) ACC learning pathways overlap with sports cardiology competencies. (B) Maron gray-zone.

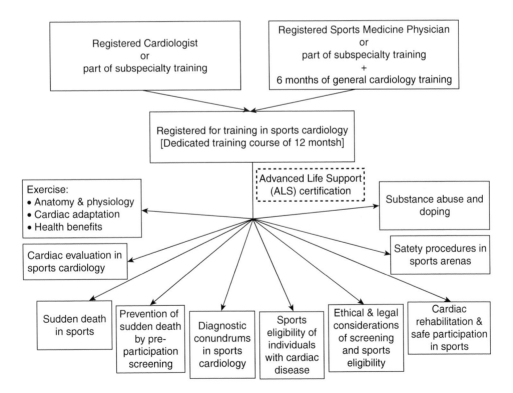

Figure 4.   ESC proposed curriculum in sports cardiology.

References

1. Heidbuchel H, Papadakis M, Panhuyzen-Goedkoop N, *et al*. Position paper: Proposal for a core curriculum for a European Sports Cardiology qualification. *Eur J Prev Cardiol* 2013;20:889–903.
2. Lawless CE, Olshansky B, Washington RL, *et al*. Sports and exercise cardiology in the United States: Cardiovascular specialists as members of the athlete healthcare team. *J Am Coll Cardiol* 2014;63:1461–1472.
3. Anastasios D, *et al*. Herodicus, the father of sports medicine. *Knee Surg Sports Traumatol Arthrosc* 2007;15:315–318.
4. Park RJ. High-protein diets, "damaged hearts," and rowing men: Antecedents of modern sports medicine and exercise science, 1867–1928. *Exerc Sport Sci Rev* 1997;25:137–169.
5. Thompson PD, Buchner D, Pina IL, Balady GJ, Williams MA, Marcus BH, Berra K, Blair SN, Costa F, Franklin B, Fletcher GF, Gordon NF, Pate RR, Rodriguez BL, Yancey AK, Wenger NK. Exercise and physical activity in the prevention and treatment of atherosclerotic cardiovascular disease: A statement from the Council on Clinical Cardiology (Subcommittee on Exercise, Rehabilitation, and Prevention) and the Council on Nutrition, Physical Activity, and Metabolism (Subcommittee on Physical Activity). *Circulation* 2003;107:3109–3116.
6. Martin D, Benarion H, Gynn R. Development of the marathon from Pheidippides to the present, with statistics of significant races. *Ann N Y Acad Sci* 1977;301:820–857.
7. Thompson PD. Historical concepts of the athlete's heart. *Med & Sci Sports Exer* 2004;36(3):363–370.
8. Opie LH. Sudden death and sport. *Lancet* 1975;1:263–266.
9. Maron BJ, Roberts WC, McAllister HA, *et al*. Sudden death in young athletes. *Circulation* 1980;62:218–229.
10. Thompson PD, Stern MP, Williams P, *et al*. Death during jogging or running: A study of 18 cases. *J Am Med Assoc* 1979;242:1265–1267.
11. Thompson PD, Funk EJ, Carleton RA, *et al*. Incidence of death during jogging in Rhode Island from 1975 through 1980. *J Am Med Assoc* 1982;247:2535–2538.
12. Sikovich DS, Weiss NS, Fletcher RH, *et al*. The incidence of primary cardiac arrest during vigorous exercise. *N Engl J Med* 1984;311:874–877.
13. Mittlemen MA, MaClure M, Tofler GH, *et al*. Triggering of acute myocardial infarction by heavy physical exertion. Protection against triggering by regular exertion. Determinants of Myocardial Infarction Onset Study Investigators. *N Engl J Med* 1993;329:1677–1683.
14. Willich SN, Lewis M, Lowel H, *et al*. Physical exertion as a trigger of acute myocardial infarction: Triggers and mechanisms of Myocardial Infarction Study Group. *N Engl J Med* 1993;329:1684–1690.
15. Farahmand B, Hållmarker U, Brobert GP, Ahlbom A. Acute mortality during long-distance ski races (Vasaloppet). *Scand J Med Sci Spor* 2007;17(4):356–361.

16. Farahmand BY, Ahlbom A, Ekblom O, *et al*. Mortality amongst participants in Vasaloppet: A classical long-distance ski race in Sweden. *J Intern Med* 2003;253(3): 276–283.

17. Marijon E, Tafflet M, Antero-Jacquemin J, El Helou N, Berthelot G, Celermajer DS, *et al*. Mortality of French participants in the Tour de France (1947–2012). *Eur Heart* 2013;34:3145–3150.

18. Van Camp SP, Bloor CM, Mueller FO, *et al*. Nontraumatic sports death in high school and college athletes. *Med Sci Sports Exerc* 1995;27:641–647.

19. Maron BJ, Haas TS, Ahluwalia A, Rutten-Ramos SC. Incidence of cardiovascular sudden deaths in Minnesota high school athletes. *Heart Rhythm* 2013;10:374–377.

20. Roberts WO, Stovitz SD. Incidence of sudden cardiac death in Minnesota high school athletes 1993–2012 screened with a standardized pre-participation evaluation. *J Am Coll Cardiol* 2013;62:1298–1301.

21. Harmon KG, Asif IM, Klossner D, Drezner JA. Incidence of sudden cardiac death in National Collegiate Athletic Association athletes. *Circulation* 2011;123: 1594–1600.

22. Kim JH, Malhotra R, Chiampas G, *et al*. Race associated cardiac arrest event registry (RACER) study group. Cardiac arrest during long-distance running races. *N Engl J Med* 2012;366:130–140.

23. Harris KM, Henry JT, Rohman E, Haas TS, Maron BJ. Sudden death during the triathlon. *J Am Med Assoc* 2010;303:1255–1257.

24. Abdulla J, Nielsen JR. Is the risk of atrial fibrillation higher in athletes than in the general population? A systematic review and meta-analysis. *Europace* 2009;11: 1156–1159.

25. Shave R, Baggish A, George K, *et al*. Exercise-induced cardiac troponin elevation evidence, mechanisms, and implications. *Am Coll Cardiol* 2010;56:169–176.

26. La Gerche A, Burns AT, Mooney DJ, *et al*. Exercise-induced right ventricular dysfunction and structural remodelling in endurance athletes. *Eur Heart J* 2012;33: 998–1006.

27. Osler W. *The Principles and Practice of Medicine*. New York: Appleton, 1892:635.

28. Rost R. The athlete's heart. Historical perspectives. *Cardiol Clin* 1992;10(2): 197–207.

29. Henschen S. Skilanglauf und skiwettlauf: Eine medizinische sportstudie. *Mitt Med Klin Upsala* (Jena). 1899;2:15–18.

30. Gott PH, Roselle HA, Crampton RS. The athletic heart syndrome. *Arch Intern Med* 1968;122:340–344.

31. Morganroth J, Maron BJ, Henry WL, Epstein SE. Comparative left ventricular dimensions in athletes. *Ann Intern Med* 1975;82:521–524.

32. Pelliccia A, Maron BJ, Spataro A, *et al*. The upper limit of physiologic cardiac hypertrophy in highly trained elite athletes. *N Engl J Med* 1991;324:295–301.

33. Basavarajaiah S, Boraita A, Whyte G, *et al*. Ethnic differences in left ventricular remodeling in highly trained athletes: Relevance to differentiating physiologic left

ventricular hypertrophy from hypertrophic cardiomyopathy. *J Am Coll Cardiol* 2008;51:2256–2262.

34. Zaidi A, Ghani S, Sharma R, *et al*. Physiological right ventricular adaptation in elite athletes of African and Afro-Caribbean origin. *Circulation* 2013;127:1783–1792.

35. Di Paolo FM, Schmied C, Zerguini YA, *et al*. The athlete's heart in adolescent Africans: An electrocardiographic and echocardiographic study. *J Am Coll Cardiol* 2012;59:1029–1036.

36. Magalski A, Maron BJ, Main ML, *et al*. Relation of race to electrocardiographic patterns in elite American football players. *J Am Coll Cardiol* 2008;51: 2250–2255.

37. Pela G, Bruschi G, Montagna L, *et al*. Left and right ventricular adaptation assessed by Doppler tissue echocardiography in athletes. *J Am Soc Echocardiogr* 2004;17: 205–211.

38. Kato TS, Noda A, Izawa H, *et al*. Discrimination of nonobstructive hypertrophic cardiomyopathy from hypertensive left ventricular hypertrophy on the basis of strain rate imaging by tissue Doppler ultrasonography. *Circulation* 2004;110:3808–3814.

39. Galderisi M, Lomoriello VS, Santoro A, *et al*. Differences of myocardial systolic deformation and correlates of diastolic function in competitive rowers and young hypertensives: A speckle-tracking echocardiography study. *J Am Soc Echocardiogr* 2010;23:1190–1198.

40. Corrado D, Pelliccia A, Heidbuchel H, *et al*., on behalf of the Section of Sports Cardiology, European Association of Cardiovascular Prevention and Rehabilitation. Recommendations for interpretation of 12-lead electrocardiogram in the athlete. *Eur Heart J* 2010;31:243–259.

41. Uberoi A, Stein R, Perez MV, *et al*. Interpretation of the electrocardiogram of young athletes. *Circulation* 2011;124:746–757.

42. Drezner JA, Ackerman MJ, Anderson J, *et al*. Electrocardiographic interpretation in athletes: The "Seattle Criteria." *Brit J Sports Med* 2013;47:122–124.

43. Breuckmann F, Möhlenkamp S, Nassenstein K, *et al*. Myocardial late gadolinium enhancement: Prevalence, pattern, and prognostic relevance in marathon runners. *Radiology* 2009;251(1):50–57.

44. Corrado D, Basso C, Pavei A, Michieli P, Schiavon M, Thiene G. Trends in sudden cardiovascular death in young competitive athletes after implementation of a preparticipation screening program. *J Am Med Assoc* 2006;296:1593–1601.

45. Ljungqvist A, Jenoure PJ, Engebretsen L, *et al*. The International Olympic Committee (IOC) consensus statement on periodic health evaluation of elite athletes. *Clin J Sport Med* 2009;19:347–365.

46. Dvorak J, Grimm K, Schmied C, Junge A. Development and implementation of a standardized precompetition medical assessment of international elite football players—2006 FIFA World Cup Germany. *Clin J Sport Med* 2009;19:316–321.

47. Maron BJ, Freidman R, Kligfield P, *et al*. Assessment of the 12-lead ECG as a screening test for detection of cardiovascular disease in healthy general populations of young people (12–25 years of age): A scientific statement from the American Heart

Association and the American College of Cardiology. *Circulation* 2014;130: 1303–1334.

48. Harris KM, Sponsel A, Hutter AM Jr, Maron BJ. Brief Communication: Cardiovascular screening practices of major North American professional sports teams. *Ann Intern Med* 2006;145:507–511.

49. Asplund C, Asif IM. Cardiovascular preparticipation screening practices among college team physicians. *Clin J Sport Med* 2014;24:275–279.

50. Maron BJ, Thompson PD, Ackerman MJ, *et al*. Recommendations and considerations related to preparticipation screening for cardiovascular abnormalities in competitive athletes: 2007 update: A scientific statement from the American Heart Association Council on Nutrition, Physical Activity, and Metabolism: Endorsed by the American College of Cardiology Foundation. *Circulation* 2007;115:1643–455.

51. Maron BJ, Pelliccia A. The heart of trained athletes: Cardiac remodeling and the risks of sports, including sudden death. *Circulation* 2006;114:1633–1644.

52. Sheikh N, Papadakis M, Schnell F, *et al*. Clinical Profile of Athletes With Hypertrophic Cardiomyopathy. *Circ Cardiovasc Imaging* 2015;8:e003454.

53. Biffi A, Pelliccia A, Verdile L, *et al*. Long-term clinical significance of frequent and complex ventricular tachyarrhythmias in trained athletes. *J Am Coll Cardiol* 2002; 40:446–452.

54. Lawless CE, Winicur ZM, Bellande B. Preparedness of US physician workforce to screen competitive athletes for sports participation. *Circulation* 2009;120:S672.

55. Lawless CE, Asplund C, Asif I, *et al*. Protecting the heart of the American athlete: Proceedings of the American College of Cardiology Sports and Exercise Cardiology Think Tank, October 18th, 2012, Washington, DC. *J Am Coll Cardiol* 2014;64: 2146–2171.

56. Saxon LA, Tun H, Riva G, *et al*. Dynamic heart rate behavior of elite athletes during football. Paper presented at Heart Rhythm 33rd Annual Scientific Sessions; May 10, 2012; Boston, MA.

57. Rossano J, Bloemers B, Sreeram N, *et al*. Efficacy of implantable loop recorders in establishing symptom-rhythm correlation in young patients with syncope and palpitations. *Pediatrics* 2003;112:e228–e233.

58. Müssigbrodt A, Richter S, Wetzel U, *et al*. Diagnosis of arrhythmias in athletes using leadless, ambulatory HR monitors. *Med Sci Sports Exer* 2013;45:1431–1435.

59. Bowie L. Smart shirt moves from research to market; goal is to ease healthcare monitoring. Georgia Institute of Technology. Available at: http://www.gatech.edu/newsroom/archive/news_releases/sensatex.html. Accessed February 28, 2014.

60. Gopinathannair R, Olshansky B. Electrophysiological approach to syncope and near-syncope in the athlete. In: Lawless CE, (ed)., *Sports Cardiology Essentials: Evaluation, Management and Case Studies*. 1st (edn.), New York: Springer Science+Business Media, 2010:181–212.

61. Baggish AL, Wood MJ. Athlete's heart and cardiovascular care of the athlete: Scientific and clinical update. *Circulation* 2011;123:2723–2735.

62. Tesch PA. Exercise performance and beta-blockade. *Sports Med* 1985;2:389–412.

63. Blomström-Lundqvist C, Scheinman MM, Aliot EM, *et al.* ACC/AHA/ESC guide-lines for the management of patients with supraventricular arrhythmias-executive summary: A report of the American College of Cardiology/American Heart Association Task Force on Practice Guidelines and the European Society of Cardiology Committee for Practice Guidelines (Writing Committee to Develop Guidelines for the Management of Patients With Supraventricular Arrhythmias). *J Am Coll Cardiol* 2003;42:1493–531.

64. Bennekers JH, van Mechelen R, Meijer A. Pacemaker safety and long-distance run-ning. *Neth Heart J* 2004;12:450–454.

65. Liberthson RR. Sudden death from cardiac causes in children and young adults. *N Engl J Med* 1996;334:1039–1044.

66. Schwartz PJ, Priori SG, Spazzolini C, *et al.* Genotype-phenotype correlation in the long-QT syndrome: Gene-specific triggers for life-threatening arrhythmias. *Circulation* 2001;103:89–95.

67. Tretter JT, Kavey RW. Distinguishing cardiac syncope from vasovagal syncope in a referral population. *J Pediatr* 2013;163:1618–1623.

68. Maron BJ, Zipes DP. 36th Bethesda Conference: Eligibility recommendations for competitive athletes with cardiovascular abnormalities. *J Am Coll Cardiol* 2005;45: 1313–1375.

69. Longmuir PE, Brothers JA, de Ferranti SD, *et al.* Promotion of physical activity for children and adults with congenital heart disease. *Circulation* 2013;127: 2147–2159.

70. Lampert R, Olshansky B, Heidbuchel H, Lawless C, *et al.* Safety of sports for athletes with implantable cardioverter-defibrillators: Results of a prospective, multinational registry. *Circulation* 2013;127:2021–2030.

71. Johnson JN, Ackerman MJ. Competitive sports participation in athletes with congeni-tal Long QT Syndrome. *J Am Med Assoc* 2012;308:764–765.

72. Maron BJ, Zipes DP, Kovacs RJ, *et al.* Eligibility and disqualification recommenda-tions for competitive athletes with cardiovascular abnormalities: Preamble, principles, and general considerations: a scientific statement from the American Heart Association and American College of Cardiology. *J Am Coll Cardiol.* 2015;66(21):2343–2349.

73. Stolen T, Chamari K, Castagna C, Wisloff U. Physiology of soccer: An update. *Sports Med* 2005;35:501–536.

74. Fukuoka Y, Gwon O, Sone R, Ikegami H. Characterization of sports by the VO_2 dynamics of athletes in response to sinusoidal work load. *Acta Physiol Scand* 1995; 153(2):117–124.

75. Carli G, Bonifazi M, Lodi L, *et al.* Hormonal and metabolic effects following a foot-ball match. *Int J Sports Med* 1986;7:36–38.

76. Haneishi K, Fry AC, Moore CA, *et al.* Cortisol and stress responses during a game and practice in female collegiate soccer players. *J Strength Cond Res* 2007;21: 583–588.

77. Löwbeer C, Seeberger A, Gustafsson SA, *et al.* Serum cardiac troponin T, troponin I, plasma BNP and left ventricular mass index in professional football players. *J Sci Med Sport* 2007;10(5):291–296. Epub Feb 6.

78. Akyuz M. Changes in serum cardiac troponin T levels in professional football players before and after the game. *Afr J Pharm Pharmacol* 2011;5(11):1365–1368.
79. Ozgunen KT, Kurdak SS, Maughan RJ, *et al.* Effect of hot environmental conditions on physical activity patterns and temperature response of football players. *Scand J Med Sci Spor* 2010;20(3):140–147.
80. Godek SF, Bartolozzi AR, Burkholder RJ, *et al.* Core temperature and percentage of dehydration in professional football linemen and backs during preseason practices. *J Athl Train* 2006;41(1):8–14.
81. Thunenkotter T, Schmied C, Dvorak J, Kindermann W. Benefits and limitations of cardiovascular pre-competition screening in international football. *Clin Res Cardiol* 2010;99(1):29–35.
82. Abernethy WB, Choo JK, Hutter AM. Echocardiographic characteristics of professional football players. *J Am Coll Cardiol* 2003;41(2):280–284.
83. Lincoln A, Vogel R, Tucker A, *et al.* Aortic size in national football league scouting combine participants. *Circulation* 2013;128:A16812.
84. Baquet G, van Praagh E, Berthoin S. Endurance training and aerobic fitness in young people. *Sports Med* 2003;33:1127–1143.
85. Makan J, Sharma S, Firoozi S, *et al.* Physiological upper limits of ventricular cavity size in highly trained adolescent athletes. *Heart* 2005;91(4):495–499.
86. Sharma S, Maron B, Whyte G, *et al.* Physiologic Limits of left ventricular hypertrophy in elite junior athletes: Relevance to differential diagnosis of athlete's heart and hypertrophic cardiomyopathy. *J Am Coll Cardiol* 2002;40:1431–1436.
87. La Gerche A, Baggish A, Knuuti J, *et al.* Cardiac imaging and stress testing asymptomatic athletes to identify those at risk of sudden cardiac death. *JACC Cardiovasc Imaging* 2013;6:993–1007.

Chapter 2

Exercise Physiology for the Clinician

Satyam Sarma and Benjamin D. Levine

Institute for Exercise and Environmental Medicine
Texas Health Presbyterian Hospital
Dallas, TX, USA

Division of Cardiology
Department of Internal Medicine
University of Texas Southwestern Medical Center
Dallas, TX, USA

Exercise physiology, and its practical application during exercise testing, is an essential tool for quantifying the functional capacity of patients and examining the integrity of the cardiorespiratory system. As such, it plays an important role for clinicians in optimizing the quality of life, independent of its ability to "diagnose" coronary artery disease.

Oxygen Uptake and the Oxygen Cascade

In order to perform physical work, the uptake and transport of oxygen is required for oxidative phosphorylation and the efficient production of adenosine triphosphate (ATP) to support the metabolic demands of the body. A simplified diagram of the components of the "oxygen cascade," or the steps of the respiratory chain through which oxygen must pass from the atmosphere to the mitochondria, is shown in Figure 1. This includes

1. Atmospheric partial pressure of oxygen determined by the environment
2. The interface between the environment and the body via the lungs and ventilation

3. Diffusion across the pulmonary capillary into the blood
4. Allosteric binding of oxygen to hemoglobin
5. Bulk transport of oxygen via the cardiovascular system
6. Diffusion at the muscle capillary into skeletal muscle
7. Oxidation in the mitochondria for energy production.[1]

At rest, this metabolic demand is dominated by the relatively high aerobic requirements of tissues such as the brain, heart, and kidney. For most individuals, on average, resting metabolic rate is approximately 3.5 mL O_2/min/kg, which has been termed 1 MET, or metabolic equivalent. Resting skeletal muscle has a very low metabolic demand and consequently a very low resting blood flow. However, during exercise, skeletal muscle has the capacity to augment its metabolic demand >10-fold (>20-fold in endurance athletes; Figure 1), leading to a large increase in systemic oxygen flux.

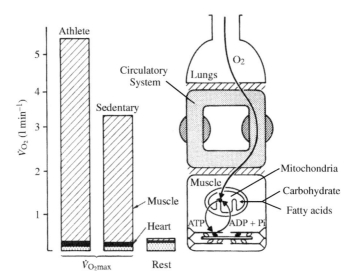

Figure 1.   The figure on the right represents a stylized depiction of the essential elements of the "oxygen cascade." Oxygen, the partial pressure of which is determined by the ambient altitude, enters the body via pulmonary ventilation; it then diffuses across the pulmonary capillary where it binds to hemoglobin and is transported by bulk flow via the cardiovascular system; a second diffusion step occurs at the muscle capillary where O_2 passes into the muscle cell and then is transported intracellularly to the mitochondria where it is used for oxidative phosphorylation and energy transduction. The left side of the figure demonstrates the large variation in oxygen uptake ($\dot{V}O_2$) from rest (right bar) to peak exercise in either a sedentary (middle bar) or athletic (left bar) human. Note that the majority of the increase in oxygen uptake during exercise comes from skeletal muscle. From Ref. 1.

As the external work performed by skeletal muscle increases (e.g. speed and grade on a treadmill, or Watts on a cycle ergometer), the amount of oxygen that passes along the oxygen cascade is increased, and the volumetric rate of oxygen uptake, or $\dot{V}O_2$, can be measured (Figure 2).

The slope of the line relating $\dot{V}O_2$ to work rate is termed the economy and is very different for different types of exercise. For example, walking is very economical, as is cycling, and the economy of the activities varies relatively little among individuals. In contrast, running is less efficient, and activities such as swimming may convert only 10% of energy production into useful work.[2,3] Eventually, there reaches a point beyond which further increases in work rate do not lead to additional increases in oxygen uptake, and this value represents $\dot{V}O_2$ max, or the maximal volumetric rate of oxygen uptake.[4]

$\dot{V}O_2$ max is the best objective measure of fitness and is a widely used index of the integrity of cardiovascular function.[5–7] According to the Fick Principle, $\dot{V}O_2$ is the product of cardiac output multiplied by the arteriovenous oxygen difference across the body. Thus, there are both central (oxygen delivery) and peripheral (oxygen extraction) factors that determine systemic oxygen utilization. However, except in some disease states that impair the ability of skeletal muscle to utilize oxygen,[8] the single most important factor that limits $\dot{V}O_2$ max in normal individuals at sea level is the maximal cardiac output.[9]

One of the most inviolate relationships in all of exercise physiology is that between oxygen uptake and cardiac output. Regardless of age, gender, or the presence of various disease states, in general, about 5–6 L/min of cardiac output are required for every liter of oxygen uptake above rest (Figure 3).[10] When this relationship breaks down, it may be a sign of severe underlying disease with

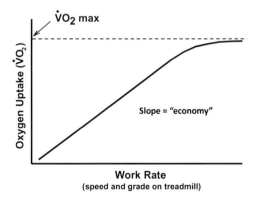

Work Rate
(speed and grade on treadmill)

Figure 2.   Idealized representation of the relationship between work rate (speed and grade on a treadmill, Watts on a cycle ergometer) and oxygen uptake ($\dot{V}O_2$). When work rate is increased, oxygen uptake increases with a slope equal to the economy of the particular activity. When work rate increases, but oxygen uptake can no longer increase, $\dot{V}O_2$ max is achieved.

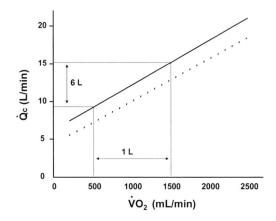

Figure 3.   This figure represents one of the key principles in exercise physiology: that is, the remarkably constant relationship between the increase in oxygen uptake ($\dot{V}O_2$) and the corresponding increase in cardiac output ($\dot{Q}c$), which in most cases is 5 to 6/1.

impending decompensation. For example, in patients with heart failure, regardless of any other clinically measured variable, the maintenance of a normal relationship between cardiac output and oxygen uptake identifies patients with relatively good short-term prognosis. In contrast, when the relationship breaks down, urgent transplantation may be required.[11] Thus, the measure of maximal exercise capacity, or $\dot{V}O_2$ max, may be viewed as a surrogate for the measure of maximal cardiac output.

Submaximal Exercise and the Maximal Steady State

Important clues to functional capacity and the ability to perform and sustain tasks of daily living also can be found in the submaximal responses to exercise (Figure 4). The most common and easy to measure variable is heart rate, which increases linearly with oxygen uptake. The slope of this line is dependent on a number of factors, particularly cardiorespiratory fitness. In unfit subjects, there is a more rapid increase in heart rate at low levels of work than more fit individuals for whom this increase is substantially delayed. Moreover, the relationship may be importantly affected by medications such as beta-blockers, or calcium channel blockers, which will blunt the heart rate response to exercise. Conversely, diseases that diminish the diastolic reserve and limit the ability to increase stroke volume during exercise (see later) will also influence the heart rate response since the relationship between oxygen uptake and cardiac output is relatively fixed.[12] As exercise intensity increases, there comes a point at which the rate of increase of

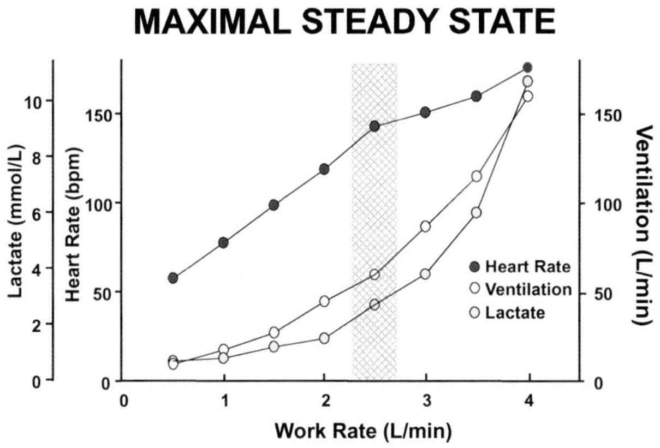

MAXIMAL STEADY STATE

Figure 4.   Graph shows the increase in heart rate, ventilation, and lactate level during incremental increases in work rate. At a specific physiological work rate, shown as a hatched bar, the rate of increase in heart rate slows (heart rate break point), ventilation increases out of proportion to oxygen uptake (ventilator threshold), and lactate begins to accumulate in the blood (lactate threshold). Because exercise intensities beyond this work rate cannot be sustained for prolonged periods of time, it is termed the "maximal steady state."

heart rate begins to slow as maximal exercise capacity is approached. This is termed the heart rate break point, or Conconi heart rate.[13]

What can also be measured is ventilation (Ve), and Ve is relatively low at low levels of exercise. As exercise intensity increases, there is a point beyond which the rate of increase in Ve is greater than the rate of increase in $\dot{V}O_2$.[14] This point is most precisely termed the ventilatory threshold. Although the regulation of breathing during exercise is beyond the scope of this chapter, a few points deserve comment. First of all, there is substantial reserve in the pulmonary system, both structurally and functionally, so that in normal individuals at sea level, the pulmonary system rarely provides any limitations to oxygen transport.[1,15]

In Figure 5, the left graph shows a typical flow-volume loop at rest (small, inside loop) and during exercise (middle loop) in a normal, healthy individual. This demonstrates a decrease in end-expiratory lung volume and an increase in end-inspiratory lung volume during exercise, both of which are well within the reserve capacity of the maximal flow-volume loop (outer loop). In contrast to this young individual, the curve on the right shows what happens to an elderly individual during exercise. Although little difference is evident at rest, the elderly individual during exercise cannot decrease end-expiratory lung volume due to decreased maximal expiratory flow and reduced lung volumes. Thus, in

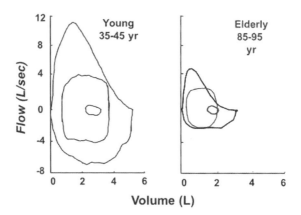

Figure 5.   Flow volume loops in a young and elderly individual at rest (small inside loop), and at peak exercise (middle loop); both loops are subtended by a maximal flow volume loop. Note that for the young individual, there is substantial inspiratory and expiratory reserve, even at peak exercise. However for the elderly person, there is prominent flow limitation on both the inspiratory and expiratory side, as well as markedly reduced peak flows.

order to increase ventilation sufficiently during exercise, end-inspiratory lung volume must increase markedly, using virtually all the inspiratory reserve available to this individual and resulting in a prominent sensation of dyspnea, even without hypoxemia. These curves demonstrate a common misconception among clinicians — that if arterial oxyhemoglobin saturation is normal, then exertional dyspnea cannot be pulmonary in origin. This conclusion is not true and for many patients, particularly the elderly, those with emphysema, or even obese patients, pulmonary limitations to exercise performance become manifest and lead to prominent dyspnea.[16–18]

Similar to the ventilatory response during exercise, as shown in Figure 4, blood lactate, the product of glycolytic metabolism, remains near resting levels at low-to-moderate intensities of exercise because lactate production is balanced by clearance in active and inactive skeletal muscle as well as heart and liver.[19] However, during graded exercise protocols in which lactate production increases more rapidly than disposal mechanisms can compensate, a certain exercise intensity is reached at which the blood lactate concentration begins to rise. This inflection in blood lactate concentration during graded exercise protocols is most precisely termed the lactate threshold, or the onset of blood lactate accumulation (OBLA). The term anaerobic threshold has been applied to this level of exercise intensity and has achieved widespread, popular appeal.[20,21]

However, current understanding of the biochemistry of exercise has made it clear that there is no "threshold" where a shift from "aerobic" to "anaerobic" metabolism occurs.[22-24] Rather, at high rates of energy requirements, substrate level phosphorylation (ATP production via glycolysis, creatine kinase, adenylate kinase, and succinyl-CoA synthetase) plays an increasingly important role in supplying ATP for contractile function, even though the rate of energy supply via oxidative phosphorylation is not exceeded.[25,26] As opposed to a shift from oxidative to glycolytic pathways, the lactate threshold during progressive exercise protocols is due to (a) the energetics of substrate utilization, which by mass action lead to an increased rate of pyruvate production and thus inevitably result in lactate production as both a product of glycolysis and for direct oxidation via the lactate shuttle; (b) an increased rate of glycolytic flux as exercise intensity increases; and (c) the efficiency of lactate clearance mechanisms.[27,28] Hence, from an organ-systems perspective, the rise in blood lactate provides useful information on compensatory mechanisms possessed by sets of distributed, but interrelated, functions. It must also be recognized that maximal or near-maximal levels of oxidative flux continue during exercise at intensities that equal or even exceed maximal oxygen uptake. Moreover, with the rapid initiation of exercise of any intensity, substrate level phosphorylation is required for energy supply. Thus, the concept of an "anaerobic threshold" is not correct and more precise physiological terminology should be encouraged.

Regardless of terminology, however, it is important to recognize that practically there exists a level of exercise intensity for every individual, beyond which exercise cannot be sustained for prolonged periods of time. The term maximal steady state is, therefore, preferred when focusing on this clinically relevant level of activity. This work rate can be identified by any of the techniques mentioned earlier (i.e. Conconi heart rate, ventilatory threshold, onset of blood lactate accumulation) and represents a discrete physiological substrate (hatched bar in Figure 4), which occurs when a certain percentage of maximal oxygen uptake is reached.[13,24] For most normal individuals, it usually occurs at 50–70% of maximal oxygen uptake, although in elite athletes, it may be as high as 90–95% of $\dot{V}O_2$ max. The maximal steady state is an important physiological parameter to identify since most sustained activities in non-athletes are performed substantially below maximal capacity. Moreover, the majority of exercise prescribed for patients for training purposes should take place at intensities below the maximal steady state.

Although an "anaerobic threshold" does not exist, maximal capacity for glycolytic flux, or "anaerobic capacity," which can be considered to mean the rate and magnitude of the absolute quantity of energy available through substrate level phosphorylation, plays an important role in high-intensity, short duration activities lasting 1–2 min in duration and may be an extremely important characteristic to identify in sprint or middle-distance athletes. Although the optimal method to measure this characteristic is still a matter of some debate, probably the best approach is that described by Medbo *et al.*, which employs the maximal accumulated oxygen deficit.[29] In essence, if high intensity exercise at an intensity above that which can be supported by maximal oxygen uptake is initiated suddenly, substrate level phosphorylation will be required to generate ATP for muscular contraction and, particularly within the 1st minute of exercise, will provide the dominant source of energy. The difference between the energy that would be required if all the exercise were performed "aerobically," or with energy supplied by oxidative sources, and the actual oxygen uptake is termed the oxygen deficit. Such high intensity effort can rarely be sustained for more than 2–4 min, and the total oxygen deficit achieved during exhaustive effort is termed the anaerobic capacity.[30,31] If the (a) maximal oxygen uptake; (b) economy; (c) maximal steady state; and (d) anaerobic capacity are measured, a comprehensive evaluation of performance capability of any competitive or recreational athlete can be obtained.

Clinical Application of Maximal Oxygen Transport During Exercise Testing

The primary unit of oxygen uptake is liters of oxygen per minute (L/min), and, in absolute terms, is a direct function of body size. However, as a measure of work capacity, or the ability to move a human body through space, it is usually normalized to body mass, and in its most familiar form is expressed as milliliters per kilogram per minute (mL/kg/min). Clinically, $\dot{V}O_2$ is normalized again to metabolic equivalents, which, as described earlier, represents an average value of resting energy expenditure of 3.5 mL/kg/min. The amount of fitness, or cardiovascular function, required to perform various occupational, recreational, or physical conditioning activities then can be represented by the number of metabolic equivalents, or the systemic oxygen transport above rest required for their pursuit (Table 1). Thus, both the achievable and sustainable metabolic equivalents are key factors in determining a patient's functional capacity.

Maximal oxygen uptake changes with respect to a number of variables such as training status, gender, and age.[5] On average, $\dot{V}O_2$ max normalized to total body weight decreases by approximately 10% per decade (0.4–0.5 mL/min/kg/year),[32,33] though this decline may be slowed by maintaining both a high level of physical activity and ideal body weight.[34,35] When absolute $\dot{V}O_2$ max is considered, or it is normalized to fat-free mass (FFM), the decline is much less (4–5% per decade, or 0.2 mL/min/kg FFM/year). The American Heart Association has established gender and age-specific guidelines that can be used to broadly characterize a patient's functional capacity (Table 2).

Table 1. Amount of oxygen uptake/energy production required for various activities.

Category	Self-care or home	Occupational	Recreational	Physical condition
Very light <3 METs <10 mL/kg/min <4 kcal	Washing, shaving, dressing Desk work, writing Washing dishes Driving auto	Sitting (clerical, assembly) Standing (store clerk, bartender) Driving truck Operating crane	Shuffleboard Horseshoes Bait casting Billiards Archery Golf (cart)	Walking (2 mi/h) Stationary bicycle (very low resistance) Very light calisthenics
Light 3–5 METs 11–18 mL/kg/min 4–6 kcal	Cleaning windows Raking leaves Weeding Power lawn mowing Waxing floors (slow) Painting Carrying objects (15–30 lb)	Stocking shelves (light objects) Light welding Light carpentry Machine assembly Auto repair Paper hanging	Dancing (social and square) Golf (walking) Sailing Horseback riding Volleyball (6-man) Tennis (doubles)	Walking (3–4 mi/h) Level bicycle (6–8 mi/h) Light calisthenics
Moderate 5–7 METs 18–25 mL/kg/min 6–8 kcal	Easy digging in garden Level hand lawn mowing Climbing stairs (slow) Carrying objects (30–60 lb)	Carpentry (exterior home building) Shoveling dirt Using pneumatic tools	Badminton (comp.) Tennis (singles) Snow skiing (downhill) Light backpacking Basketball Football Skating (ice/roller) Horseback riding (glp)	Walking (4.5–5 mi/h) Bicycle (9–10 mi/h) Swimming (breast stroke)
Heavy 7–9 METs 25–32 mL/kg/min 8–10 kcal	Sawing wood Heavy shoveling Climbing stairs (mod.) Carrying objects (60–90 lb)	Tending furnace Digging ditches Pick and shovel	Canoeing Mountain climbing Fencing Paddleball Touch football	Jog (5 mi/h) Swim (crawl stroke) Rowing machine Heavy calisthenics Bicycling (12 mi/h)
Very Heavy >9 METs >32 mL/kg/min >10 kcal	Carrying loads upstairs Climbing stairs (fast) Carrying objects (>90 lb) Shoveling heavy snow Shoveling 10 min (16lb)	Lumberjack Heavy laborer	Handball Squash Ski touring over hills Vigorous basketball	Running (6+ mi/h) Bicycling (13+ mi/h or up steep hill) Rope jumping

Table 2.   Guidelines characterizing functional capacity.

| | | Cardiorespiratory fitness classification | | | |
| | | Maximum oxygen uptake (mL/kg/min) | | | |
Age (years)	Low	Fair	Average	Good	High
		Women			
20–29	<24	24–30	31–37	38–48	49+
30–39	<20	20–27	28–33	34–44	45+
40–49	<17	17–23	24–30	31–41	42+
50–59	<15	15–20	21–27	28–37	38+
60–69	<13	13–17	18–23	24–34	35+
		Men			
20–29	<25	25–33	34–42	43–52	53+
30–39	<23	23–30	31–38	39–48	49+
40–49	<20	20–26	27–35	36–44	45+
50–59	<18	18–24	25–33	34–42	43+
60–69	<16	16–22	23–30	31–40	41+

Source: Adapted from Ref. 136.

The quantification of $\dot{V}O_2$ max, or maximal metabolic equivalent level, is a key variable in determining functional capacity, with inherent clinical relevance (Table 3). For example, most activities of daily living require energy expenditures ≤4 METs.[36,37] For a patient with congestive heart failure, if this level of oxygen transport exceeds $\dot{V}O_2$ max, the short-term prognosis is extremely poor. Heart transplant specialists use this level as a critical determinant of whether a patient is in imminent need of cardiac transplantation or mechanical circulatory support.[38] In contrast, for a patient with coronary heart disease, the ability to exercise to 10 METs without ischemia places the patient in an extremely low risk subgroup, with a 1-year mortality of <2%.[39] A maximal exercise capacity of 13 METs, regardless of other comorbidities or the presence and extent of ischemia, predicts a similarly excellent short-term prognosis.

Thus, the ability to measure exercise capacity precisely is an essential component of an exercise tolerance test. Unfortunately, habit and economics have conspired to reduce the precision with which most clinical exercise tests provide this information, based on the widespread use of the Bruce protocol for exercise tolerance testing. Developed by Robert Bruce at the University of Washington in the late 1960s, the speeds and grades used in the protocol were not determined by reasonable consideration and physiological principles, but by the fixed gear

Table 3. Maximal metabolic equivalent level in determining functional capacity.

METs	Functional capacity
1	Resting
2	Level walking at 2 mi/h
3	Level walking at 4 mi/h
<4	Poor prognosis; usual limit immediately after MI; peak cost of basic activities of daily living
10	Prognosis with medical therapy as good as coronary artery bypass surgery
13	Excellent prognosis regardless of other exercise responses
18	Endurance athletes
>20	World class athletes

Source: Adapted from Ref. 137.

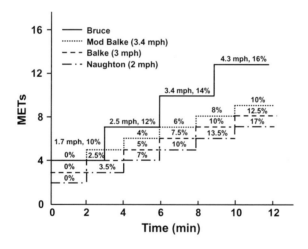

Figure 6.   Idealized representation of common clinical protocols. The Bruce protocol is unique in that large increases in work rate (accomplished by changing both speed and grade on the treadmill) occur with each stage, so that for relatively deconditioned patients, maximal work capacity is rapidly exceeded. Other protocols establish a basic treadmill speed, and increase by approximately 1 MET every 2 min exclusively by increases in grade.

ratios available on the treadmill used for the initial development and validation of the concept.[40] The biggest problem with using the Bruce protocol for testing of patients with cardiovascular disease is the relatively large increments in $\dot{V}O_2$ required to make the transitions between the early stages. Why is this such an important issue?

It is an inherent principle in medicine and science that the sampling frequency of any measure determines the maximal resolution of the measuring instrument

(Nyqvist limit). A well-known example of this phenomenon is the ability of the human eye to determine the direction of motion of a rapidly spinning airplane propeller. As the rate of rotation of the propeller increases to the point where it makes slightly less than a full rotation during a single sampling period and falls below the sampling frequency of the human eye (1/35 s), the propeller looks as if it changes direction. This process is called aliasing and represents the loss of discriminatory power of the technique.

For exercise testing, one of the most important pieces of clinical information comes from the ability to discriminate at least 1 MET increments in functional capacity. Especially at low levels of physical activity, 1 MET may be a substantial fraction of a patient's maximal aerobic power. Simplified examples of some common clinical protocols are shown in Figure 7.[37]

The Bruce protocol is unique among these by beginning at about 4 METs and progressing with relatively large increments in aerobic requirements of 3 METs

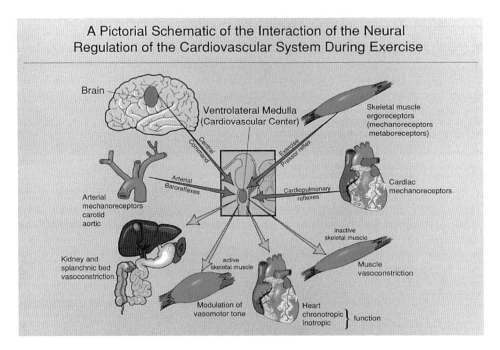

Figure 7.   Pictorial representation of the cardiovascular response to exercise. Central command initiates the exercise pressor response, which is maintained and augmented via feedback from cardiopulmonary and arterial baroreceptors, as well as by stimulation of skeletal muscle mechanically sensitive and metabolically sensitive receptors. After integration in the brain, efferent responses via the parasympathetic (vagal) and sympathetic nervous systems result in increased heart rate and contractility, vasoconstriction in inactive skeletal muscle, and vasodilation in active muscle beds mediated by release of local vasodilating substances ("functional sympatholysis").

every 3 min by an increase in both speed and grade. The first change in stage thus involves nearly a doubling of the work requirements (from 4 to 7 METs) and is not very useful in determining true functional capacity at the level that most patients with cardiovascular disease can achieve. Alternative protocols shown in the figure begin at different intensities and walking speeds, which can be estimated by watching the patient walk in the treadmill room. Each, in general, involves a fixed walking speed, with increments in grade that add approximately 1 MET every 2 min. Such protocols should be the rule rather than the exception, unless the patient is young, fit, and the clinical expectation is that his or her capacity exceeds 10 METs. For the testing of competitive athletes, similar considerations apply. Thus, an initial speed should be chosen. This speed should reflect a comfortable base training pace (e.g. 9–10 mi/h for collegiate middle-distance runners with a VO_2 max of 65–75 mL/kg/min), with increments in grade of 2% every 2 min. Such protocols invariably result in exhaustion in 10–12 min and provide an appropriate testing environment for the athlete.[41]

Finally, since maximal work capacity provides such important, clinically relevant information, clinical exercise tests should never be stopped arbitrarily by the test administrator for fixed endpoints such as a specific work rate or percentage of predicted maximal heart rate. The latter is so variable, with a standard deviation of ±10 bpm, as to be essentially useless for individual patients.[42] Patient-specific criteria, such as fatigue, dyspnea, hemodynamics, development of signs or symptoms of ischemia, or arrhythmias, are more appropriate endpoints, the threshold for which may be altered depending on the specific clinical situation.

Cardiovascular Regulation During Exercise: From External to Internal Work

The previous sections of this chapter have focused on the integrative, systemic responses of the body during exercise with an emphasis on oxygen uptake. The majority of the increase in oxygen demand during exercise comes from skeletal muscle, which must be met by appropriate increases in oxygen transport along the oxygen cascade.[1,43] The following section of this chapter will focus on the specific mechanisms by which the cardiovascular system mediates this increase in oxygen transport, both to the skeletal and cardiac muscles. Neural mechanisms, mediated by the autonomic nervous system, and local mechanisms, mediated by the mechanical function of the heart, and regional regulation of vascular resistance are essential to this coordinated response. An overview of the cardiovascular response to exercise is shown diagrammatically in Figure 8.

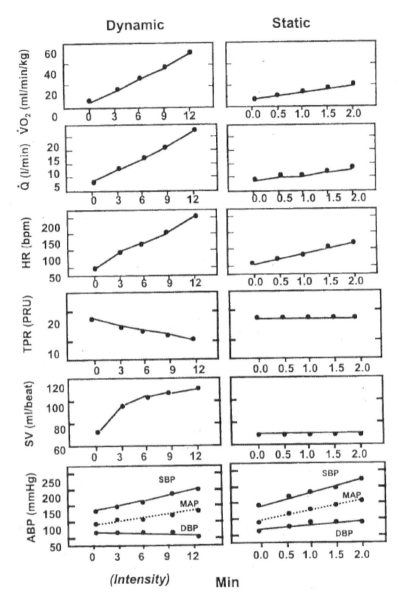

Figure 8.   Hemodynamic responses to dynamic (regular, rhythmic contraction of large muscle groups) and static (isometric or high intensity sustained contraction) exercise. Reproduced from Ref. 49.

During dynamic exercise, involving rhythmic contractions of large muscle groups (such as running, swimming, or cycling), the cardiovascular response to exercise is initiated by higher order centers in the brain, termed *central command*.[44–46] As exercise continues, both mechanical and metabolic signals from the active skeletal muscle provide feedback to cardiovascular centers in the brain to

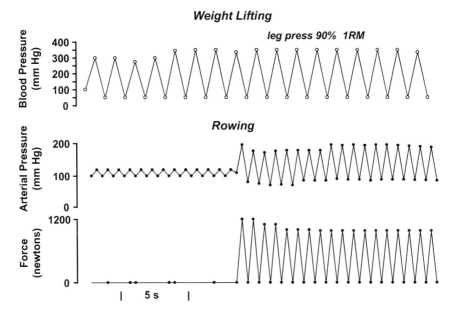

Figure 9.   Top graph shows the dramatic hypertension (systolic blood pressure 300–400 mmHg) which occurs during weight lifting at 90% of a single repetition maximum (RM) leg press. From Ref. 51. Bottom graph shows similar hypertension with mean blood pressures nearly 200 mmHg which occurs during each stroke on a rowing ergometer. From Ref. 50.

precisely match systemic oxygen delivery with metabolic demand.[47,48] Vascular resistance decreases to facilitate increases in muscle perfusion, and cardiac output increases proportionate with oxygen uptake, thus allowing the maintenance or even increase in mean arterial pressure.

The cardiovascular responses to dynamic exercise and static exercise are significantly different. Static exercise (high-intensity, sustained muscle contractions limiting muscle blood flow such as weight lifting or isometric exercise) is associated with smaller increases in oxygen uptake, cardiac output, and stroke volume than dynamic exercise, but with equivalent increases in blood pressure[49] (Figure 8). Many activities include a combination of both static and dynamic exercise. Under such circumstances, such as rowing, high-resistance cycling, or jumping sports, increases in blood pressure may be particularly dramatic[50,51] (Figure 9).

Blood Pressure Regulation During and After Exercise: The Concept of the "Triple Product"

Arterial pressure is a function of the product of heart rate × stroke volume (i.e. cardiac output) × total peripheral resistance.[52] Increases in both heart rate and

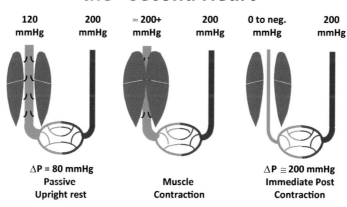

**MUSCLE PUMP
the "Second Heart"**

| 120 mmHg | 200 mmHg | ≈ 200+ mmHg | 200 mmHg | 0 to neg. mmHg | 200 mmHg |

ΔP = 80 mmHg
Passive
Upright rest

Muscle
Contraction

ΔP ≅ 200 mmHg
Immediate Post
Contraction

Figure 10.   In the upright position, large hydrostatic gradients exist in the lower extremities with a perfusion pressure of approximately 80 mmHg in leg skeletal muscle. During muscle contraction, the veins are transiently occluded resulting in a rise in pressure (middle figure); when the muscle relaxes, intact valves lead to a negative pressure in the veins markedly increasing the effective perfusion pressure. From Ref. 10.

stroke volume contribute to the increase in cardiac output, though body posture markedly influences the relative importance of changes in stroke volume.

Gravity plays a critical role in determining the distribution of pressure and volume within the cardiovascular system.[53] In the upright position, stroke volume is only about one-half its value in the supine position, due to peripheral pooling and a reduction in left ventricular end-diastolic volume. At the onset of exercise, the pumping action of skeletal muscle[54,55] (Figure 11) acts to augment venous return substantially, and stroke volume normally increases >50% via the Starling mechanism.[56]

Maximal stroke volume is achieved at relatively low levels of exercise intensity (approximately 50% of $\dot{V}O_2$ max), as pericardial constraint serves to limit left ventricular end-diastolic volume. Evidence in support of this concept may be seen during supine exercise, when left ventricular end-diastolic volume and consequently stroke volumes do not increase during graded exercise.[56] Moreover, if the pericardium is surgically removed, maximal stroke volume, maximal cardiac output, and maximal oxygen uptake may be increased in experimental animals.[57] Elite athletes have a marked increase in the ability to use the Starling mechanism during exercise, which is the primary adaptation allowing the very high maximal cardiac outputs and oxygen uptakes of endurance athletes.[58] In contrast, patients with

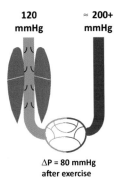

120
mmHg

≈ 200+
mmHg

ΔP = 80 mmHg
after exercise

Figure 11.   During exercise there is a marked redistribution of the cardiac output to skeletal muscle due to metabolic vasodilation. After exercise, without the muscle pump to increase venous return, cardiac filling may fall dramatically due to a reduction in LVEDV and SV leading to hypotension and syncope.

congestive heart failure with reduced ejection fraction have diminished diastolic reserve and stroke volume may not increase appreciably, even during upright exercise.[59]

At very high work rates, when a large amount of active muscle mass is engaged, the capacity for muscle vasodilation may exceed the cardiac pump capacity and blood pressure may decrease unless sympathetically mediated vaso-constriction occurs in active muscle as well as other vascular beds.[9,60,61] If exercise and muscle contraction cease abruptly, the pumping action of skeletal muscle is lost despite persistent vasodilatation. The importance of this redistribution of the cardiac output into the venous capacitance was recognized more than 300 years ago by Richard Lower who wrote in *Tractatus De Corde* in 1669:

> A defective pulse and languor of the spirit are thus the sequel to over-dilation of these veins — venous dilation anywhere diminishes the movement of the heart very appreciably by diverting the due supply and inflow of blood.[62]

It should be no surprise therefore that blood pressure may fall acutely under such circumstances. Syncope is relatively common in athletes or exercising individuals, who stand still immediately *following* a bout of intensive exercise such as occurs after a road or track race or at the foul line on a basketball court. Originally described by Gordon in 1907,[63] this process of post-exercise hypotension was first systematically investigated in the 1940s by Ludwig Eichna, who performed tilt studies on soldiers after marching or treadmill exercise, at the Armored Medical

Research Laboratory in Fort Knox, Kentucky.[64] The *key observations* from these studies included the following:

1. Slightly more than 50% of the soldiers experienced post-exertional orthostatic hypotension.
2. Of these, an additional 50% (27% of the total) developed true syncope and were unable to remain in the tilt position for a full 5 min.
3. Repeat testing in susceptible individuals revealed continued syncope and orthostatic hypotension for an average of 1 and 2 h, respectively. In one subject, after a 32 mi hike, orthostatic hypotension was still present 12 h after completion of the exercise.
4. Simple maneuvers such as moving the legs were sufficient to restore blood pressure to normal during acute hypotension, emphasizing the importance of both peripheral redistribution of blood volume and the muscle pump.

Studies by Holtzhausen and Noakes before and after an ultra-marathon of 80 km (50 mi) revealed that 68% of runners experienced orthostatic hypotension during quiet standing.[65] Although none of their subjects actually became syncopal, 23% had blood pressures below 90 mmHg and all of these had symptoms of dizziness and nausea. Interestingly, the magnitude of the post-race hypotension could not be related to the degree of plasma volume lost during the race, despite that on average the runners had lost nearly 5% of body weight. Thus, although dehydration probably contributed to reducing left ventricular filling and orthostatic hypotension, it appears likely that other factors regulating distribution of cardiac output such as thermoregulation may be more important. During severe heat stress, nearly one-third of the cardiac output may be redirected to the skin to facilitate cooling.[66] This redistribution of pre-load with heat stress can have significant implications in elite athletes. Largely as a result of operating on the "steeper portion" of the Starling curve, athletes are very sensitive to changes in pre-load such that for any given change in filling pressure, there is a much larger drop in ventricular end-diastolic volumes leading to orthostatic intolerance.[67]

Heart Rate Regulation

At low levels of exercise, heart rate increases almost exclusively via vagal withdrawal, with little evidence for systematic increases in sympathetic nerve activity until the intensity of exercise is at or above the maximal steady state.[68,69] Central command plays an essential role in the increase in heat rate during exercise, in contrast to sympathetic nerve activity and the regulation of systemic vascular resistance, which is adjusted to feedback from muscle metabo-receptors.[46] Three (extensive) lines of evidence support this conceptual framework. First, cardioac-celeration actually precedes the onset of muscle contraction during voluntary exercise.[44,70] Second, when neuromuscular blocking agents such as curare are administered to reduce muscle force and metabolic stimulation, but subjects are instructed to try to maintain force (increased effort and central command but decreased feedback from exercising muscle), the heart rate response is increased.[46,71] Third, if a blood pressure cuff is inflated to supra-systolic levels at peak exercise and subjects stop exercising, thereby trapping muscle metabolites and sustaining metabo-receptor stimulation but eliminating central command and mechano-receptor stimulation, heart rate returns immediately to baseline, while blood pressure and sympathetic nerve activity remain high.[72]

The key determinant of the magnitude of the heart rate and blood pressure response to exercise is the *relative intensity* — that is, the fraction of maximal voluntary contraction for static exercise, or the percentage of $\dot{V}O_2$ max for dynamic exercise, as well as the absolute amount of muscle mass engaged.[73,74] For example, consider two different individuals: a 30-year-old competitive marathon runner and a 50-year-old sedentary male executive. If each goes for an easy jog — the marathon runner at 10 mi/h and the executive at 5 mi/h — each may be running at 70% of $\dot{V}O_2$ max and each might have a heart rate of 150 or 85% of maximal heart rate. In contrast, if the executive tried to run at 10 mi/h, he might easily achieve his maximal heart rate of 180 and be unable to sustain this absolute work rate for more than a few seconds. Similarly, if the marathon runner ran at 5 mi/h, this might be perceived as no more than minimal exertion and heart rate would be only slightly above rest. Moreover, if the executive performed exercise training for 6 months, he would increase his $\dot{V}O_2$ max and be able to run at substantially faster absolute speeds, even though his heart rate would remain approximately 150 bpm at 70% of $\dot{V}O_2$ max. A similar example could be given for static exercise. A 250-lb bodybuilder might be able to lift 500 lbs of weight with a maximal voluntary con-traction (MVC), while the same executive could only lift 150 lbs. However, at 30% of MVC (150 lbs for the bodybuilder, 45 lbs for the executive), the heart rate and blood pressure response would essentially be the same. Weight training would reduce the relative cardiovascular stress at any given absolute workload in a fash-ion similar to endurance training as described earlier.

Myocardial Oxygen Demand and Supply

The magnitude of the cardiovascular response to exercise will determine the mag-nitude by which blood flow to the heart must increase to meet its own oxygen requirements, *regardless of the absolute level of external work being performed*. Myocardial oxygen uptake ($\dot{M}O_2$), or the *internal* work of the heart, will depend

DETERMINANTS OF
MYOCARDIAL OXYGEN DEMANDS ($\dot{M}O_2$)

WALL STRESS: <u>LV PRESSURE * LV VOLUME</u>
WALL THICKNESS

HEART RATE

CONTRACTILITY

Figure 12.   The primary determinants of myocardial oxygen demands, including wall stress immediately before the onset of contraction (pre-load), wall stress immediately after and during contraction (afterload), heart rate (chronotropic work), and contractility.

$$RPP\ =\ HR_{max} * SBP_{max}$$

$$HR * (Q_c * TPR)$$

$$HR * (HR * SV) * TPR$$

$$RPP \approx HR^2 * SV * TPR$$

Figure 13.   Derivation of the rate-pressure product (RPP) as an index of myocardial oxygen consumption during exercise. HR = heart rate, SBP = systolic blood pressure, TPR = total peripheral
resistance, Q_c = cardiac output. Thus, the RPP is weighted in favor of chronotropic work, but also
includes components reflecting both pressure and volume work of the heart.

on the extent to which the well-known determinants of myocardial oxygen
requirements increase during exercise (Figure 12). *It is important to emphasize
that the* $\dot{M}O_2$, *rather than the* $\dot{V}O_2$ *is what determines the degree to which myocardial blood flow must increase during exercise.*

Although direct measures of $\dot{M}O_2$ are difficult to make, it can be estimated
using simple clinical parameters measured during routine exercise tests. Figure 13
shows the derivation of the "rate pressure product," which provides a remarkably
good estimate of $\dot{M}O_2$[75] and which is weighted heavily towards the contribution of
heart rate and chronotropic work, but also incorporates the significant contribution
of inotropic, pressure, and volume work of the heart.

A form of the Fick equation, similar to that for *systemic* oxygen uptake
emphasizes that *myocardial* oxygen uptake ($\dot{M}O_2$) is a function of myocardial
blood flow multiplied by the arteriovenous oxygen difference across the heart.
However, the heart is unique in that it extracts the majority of oxygen that it
receives even at rest. Thus, the ability of the heart to augment oxygen utilization

to meet increased energy demand must be met predominantly by increasing myocardial blood flow. Normally, coronary blood flow can increase by at least 5-fold both via vasodilation of small, peripheral resistance arterioles, as well as by flow mediated vasodilation of the large conduit arteries. This process is called *coronary flow reserve* and is the essential physiological factor that determines whether exercise will result in myocardial ischemia in patients with atherosclerosis. When atherosclerosis involves the epicardial vessels, both their conduit function and their vascular responsiveness may be impaired. A waterfall effect begins to become physiologically significant when the total luminal cross-sectional area is reduced approximately 75% (>50% cross-sectional diameter).[76] In addition, even modest degrees of atherosclerosis may impair the normal endothelium-dependent vasodilation of the coronary arteries leading to vasoconstriction, rather than vasodilation during exercise.[77] Ultimately, if the ability to augment coronary blood flow is inadequate to meet myocardial oxygen demands at a given level of both systemic and myocardial work, then ischemia will develop.

Cardiac Contractility and Contractile Reserve

The ability of the heart to generate adequate circulatory power depends on effective and efficient contraction of the cardiac myocyte. In a healthy heart, ejection fraction can increase up to 30% during exercise.[78] Independent of changes in afterload and pre-load, contractility refers to the intrinsic capacity of the myocyte to generate force. At a cellular level, as heart rate rises the flux of calcium ions through the cytosol increases due to increasing frequency of L-type calcium channel depolarization and calcium induced calcium release from the sarcoplasmic reticulum.[79] Termed the force-frequency relationship (FFR), this increase in systolic cytosolic calcium concentrations leads to stronger actin–myosin cross-bridge interactions and more forceful myocyte shortening.[80]

Increasing cardiac contractility is a highly energy intensive process with large amounts of ATP necessary to restore diastolic calcium gradients between the sarcoplasmic reticulum and cytosol (~1,000–10,000-fold) to pre-contraction levels.[81] The loss of contractile reserve, either through myocardial ischemia leading to a decrease in oxidative potential and ATP production or chronic sympathetic activation causing abnormalities in calcium flux as occurs in systolic heart failure,[82] hinders the amount of "internal" work the heart can perform. Thus in patients with cardiovascular disease, a decline in contractile reserve can affect stroke volume response during exercise, limiting $\dot{V}O_2$ max and aerobic performance.

While contractile function is linearly correlated with myocardial oxygen uptake,[83] there are less energy intensive means of augmenting contractility and stroke volume. In highly trained athletes, stroke volume increases primarily from increases in end-diastolic volume.[84] From a cardiac mechanics standpoint, this reliance on the Frank–Starling mechanism is an efficient means of increasing stroke volume via "passive" filling of a large and compliant ventricle. As the cardiac myofilament is stretched, its sensitivity for calcium increases which in turn allows for the development of greater tensile force.[85] In contrast, untrained or sedentary individuals who are unable to augment end-diastolic volumes as effectively as trained athletes, rely more on increases in cardiac contractility, a higher energy consuming process of increasing stroke volume by reducing end-systolic volume.[84]

Cardiac contractility can be quantified at the organ level, beyond the individual myofilament, using pressure volume loops. By manipulating afterload, the end-systolic pressure-volume relationship (ESPVR) can be constructed and directly reflects the intrinsic contractile performance of the left ventricle (Figure 14). With increasing afterload or end-systolic pressure (ESP), end-systolic volume (ESV)

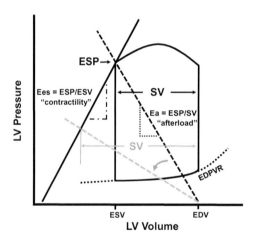

Figure 14.   Idealized left ventricular pressure–volume during a cardiac cycle. At end systole, pressure rapidly falls and ventricular volume increases. During this portion of the cardiac cycle, the relationship between LV pressure and volume is defined as the end-diastolic pressure-volume relationship (EDPVR). Stroke volume can be calculated as the difference between end-diastolic and end-systolic volumes. At end systole, the relationship between end-systolic pressure and end-systolic volume can be measured as the slope of ESP and ESV and reflects the intrinsic contractility or end-systolic elastance (Ees) of the ventricle. Arterial afterload can also be estimated as the slope of end-systolic pressure and stroke volume. The intersection of these two slopes represents ventriculoarterial (VA) coupling. As afterload is reduced, shown by the dashed gray line, a new VA coupling equilibrium point is reached and SV increases assuming cardiac contractility is unchanged. ESP: end-systolic pressure; SV: stroke volume; Ees: elastance end systole; Ea: elastance arterial; EDPVR: end-diastolic pressure-volume relationship; ESV: end-systolic volume; EDV: end-diastolic volume.

increases (pressure–volume curve shifts rightwards), while decreasing afterload decreases ESV and increases stroke volume (pressure–volume curve shifts leftwards). The slope of this relationship between end-systolic pressure and end-systolic volume, also known as end-systolic cardiac elastance (Ees), represents the degree to which the ventricle "stiffens" (i.e. contracts) in order to expel blood into the periphery.[86] A ventricle operating under high elastance performs more internal myocardial work, consuming more oxygen in order to maintain or augment stroke volume and is less energetically efficient than one operating under lower elastance. At rest, there is little difference in baseline ventricular systolic elastance in healthy individuals. However, age and sex (female) correlate with increased Ees, largely related to a reduction in LV chamber size.[87,88]

Ventriculo–Arterial Coupling

The increase in cardiac output during exercise is achieved both by increases in heart rate as well as stroke volume. As described in the previous section, increases in cardiac contractility, or end-systolic elastance (Ees), help to reduce end-systolic volume, increase ejection fraction and, thus increase stroke volume. However, an additional mechanism helps aid increases in stroke volume: vasodilation of exercising skeletal muscle vascular beds which leads to reductions in cardiac afterload. This decrease in cardiac afterload is achieved primarily by decreasing total peripheral resistance, but afterload is comprised of more than just total peripheral resistance (i.e. static load) and includes both aortic pressure and arterial impedance (i.e. pulsatile or time varying loads). Arterial elastance (Ea) provides an approximation of effective afterload by integrating both static and pulsatile components of load imposed on the left ventricle and, in contrast to total peripheral resistance, often rises or remains unchanged during exercise as heart rate increases.[89,90] Similarly to calculating Ees, Ea can be estimated from the pressure–volume loop and represents the slope of the end-systolic pressure and stroke volume relationship (ESP/SV) (Figure 14).

The intersection between Ees and Ea represents the coupling or impedance interaction between two systems, the left ventricle and systemic arterial tree, respectively. Termed ventriculoarterial coupling, the Ea/Ees ratio describes the interaction between these two systems and the changes in stroke volume and end-systolic pressure that result as ventricular load is changed.[91] When the impedances between the two systems are harmonized or the Ea/Ees ratio is close to 1, there is effective coupling between the left ventricle and arteries allowing for efficient ejection of blood to the body. If the impedance of the arterial system is higher than the ventricle, as can occur with acute rises in arterial pressure, there is a decrease in stroke volume unless the contractility or end-systolic elastance of the ventricle increases. With exercise, the increase in Ees leads to a decrease in Ea/Ees coupling ratio with a concomitant increase in stroke volume. The greater increase in Ees or contractility however comes at a cost; sacrificing energetic efficiency (increasing internal myocardial work and oxygen consumption) in order to gain cardiac mechanical efficacy (increasing stroke volume).[92]

Personal Perspective: Application of Exercise Physiology Principles Clinically — Beyond Coronary Ischemia Testing

The application of exercise physiology principles within the clinical realm is often limited to exercise testing for the detection of ischemic heart disease. Many clinicians are unfamiliar with $\dot{V}O_2$ testing variables and the interpretation of cardiopulmonary exercise tests. This can lead to a fragmented process for evaluating exertional dyspnea with diagnoses assigned either as a "primary" cardiac or pulmonary cause. The lack of an integrative approach to assessing limitations in exercise tolerance can be frustrating for both the clinician and patient. Dyspnea is a common complaint with prevalence close to 10% of the general population driven largely by aging, obesity, and inactivity.[93] The use of exercise testing primarily to rule out ischemic heart disease is a missed opportunity to comprehensively assess aerobic fitness and the potential etiology for breathlessness.

One disease in particular that benefits from this integrative approach in terms of diagnosis and management is heart failure with preserved ejection fraction (HFpEF). The HFpEF syndrome is characterized by a multitude of deficits within the "oxygen cascade" and represents a chance to revive the principles of exercise physiology testing which clinically is quickly becoming a lost art.

Exercise Intolerance in Heart Failure with Preserved Ejection Fraction

Heart failure with preserved ejection fraction (HFpEF) is increasing in prevalence and accounts for nearly 50% of hospital admissions for heart failure.[94] With similar mortality rates as heart failure with reduced ejection fraction (HFrEF), there are no proven therapies for the syndrome with considerable controversy around the key pathophysiologic mechanisms responsible for limitations in exercise tolerance.[95] Peak $\dot{V}O_2$ can be as low as levels observed in patients with HFrEF underscoring the degree of cardiorespiratory limitations.[96] Identifying mechanisms responsible for exercise intolerance in these patients is an important step in identifying novel therapeutic pathways and interventions for a disease that is common and currently untreatable.

Cardiac Limitations

Systolic function

As described earlier, cardiac output is the primary determinant of cardiorespiratory fitness and exercise capacity. Decreases in either chronotropic or contractile reserve (change from rest to peak) can blunt increases in cardiac output. While ejection fraction at rest is by definition "preserved" in patients with HFpEF, subtle systolic dysfunction can be detected and reflect abnormalities in either intrinsic ventricular contractility or ventricular–arterial coupling. Impairments in left ventricular longitudinal strain, twist mechanics (torsion), and tissue Doppler velocities suggest systolic deformation in the hearts of HFpEF patients is not normal despite a preserved EF.[97–99]

These findings of impaired contractility at rest conflict somewhat with the observation of increased end-systolic elastance in HFpEF.[100] As described earlier, end-systolic elastance reflects the intrinsic contractility of the ventricle. However, if systolic elastance is compartmentalized into its two component parts, passive systolic stiffening and myocardial contractility, the discrepant finding of high ventricular elastance but *low* contractility can be resolved. Compared to patients with hypertension but no history of heart failure, HFpEF patients have similar end-systolic elastances but impaired myocardial contractility, suggesting that high Ees is driven primarily by increased passive chamber stiffness.[101] Decreased contractile function likely contributes to the diminished stroke volume reserve of the left ventricle during physical exertion.[102–104] Despite similar end-diastolic reserve (the increase in LV end-diastolic volume with exercise) compared to healthy controls,[105] HFpEF patients are unable to augment stroke volume to the same degree as hypertensive controls. Thus while ejection fraction is nominally "preserved" under resting conditions, subtle abnormalities in systolic deformation likely persist during exercise and translate to impairments in peak contractile force generation.

The high LV chamber elastance also helps explain why vasodilators are of limited benefit in HFpEF patients. Figure 15 shows the effect of raising or lowering arterial afterload in a ventricle with high end-systolic elastance. Changes in Ea lead to sharp drops or increases in end-systolic pressure with very little change in stroke volume. This highly labile blood pressure fluctuation in response to changes in afterload is in stark contrast to patients with HFrEF.[106] HFrEF patients, because of low Ees, have small changes in arterial pressure and much larger increases in

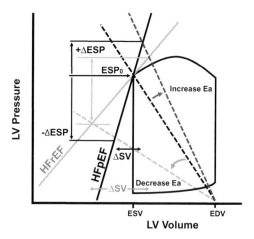

Figure 15.   Changes in afterload have different hemodynamic effects depending on heart failure subtype. Patients with heart failure with preserved ejection fraction (HFpEF; black line) have higher end-systolic elastance (slope of ESP and ESV relation) compared to patients with heart failure with reduced ejection fraction (HFrEF; gray line). For similar changes in afterload (dashed lines), there is more of a change in end-systolic pressures and less of a change in stroke volume in HFpEF vs. HFrEF. ESP: end-systolic pressure; Ea: elastance arterial; SV: change in stroke volume from low Ea to high Ea.

stroke volume after vasodilator administration highlighting the fundamental differences in cardiac physiology between these two types of heart failure.

Ventriculoarterial coupling

In addition to decreased myocardial contractility, stroke volume reserve may also be diminished as a result of inefficient ventriculoarterial (VA) coupling.[107] At rest VA coupling, calculated as the ratio of arterial and end-systolic elastances (Ea/Ees), is comparable to age matched controls due to similar elevations in arterial and ventricular stiffness.[100] In a healthy individual, Ees increases with exercise while Ea remains the same or decreases leading to a fall in the coupling ratio. A low Ea allows for a relatively large increase in stroke volume, but in patients with HFpEF, high baseline arterial stiffness in conjunction with high ventricular elastance limits stroke volume responsivness[108] which in turn affects aerobic performance[109] (Figure 15).

Chronotropic incompetence

"Chronotropic incompetence" (CI) during exercise, or an inability to augment heart rate, is another prominent feature observed in HFpEF occurring in approximately 30–60% of patients.[110,111] Heart rate response is the strongest determinant for raising cardiac output during exercise and limitations in heart rate response can thus affect peak $\dot{V}O_2$. Compared to age matched and hypertensive controls, HFpEF patients have blunted peak heart rate at maximal exercise.[110,112] While there are no consensus guidelines for defining chronotropic competence, arbitrary cut-points of failure to reach 70–85% of age-predicted maximum heart rate during incremental exercise to fatigue are commonly used.[113] However, it is important to ascertain whether an individual has truly given a maximal cardiorespiratory effort before CI can be diagnosed. Subjective ratings of perceived exertion as well as objective measures of respiratory rate, respiratory exchange ratio (RER), and ventilatory equivalent ratio for carbon dioxide (Ve/VCO$_2$) can be used.

The relationship between heart rate response and dyspnea may be particularly important in the HFpEF syndrome. With increasing heart rates, a myocardium with impaired lusitropy has much higher elevations in end-diastolic filling pressures compared to a ventricle that is able to relax more vigorously.[114] A hallmark finding in HFpEF is the rapid elevation of pulmonary capillary wedge pressure occurring with low-level exercise and persisting to peak.[115,116] Even in patients who are euvolemic and otherwise have normal *resting* hemodynamics, exercise induced elevations in pulmonary pressures can be quite dramatic and limit peak cardiac performance as measured by maximal heart rate and cardiac output response.[117]

The etiology for chronotropic incompetence is not entirely clear, but at least in HFrEF appears to be associated with more advanced disease.[118] HFpEF patients may have decreased beta-adrenergic receptor sensitivity and down regulation in the setting of chronic sympathetic activation,[119] blunted central command responses, or stop exercising prematurely due to the sensation of significant dyspnea as a result of excessive rise in pulmonary capillary pressures. Chronotropic incompetence may thus actually reflect non-chronotropic limitations to exercise rather than true functional deficits in heart rate response during exercise as regulated by central command and muscle mechano- and metabo-receptor feedback (see heart rate regulation earlier in this chapter).

Diastolic function

As the original name for the syndrome implies, the presence of diastolic dysfunction is the *sine qua non* for diagnosing HFpEF. However, there is significant controversy regarding the characteristics of diastolic dysfunction that are diagnostic for HFpEF. Diastolic abnormalities can be subdivided into either (1) active mechanisms, occurring early in diastole as the ventricle relaxes or untwists, or (2) passive mechanisms typically characterized at end or late diastole after the ventricle has completely filled.

Abnormalities in lusitropy, measured by impaired tissue relaxation and tor-sion, are evident both at rest and during exercise in HFpEF patients[98] although the sensitivity for diagnosis is lessened when solely measured under resting condi-tions. Indeed, up to a third of HFpEF patients have normal diastolic "relaxation" by echocardiography despite significant left ventricular hypertrophy and left atrial enlargement.[120] The consequences of impaired relaxation are most likely evident during physical activity with faster heart rates leading to a greater rise in left ven-tricular filling pressures.[114]

While traditional assessments of diastolic function have focused primarily on the active components of impaired relaxation and decreased ventricular suction, passive chamber stiffness likely plays an important role but can be challenging to quantify in the clinical setting.[121] Increased left ventricular mass and left atrial size appear to be better markers for mortality and morbidity risk compared to echocardiography markers of relaxation and likely reflect the degree of end-diastolic chamber elastance or stiffness.[122] As cardiac stiffness increases, the ventricle becomes less distensible during diastole, where for a given volume end-diastolic pressure is higher.[123] During exercise, when pre-load and heart rate are both elevated, the decrease in distensibility in conjunction with impaired lusitropy lead to rapid rises in pulmonary filling pressures.

The factors leading to a slowly relaxing and less distensible ventricle are not completely understood. Aging, hypertension, and obesity are common precursors to HFpEF but likely affect ventricular function through different mechanisms. Aging is marked by reductions in ventricular relaxation and diastolic suction.[124] Many elderly individuals are misclassified as having HFpEF on the basis of decreased tissue Doppler relaxation patterns. These characteristics are independ-ent of fitness status and co-morbid conditions; even elite senior athletes who are otherwise healthy and have large compliant ventricles exhibit myocardial tissue relaxation patterns similar to sedentary age-matched controls.[12] In contrast, hyper-tension and obesity independently lead to changes in *both* ventricular morphology as well as functional changes in diastolic tissue relaxation.[125–127] Patients with hypertension or obesity have increased LV mass, decreased diastolic recoil, and diminished diastolic relaxation. Thus, the interaction between aging and its associ-ated impairments in lusitropy, in conjunction with hypertension and obesity-related ventricular hypertrophy and end-diastolic stiffness, results in a cardiac phenotype at risk for the development of HFpEF.

Peripheral Limitations

While cardiac output is the primary determinant of aerobic fitness and oxygen uptake during exercise, peripheral factors can also affect peak $\dot{V}O_2$ and exercise intolerance. Peripheral factors have often been ignored owing to the difficulty in measuring cardiac output or sampling mixed venous blood during exercise. In HFpEF patients, both indirect[128] and direct[129] measures of $AV - O_2$ difference have been shown to be low and independently correlate with decreased aerobic performance. The mechanisms that limit peripheral oxygen uptake and consumption are not entirely known but thought to be a result of decreased skeletal muscle mass, decreased capillary density and endothelial function, low numbers of oxidative myofibers, and decreased mitochondrial oxidative potential. The importance of peripheral determinants of $\dot{V}O_2$ cannot be underestimated as many of the benefits of exercise training in HFpEF appear to be primarily due to improvements in $AV-O_2$ difference, rather than changes in cardiac compliance and diastolic function.[130]

Sarcopenia

Decreased skeletal muscle mass, or sarcopenia, is common in elderly and sedentary individuals. During exercise, oxygen uptake by active muscle is responsible for nearly all the increase observed in $\dot{V}O_2$ and low amounts of muscle mass can limit maximal $\dot{V}O_2$ response. Compared to age matched controls, HFpEF patients have lower overall lean body mass and in particular, low leg muscle mass.[131] It is unclear if the decrease is due to disuse or cachectic atrophy but may be related to obesity and body weight. In a longitudinal study of healthy senior adults, high fat mass initially correlated with increased lean leg mass and greater lower body muscle strength, but over time was associated with an eventual decrease in lean mass and muscle quality.[132] In HFpEF patients, many of whom are obese, the challenge of physically mobilizing a large body mass in conjunction with exertional dyspnea likely leads to a progressive cycle of disuse atrophy. Therapies to improve lower leg muscle mass may therefore improve functional capacity and quality of life by lessening muscle fatigue.

Sarcopenia may also confound assessments of cardiorespiratory fitness. Peak $\dot{V}O_2$ is often adjusted for total body mass in kilograms to account for differences in body weight between individuals. A conundrum exists however, in the assessment of relative $\dot{V}O_2$ max in individuals who are obese and have larger body mass due to an increase in fat mass, a less metabolically active tissue than muscle during exercise. In the presence of sarcopenia or high body fat percentage, scaling $\dot{V}O_2$ to total body mass (mL/min/kg) may underestimate aerobic fitness. Two individuals with similar absolute $\dot{V}O_2$ (mL/min) can have very different relative $\dot{V}O_2$ depending on body composition, with the more obese individual registering a low $\dot{V}O_2$ when indexed to total body weight. The degree to which the obese individual is classified as unfit, and possibly even being diagnosed as HFpEF, may be out of proportion to actual cardio-pulmonary limitations. In this instance, $\dot{V}O_2$ scaled to lean body (i.e. non-fat) mass or ideal body weight, may be the better marker of fitness and a normally functioning "oxygen cascade."[133]

Microvascular function and oxidative potential

In addition to low muscle mass, patients with HFpEF also have abnormalities in skeletal muscle composition. Muscle biopsies from these patients show decreased capillary density and reduced numbers of type 1 slow twitch (or aerobic) fibers compared to age matched controls.[134] The combination of low capillary density and reduced bulk delivery of oxygen to exercising muscle along with decreased proportion of aerobic fibers limits the oxidative potential of skeletal muscle. In a small study measuring skeletal muscle oxidative phosphorylation using[31] phophatc nuclear magnetic resonance spectroscopy, HFpEF patients had lower ATP production rates, quicker depletion of phosphocreatine stores, as well as slower phosphocreatine regeneration rates.[135]

Conclusions

Exercise testing is a valuable tool for detecting coronary ischemia and evaluating exertional dyspnea. While the principles of exercise physiology have been primarily relegated to the training of elite athletes or confined to the research environment, any physician involved in the evaluation of dyspnea can stand to benefit from better understanding of the oxygen cascade. The HFpEF syndrome may provide a renaissance for re-introducing the principles of cardiac physiology into the clinical realm. Improved phenotyping of the limitations in exercise tolerance may help improve both diagnostic algorithms and guide future treatment strategies in a more integrated manner.

Personal Perspectives

Satyam Sarma

As a former molecular biologist, I became interested in sports science after training for my 1st marathon. My wife, a veteran of four marathons, begrudgingly pushed me into what I thought was a feat reserved for super humans. My 1st race opened my eyes to the trainability and plasticity of the cardiovascular system and now having completed my 4th marathon and going on 5 and 6, I've learned to appreciate the factors that make human performance possible. As a clinical cardiologist, I think about these principles when I try to decipher why my patients are dyspneic just walking across the room. In particular, it has helped me manage patients with heart failure with preserved ejection fraction (HFpEF) who have a number of abnormalities in their "oxygen cascade." My research focuses on obesity and left ventricular hypertrophy and how these conditions eventually lead to a detrimental loss of aerobic power and eventually HFpEF. While a number of seminal discoveries in exercise physiology were made over 100 year ago, the field remains fresh and innovative as new tools allow us to see and understand subclinical changes that limit organ performance.

Benjamin Levine

I was a competitive athlete in college and planned to go into the orthopedic side of sports medicine. However as a resident, I found I was more passionate about the physiology of human performance (exercise, high altitude, space) than the carpentry of orthopedic surgery. Considering that cardiology is the one field in medicine where exercise is an intrinsic part of both the diagnosis and treatment of disease, I met with Bill Haskell, at the time the President of the American College of Sports Medicine, to ask his advice about where I could get great clinical training in cardiology, but also outstanding research training in exercise science; he didn't hesitate and told me he would give his right arm to train with Gunnar Blomqvist and Jere Mitchell at UT Southwestern in Dallas. So, after a year studying high altitude physiology in Japan as a Henry Luce Foundation Scholar, and a stint with the Himalayan Rescue Association in Nepal, I came to Dallas for what I thought would be a 3-year cardiology fellowship. However, I became immersed in the majesty of exercise and cardiovascular physiology, and followed Jere to Copenhagen where I was a Fulbright Scholar under Niels Secher and the late Bengt Saltin. This experience stimulated me to bring the Scandinavian model of clinical physiology to Dallas where I founded the Institute for Exercise and Environmental Medicine, which celebrated its 20th anniversary in 2012. Our mission is to explore and define the limits to human functional capacity in health and disease and in this context, I have merged my research interests in exercise physiology and sports science with a clinical practice in sports cardiology.

References

1. Hoppeler H, Weibel ER. Limits for oxygen and substrate transport in mammals. *J Exp Biol* 1998;201:1051–1064.
2. van Ingen Schenau GJ, Cavanagh PR. Power equations in endurance sports. *J Biomech* 1990;23:865–881.
3. Baudinette RV. The energetics and cardiorespiratory correlates of mammalian terrestrial locomotion. *J Exp Biol* 1991;160:209–231.

4. Mitchell JH, Blomqvist G. Maximal oxygen uptake. *N Engl J Med* 1971;284: 1018–1022.

5. Snell PG, Mitchell JH. The role of maximal oxygen uptake in exercise performance. *Clin Chest Med* 1984;5:51–62.

6. Hawkins MN, Raven PB, Snell PG, Stray-Gundersen J, Levine BD. Maximal oxygen uptake as a parametric measure of cardiorespiratory capacity. *Med Sci Sports Exerc* 2007;39:103–107.

7. Levine BD. VO$_2$ max: What do we know, and what do we still need to know? *J Physiol* 2008;586:25–34.

8. Lewis SF, Haller RG. Skeletal muscle disorders and associated factors that limit exercise performance. *Exerc Sport Sci Rev* 1989;17:67–113.

9. Saltin B. Hemodynamic adaptations to exercise. *Am J Cardiol* 1985;55:42D–47D.

10. Rowell L. *Human Circulation: Regulation During Physical Stress.* 1st (edn.), New York: Oxford University Press, 1986.

11. Chomsky DB, Lang CC, Rayos GH, Shyr Y, Yeoh TK, Pierson RN, 3rd, Davis SF, Wilson JR. Hemodynamic exercise testing. A valuable tool in the selection of cardiac transplantation candidates. *Circulation* 1996;94:3176–3183.

12. Carrick-Ranson G, Hastings JL, Bhella PS, Fujimoto N, Shibata S, Palmer MD, Boyd K, Livingston S, Dijk E, Levine BD. The effect of lifelong exercise dose on cardiovascular function during exercise. *J Appl Physiol* 2014;116:736–745.

13. Conconi F, Grazzi G, Casoni I, Guglielmini C, Borsetto C, Ballarin E, Mazzoni G, Patracchini M, Manfredini F. The Conconi test: Methodology after 12 years of application. *Int J Sports Med* 1996;17:509–519.

14. Whipp BJ, Ward SA. Cardiopulmonary coupling during exercise. *J Exp Biol* 1982;100:175–193.

15. Dempsey JA, Wagner PD. Exercise-induced arterial hypoxemia. *J Appl Physiol* 1999;87:1997–2006.

16. O'Donnell DE, Bertley JC, Chau LK, Webb KA. Qualitative aspects of exertional breathlessness in chronic airflow limitation: Pathophysiologic mechanisms. *Am J Respir Crit Care Med* 1997;155:109–115.

17. O'Donnell DE, Lam M, Webb KA. Measurement of symptoms, lung hyperinflation, and endurance during exercise in chronic obstructive pulmonary disease. *Am J Respir Crit Care Med* 1998;158:1557–1565.

18. O'Donnell DE. Dyspnea in advanced chronic obstructive pulmonary disease. *J Heart Lung Transplant* 1998;17:544–554.

19. Brooks GA. Anaerobic threshold: review of the concept and directions for future research. *Med Sci Sports Exerc* 1985;17:22–34.

20. Davis JA. Anaerobic threshold: review of the concept and directions for future research. *Med Sci Sports Exerc* 1985;17:6–21.

21. Wasserman K. Anaerobiosis, lactate, and gas exchange during exercise: the issues. *Fed Proc* 1986;45:2904–2909.

22. Connett RJ, Gayeski TE, Honig CR. Lactate accumulation in fully aerobic, working, dog gracilis muscle. *Am J Physiol* 1984;246:H120–H128.

23. Connett RJ, Honig CR, Gayeski TE, Brooks GA. Defining hypoxia: A systems view of VO$_2$, glycolysis, energetics, and intracellular PO$_2$. *J Appl Physiol* 1990;68:833–842.

24. Myers J, Ashley E. Dangerous curves. A perspective on exercise, lactate, and the anaerobic threshold. *Chest* 1997;111:787–795.

25. Katz A, Sahlin K. Regulation of lactic acid production during exercise. *J Appl Physiol* 1988;65:509–518.

26. Connett RJ, Sahlin K. 1996. *Control of Glycolysis and Glycogen Metabolism.* New York: Oxford University Press for the American Physiological Society.

27. Howlett RA, Heigenhauser GJ, Hultman E, Hollidge-Horvat MG, Spriet LL. Effects of dichloroacetate infusion on human skeletal muscle metabolism at the onset of exercise. *Am J Physiol* 1999;277:E18–E25.

28. Gibala MJ, MacLean DA, Graham TE, Saltin B. Anaplerotic processes in human skeletal muscle during brief dynamic exercise. *J Physiol* 1997;502 (Pt 3): 703–713.

29. Medbo JI, Mohn AC, Tabata I, Bahr R, Vaage O, Sejersted OM. Anaerobic capacity determined by maximal accumulated O$_2$ deficit. *J Appl Physiol* 1988;64:50–60.

30. Medbo JI, Tabata I. Relative importance of aerobic and anaerobic energy release during short-lasting exhausting bicycle exercise. *J Appl Physiol* 1989;67: 1881–1886.

31. Medbo JI, Burgers S. Effect of training on the anaerobic capacity. *Med Sci Sports Exerc* 1990;22:501–507.

32. Astrand I, Astrand PO, Hallback I, Kilbom A. Reduction in maximal oxygen uptake with age. *J Appl Physiol* 1973;35:649–654.

33. Hodgson JL, Buskirk ER. Physical fitness and age, with emphasis on cardiovascular function in the elderly. *J Am Geriatr Soc* 1977;25:385–392.

34. Astrand PO, Bergh U, Kilbom A. A 33-yr follow-up of peak oxygen uptake and related variables of former physical education students. *J Appl Physiol* 1997;82: 1844–1852.

35. Kasch FW, Boyer JL, Van Camp S, Nettl F, Verity LS, Wallace JP. Cardiovascular changes with age and exercise. A 28-year longitudinal study. *Scand J Med Sci Sports* 1995;5:147–151.

36. Fletcher GF, Balady G, Blair SN, Blumenthal J, Caspersen C, Chaitman B, Epstein S, Sivarajan Froelicher ES, Froelicher VF, Pina IL, Pollock ML. Statement on exercise: Benefits and recommendations for physical activity programs for all Americans. A statement for health professionals by the Committee on Exercise and Cardiac Rehabilitation of the Council on Clinical Cardiology, American Heart Association. *Circulation* 1996;94:857–862.

37. Fletcher GF, Balady G, Froelicher VF, Hartley LH, Haskell WL, Pollock ML. Exercise standards. A statement for healthcare professionals from the American Heart Association. Writing Group. *Circulation* 1995;91:580–615.

38. Weber KT. What can we learn from exercise testing beyond the detection of myocardial ischemia? *Clin Cardiol* 1997;20:684–696.

39. DeBusk RF, Blomqvist CG, Kouchoukos NT, Luepker RV, Miller HS, Moss AJ, Pollock ML, Reeves TJ, Selvester RH, Stason WB, *et al*. Identification and treatment of low-risk patients after acute myocardial infarction and coronary-artery bypass graft surgery. *N Engl J Med* 1986;314:161–166.

40. Bruce RA, McDonough JR. Stress testing in screening for cardiovascular disease. *Bull N Y Acad Med* 1969;45:1288–1305.

41. Levine BD, Stray-Gundersen J. "Living high-training low": Effect of moderate-altitude acclimatization with low-altitude training on performance. *J Appl Physiol* 1997;83:102–112.

42. Myers J, Froelicher VF. Exercise testing. Procedures and implementation. *Cardiol Clin* 1993;11:199–213.

43. Knight DR, Poole DC, Schaffartzik W, Guy HJ, Prediletto R, Hogan MC, Wagner PD. Relationship between body and leg VO_2 during maximal cycle ergometry. *J Appl Physiol* 1992;73:1114–1121.

44. Victor RG, Secher NH, Lyson T, Mitchell JH. Central command increases muscle sympathetic nerve activity during intense intermittent isometric exercise in humans. *Circ Res* 1995;76:127–131.

45. Williamson JW, Olesen HL, Pott F, Mitchell JH, Secher NH. Central command increases cardiac output during static exercise in humans. *Acta Physiol Scand* 1996;156:429–434.

46. Mitchell JH, Victor RG. Neural control of the cardiovascular system: Insights from muscle sympathetic nerve recordings in humans. *Med Sci Sports Exerc* 1996;28:S60–S69.

47. Rowell L. *Human Circulation: Regulation during Physical Stress.* 2nd (edn.), New York: Oxford University Press, 1996.

48. Thomas GD, Chavoshan B, Sander M, Victor RG. Invited editorial on "Effect of arterial occlusion on responses of group III and IV afferents to dynamic exercise." *J Appl Physiol* 1998;84:1825–1826.

49. Mitchell JH, Haskell WL, Raven PB. Classification of sports. *J Am Coll Cardiol* 1994;24:864–866.

50. Clifford PS, Hanel B, Secher NH. Arterial blood pressure response to rowing. *Med Sci Sports Exerc* 1994;26:715–719.

51. MacDougall JD, Tuxen D, Sale DG, Moroz JR, Sutton JR. Arterial blood pressure response to heavy resistance exercise. *J Appl Physiol* 1985;58:785–790.

52. Levine BD, Buckey JC, Fritsch JM, Yancy CW, Jr., Watenpaugh DE, Snell PG, Lane LD, Eckberg DL, Blomqvist CG. Physical fitness and cardiovascular regulation: Mechanisms of orthostatic intolerance. *J Appl Physiol* 1991;70:112–122.

53. Blomqvist CG. Cardiovascular adaptation to weightlessness. *Med Sci Sports Exerc* 1983;15:428–431.

54. Richardson RS, Poole DC, Knight DR, Kurdak SS, Hogan MC, Grassi B, Johnson EC, Kendrick KF, Erickson BK, Wagner PD. High muscle blood flow in man: Is maximal O2 extraction compromised? *J Appl Physiol* 1993;75:1911–1916.

55. Sheriff DD, Zhou XP, Scher AM, Rowell LB. Dependence of cardiac filling pressure on cardiac output during rest and dynamic exercise in dogs. *Am J Physiol* 1993;265:H316–H322.
56. Poliner LR, Dehmer GJ, Lewis SE, Parkey RW, Blomqvist CG, Willerson JT. Left ventricular performance in normal subjects: A comparison of the responses to exercise in the upright and supine positions. *Circulation* 1980;62:528–534.
57. Stray-Gundersen J, Musch TI, Haidet GC, Swain DP, Ordway GA, Mitchell JH. The effect of pericardiectomy on maximal oxygen consumption and maximal cardiac output in untrained dogs. *Circ Res* 1986;58:523–530.
58. Levine BD. VO2max: What do we know, and what do we still need to know? *J Physiol.* 2008;586(1):25–34.
59. Sullivan MJ, Cobb FR. Central hemodynamic response to exercise in patients with chronic heart failure. *Chest* 1992;101:340S–346S.
60. Secher NH, Clausen JP, Klausen K, Noer I, Trap-Jensen J. Central and regional circulatory effects of adding arm exercise to leg exercise. *Acta Physiol Scand* 1977;100:288–297.
61. Saltin B. Capacity of blood flow delivery to exercising skeletal muscle in humans. *Am J Cardiol* 1988;62:35E–30E.
62. Lower R. 1669. Tractatus de corde, item de motu et collore sanguinis, et chyli in eum transitu. In Redmayne J (ed.) *J Allestry.* London.
63. Gordan G. Observations on the effect of prolonged and severe exertion on the blood pressure in healthy athletes. *Edin Med J* 1907;22:53–56.
64. Eichna LW, Horvath SM, Bean WB. Post-exertional orthostatic hypotension. *Am J Med Sci* 1947;213:641–654.
65. Holtzhausen LM, Noakes TD. The prevalence and significance of post-exercise (postural) hypotension in ultramarathon runners. *Med Sci Sports Exerc* 1995;27:1595–1601.
66. Rowell LB. Cardiovascular aspects of human thermoregulation. *Circ Res* 1983;52:367–379.
67. Levine BD, Lane LD, Buckey JC, Friedman DB, Blomqvist CG. Left ventricular pressure-volume and Frank-Starling relations in endurance athletes. Implications for orthostatic tolerance and exercise performance. *Circulation* 1991;84:1016–1023.
68. Ray CA, Rea RF, Clary MP, Mark AL. Muscle sympathetic nerve responses to dynamic one-legged exercise: Effect of body posture. *Am J Physiol* 1993;264:H1–H7.
69. Saito M, Tsukanaka A, Yanagihara D, Mano T. Muscle sympathetic nerve responses to graded leg cycling. *J Appl Physiol* 1993;75:663–667.
70. Vissing SF, Scherrer U, Victor RG. Stimulation of skin sympathetic nerve discharge by central command. Differential control of sympathetic outflow to skin and skeletal muscle during static exercise. *Circ Res* 1991;69:228–238.
71. Leonard B, Mitchell JH, Mizuno M, Rube N, Saltin B, Secher NH. Partial neuromuscular blockade and cardiovascular responses to static exercise in man. *J Physiol* 1985;359:365–379.

72. Mitchell JH, Kaufman MP, Iwamoto GA. The exercise pressor reflex: Its cardiovascular effects, afferent mechanisms, and central pathways. *Annu Rev Physiol* 1983;45:229–242.
73. Lewis SF, Taylor WF, Graham RM, Pettinger WA, Schutte JE, Blomqvist CG. Cardiovascular responses to exercise as functions of absolute and relative work load. *J Appl Physiol Respir Environ Exerc Physiol* 1983;54:1314–1323.
74. Mitchell JH, Payne FC, Saltin B, Schibye B. The role of muscle mass in the cardiovascular response to static contractions. *J Physiol* 1980;309:45–54.
75. Rooke GA, Feigl EO. Work as a correlate of canine left ventricular oxygen consumption, and the problem of catecholamine oxygen wasting. *Circ Res* 1982;50:273–286.
76. Gould KL, Lipscomb K, Hamilton GW. Physiologic basis for assessing critical coronary stenosis. Instantaneous flow response and regional distribution during coronary hyperemia as measures of coronary flow reserve. *Am J Cardiol* 1974;33:87–94.
77. Gordon JB, Ganz P, Nabel EG, Fish RD, Zebede J, Mudge GH, Alexander RW, Selwyn AP. Atherosclerosis influences the vasomotor response of epicardial coronary arteries to exercise. *J Clin Invest* 1989;83:1946–1952.
78. Fleg JL, O'Connor F, Gerstenblith G, Becker LC, Clulow J, Schulman SP, Lakatta EG. Impact of age on the cardiovascular response to dynamic upright exercise in healthy men and women. *J Appl Physiol* 1995;78:890–900.
79. Bombardini T. Myocardial contractility in the echo lab: Molecular, cellular and pathophysiological basis. *Cardiovasc Ultrasound* 2005;3:27.
80. Piot C, Lemaire S, Albat B, Seguin J, Nargeot J, Richard S. High frequency-induced upregulation of human cardiac calcium currents. *Circulation* 1996;93:120–128.
81. Tian R. Thermodynamic limitation for the sarcoplasmic reticulum Ca(2+)-ATPase contributes to impaired contractile reserve in hearts. *Ann N Y Acad Sci* 1998;853:322–324.
82. Mulieri LA, Hasenfuss G, Leavitt B, Allen PD, Alpert NR. Altered myocardial force-frequency relation in human heart failure. *Circulation* 1992;85:1743–1750.
83. Boerth RC, Covell JW, Pool PE, Ross J, Jr. Increased myocardial oxygen consumption and contractile state associated with increased heart rate in dogs. *Circ Res* 1969;24:725–734.
84. Crawford MH, Petru MA, Rabinowitz C. Effect of isotonic exercise training on left ventricular volume during upright exercise. *Circulation* 1985;72:1237–1243.
85. de Tombe PP, Mateja RD, Tachampa K, Ait Mou Y, Farman GP, Irving TC. Myofilament length dependent activation. *J Mol Cell Cardiol* 2010;48:851–858.
86. Suga H, Sagawa K. Instantaneous pressure-volume relationships and their ratio in the excised, supported canine left ventricle. *Circ Res* 1974;35:117–126.
87. Hayward CS, Kalnins WV, Kelly RP. Gender-related differences in left ventricular chamber function. *Cardiovasc Res* 2001;49:340–350.
88. Redfield MM, Jacobsen SJ, Borlaug BA, Rodeheffer RJ, Kass DA. Age- and gender-related ventricular-vascular stiffening: A community-based study. *Circulation* 2005;112:2254–2262.

89. Park S, Ha JW, Shim CY, Choi EY, Kim JM, Ahn JA, Lee SW, Rim SJ, Chung N. Gender-related difference in arterial elastance during exercise in patients with hypertension. *Hypertension* 2008;51:1163–1169.

90. Cohen-Solal A, Faraggi M, Czitrom D, Le Guludec D, Delahaye N, Gourgon R. Left ventricular-arterial system coupling at peak exercise in dilated nonischemic cardiomyopathy. *Chest* 1998;113:870–877.

91. Little WC, Cheng CP. Left ventricular-arterial coupling in conscious dogs. *Am J Physiol* 1991;261:H70–H76.

92. Najjar SS, Schulman SP, Gerstenblith G, Fleg JL, Kass DA, O'Connor F, Becker LC, Lakatta EG. Age and gender affect ventricular-vascular coupling during aerobic exercise. *J Am Coll Cardiol* 2004;44:611–617.

93. Bowden JA, To TH, Abernethy AP, Currow DC. Predictors of chronic breathlessness: A large population study. *BMC Public Health* 2011;11:33.

94. Owan TE, Hodge DO, Herges RM, Jacobsen SJ, Roger VL, Redfield MM. Trends in prevalence and outcome of heart failure with preserved ejection fraction. *N Engl J Med* 2006;355:251–259.

95. Borlaug BA. The pathophysiology of heart failure with preserved ejection fraction. *Nat Rev Cardiol* 2014;11:507–515.

96. Kitzman DW, Little WC, Brubaker PH, Anderson RT, Hundley WG, Marburger CT, Brosnihan B, Morgan TM, Stewart KP. Pathophysiological characterization of isolated diastolic heart failure in comparison to systolic heart failure. *JAMA* 2002;288:2144–2150.

97. Kraigher-Krainer E, Shah AM, Gupta DK, Santos A, Claggett B, Pieske B, Zile MR, Voors AA, Lefkowitz MP, Packer M, McMurray JJ, Solomon SD, Investigators P. Impaired systolic function by strain imaging in heart failure with preserved ejection fraction. *J Am Coll Cardiol* 2014;63:447–456.

98. Tan YT, Wenzelburger F, Lee E, Heatlie G, Leyva F, Patel K, Frenneaux M, Sanderson JE. The pathophysiology of heart failure with normal ejection fraction: exercise echocardiography reveals complex abnormalities of both systolic and diastolic ventricular function involving torsion, untwist, and longitudinal motion. *J Am Coll Cardiol* 2009;54:36–46.

99. Yu CM, Lin H, Yang H, Kong SL, Zhang Q, Lee SW. Progression of systolic abnormalities in patients with "isolated" diastolic heart failure and diastolic dysfunction. *Circulation* 2002;105:1195–1201.

100. Kawaguchi M, Hay I, Fetics B, Kass DA. Combined ventricular systolic and arterial stiffening in patients with heart failure and preserved ejection fraction: Implications for systolic and diastolic reserve limitations. *Circulation* 2003;107:714–720.

101. Borlaug BA, Lam CS, Roger VL, Rodeheffer RJ, Redfield MM. Contractility and ventricular systolic stiffening in hypertensive heart disease insights into the pathogenesis of heart failure with preserved ejection fraction. *J Am Coll Cardiol* 2009;54:410–418.

102. Phan TT, Abozguia K, Nallur Shivu G, Mahadevan G, Ahmed I, Williams L, Dwivedi G, Patel K, Steendijk P, Ashrafian H, Henning A, Frenneaux M. Heart

failure with preserved ejection fraction is characterized by dynamic impairment of active relaxation and contraction of the left ventricle on exercise and associated with myocardial energy deficiency. *J Am Coll Cardiol* 2009;54:402–409.

103. Kitzman DW, Higginbotham MB, Cobb FR, Sheikh KH, Sullivan MJ. Exercise intolerance in patients with heart failure and preserved left ventricular systolic function: Failure of the Frank-Starling mechanism. *J Am Coll Cardiol* 1991;17:1065–1072.

104. Abudiab MM, Redfield MM, Melenovsky V, Olson TP, Kass DA, Johnson BD, Borlaug BA. Cardiac output response to exercise in relation to metabolic demand in heart failure with preserved ejection fraction. *Eur J Heart Fail* 2013;15:776–785.

105. Borlaug BA, Olson TP, Lam CS, Flood KS, Lerman A, Johnson BD, Redfield MM. Global cardiovascular reserve dysfunction in heart failure with preserved ejection fraction. *J Am Coll Cardiol* 2010;56:845–854.

106. Schwartzenberg S, Redfield MM, From AM, Sorajja P, Nishimura RA, Borlaug BA. Effects of vasodilation in heart failure with preserved or reduced ejection fraction implications of distinct pathophysiologies on response to therapy. *J Am Coll Cardiol* 2012;59:442–451.

107. Borlaug BA, Kass DA. Ventricular-vascular interaction in heart failure. *Heart Fail Clin* 2008;4:23–36.

108. Tartiere-Kesri L, Tartiere JM, Logeart D, Beauvais F, Cohen Solal A. Increased proximal arterial stiffness and cardiac response with moderate exercise in patients with heart failure and preserved ejection fraction. *J Am Coll Cardiol* 2012;59:455–461.

109. Kitzman DW, Herrington DM, Brubaker PH, Moore JB, Eggebeen J, Haykowsky MJ. Carotid arterial stiffness and its relationship to exercise intolerance in older patients with heart failure and preserved ejection fraction. *Hypertension* 2013;61: 112–119.

110. Phan TT, Shivu GN, Abozguia K, Davies C, Nassimizadeh M, Jimenez D, Weaver R, Ahmed I, Frenneaux M. Impaired heart rate recovery and chronotropic incompetence in patients with heart failure with preserved ejection fraction. *Circ Heart Fail* 2010;3:29–34.

111. Brubaker PH, Joo KC, Stewart KP, Fray B, Moore B, Kitzman DW. Chronotropic incompetence and its contribution to exercise intolerance in older heart failure patients. *J Cardiopulm Rehabil* 2006;26:86–89.

112. Borlaug BA, Melenovsky V, Russell SD, Kessler K, Pacak K, Becker LC, Kass DA. Impaired chronotropic and vasodilator reserves limit exercise capacity in patients with heart failure and a preserved ejection fraction. *Circulation* 2006;114: 2138–2147.

113. Lauer MS, Francis GS, Okin PM, Pashkow FJ, Snader CE, Marwick TH. Impaired chronotropic response to exercise stress testing as a predictor of mortality. *J Am Med Assoc* 1999;281:524–529.

114. Hay I, Rich J, Ferber P, Burkhoff D, Maurer MS. Role of impaired myocardial relaxation in the production of elevated left ventricular filling pressure. *Am J Physiol Heart Circ Physiol* 2005;288:H1203–H1208.

115. Borlaug BA, Jaber WA, Ommen SR, Lam CS, Redfield MM, Nishimura RA. Diastolic relaxation and compliance reserve during dynamic exercise in heart failure with preserved ejection fraction. *Heart* 2011;97:964–969.

116. Maeder MT, Thompson BR, Brunner-La Rocca HP, Kaye DM. Hemodynamic basis of exercise limitation in patients with heart failure and normal ejection fraction. *J Am Coll Cardiol* 2010;56:855–863.

117. Borlaug BA, Nishimura RA, Sorajja P, Lam CS, Redfield MM. Exercise hemodynamics enhance diagnosis of early heart failure with preserved ejection fraction. *Circ Heart Fail* 2010;3:588–595.

118. Benes J, Kotrc M, Borlaug BA, Lefflerova K, Jarolim P, Bendlova B, Jabor A, Kautzner J, Melenovsky V. Resting heart rate and heart rate reserve in advanced heart failure have distinct pathophysiologic correlates and prognostic impact: A prospective pilot study. *JACC Heart Fail* 2013;1:259–266.

119. Colucci WS, Ribeiro JP, Rocco MB, Quigg RJ, Creager MA, Marsh JD, Gauthier DF, Hartley LH. Impaired chronotropic response to exercise in patients with congestive heart failure. Role of postsynaptic beta-adrenergic desensitization. *Circulation* 1989;80:314–323.

120. Shah AM, Shah SJ, Anand IS, Sweitzer NK, O'Meara E, Heitner JF, Sopko G, Li G, Assmann SF, McKinlay SM, Pitt B, Pfeffer MA, Solomon SD, Investigators T. Cardiac structure and function in heart failure with preserved ejection fraction: Baseline findings from the echocardiographic study of the Treatment of Preserved Cardiac Function Heart Failure with an Aldosterone Antagonist trial. *Circ Heart Fail* 2014;7:104–115.

121. Zile MR, Baicu CF, Gaasch WH. Diastolic heart failure — abnormalities in active relaxation and passive stiffness of the left ventricle. *N Engl J Med* 2004;350: 1953–1959.

122. Zile MR, Gottdiener JS, Hetzel SJ, McMurray JJ, Komajda M, McKelvie R, Baicu CF, Massie BM, Carson PE, Investigators IP. Prevalence and significance of alterations in cardiac structure and function in patients with heart failure and a preserved ejection fraction. *Circulation* 2011;124:2491–2501.

123. Prasad A, Hastings JL, Shibata S, Popovic ZB, Arbab-Zadeh A, Bhella PS, Okazaki K, Fu Q, Berk M, Palmer D, Greenberg NL, Garcia MJ, Thomas JD, Levine BD. Characterization of static and dynamic left ventricular diastolic function in patients with heart failure with a preserved ejection fraction. *Circ Heart Fail* 2010;3: 617–626.

124. Popovic ZB, Prasad A, Garcia MJ, Arbab-Zadeh A, Borowski A, Dijk E, Greenberg NL, Levine BD, Thomas JD. Relationship among diastolic intraventricular pressure gradients, relaxation, and preload: Impact of age and fitness. *Am J Physiol Heart Circ Physiol* 2006;290:H1454–H1459.

125. Lauer MS, Anderson KM, Kannel WB, Levy D. The impact of obesity on left ventricular mass and geometry. The Framingham Heart Study. *J Am Med Assoc* 1991;266:231–236.

126. Russo C, Jin Z, Homma S, Rundek T, Elkind MS, Sacco RL, Di Tullio MR. Effect of obesity and overweight on left ventricular diastolic function: A community-based study in an elderly cohort. *J Am Coll Cardiol* 2011;57:1368–1374.

127. Mogelvang R, Sogaard P, Pedersen SA, Olsen NT, Schnohr P, Jensen JS. Tissue Doppler echocardiography in persons with hypertension, diabetes, or ischaemic heart disease: The Copenhagen City Heart Study. *Eur Heart J* 2009;30:731–739.

128. Haykowsky MJ, Brubaker PH, John JM, Stewart KP, Morgan TM, Kitzman DW. Determinants of exercise intolerance in elderly heart failure patients with preserved ejection fraction. *J Am Coll Cardiol* 2011;58:265–274.

129. Dhakal BP, Malhotra R, Murphy RM, Pappagianopoulos PP, Baggish AL, Weiner RB, Houstis NE, Eisman AS, Hough SS, Lewis GD. 2014. Mechanisms of exercise intolerance in heart failure with preserved ejection fraction: The role of abnormal peripheral oxygen extraction. *Circ Heart Fail* 2015;8(2):286–294.

130. Haykowsky MJ, Brubaker PH, Stewart KP, Morgan TM, Eggebeen J, Kitzman DW. Effect of endurance training on the determinants of peak exercise oxygen consumption in elderly patients with stable compensated heart failure and preserved ejection fraction. *J Am Coll Cardiol* 2012;60:120–128.

131. Haykowsky MJ, Brubaker PH, Morgan TM, Kritchevsky S, Eggebeen J, Kitzman DW. Impaired aerobic capacity and physical functional performance in older heart failure patients with preserved ejection fraction: Role of lean body mass. *J Gerontol A Biol Sci Med Sci* 2013;68:968–975.

132. Koster A, Ding J, Stenholm S, Caserotti P, Houston DK, Nicklas BJ, You T, Lee JS, Visser M, Newman AB, Schwartz AV, Cauley JA, Tylavsky FA, Goodpaster BH, Kritchevsky SB, Harris TB, Health ABCs. Does the amount of fat mass predict age-related loss of lean mass, muscle strength, and muscle quality in older adults? *J Gerontol A Biol Sci Med Sci* 2011;66:888–895.

133. Goran M, Fields DA, Hunter GR, Herd SL, Weinsier RL. Total body fat does not influence maximal aerobic capacity. *Int J Obes Relat Metab Disord* 2000;24:841–848.

134. Kitzman DW, Nicklas B, Kraus WE, Lyles MF, Eggebeen J, Morgan TM, Haykowsky M. Skeletal muscle abnormalities and exercise intolerance in older patients with heart failure and preserved ejection fraction. *Am J Physiol Heart Circ Physiol* 2014;306:H1364–H1370.

135. Bhella PS, Prasad A, Heinicke K, Hastings JL, Arbab-Zadeh A, Adams-Huet B, Pacini EL, Shibata S, Palmer MD, Newcomer BR, Levine BD. Abnormal haemodynamic response to exercise in heart failure with preserved ejection fraction. *Eur J Heart Fail* 2011;13:1296–1304.

136. American Heart Association: Exercise Testing and Training of Apparently Healthy Individuals. *A Handbook for Physicians.* 15th (edn.), Dallas, TX, 1972;40.

137. Fletcher GF, Balady G, Froelicher VF, *et al.* Exercise standards: A statement of healthcare professionals from the American Heart Association Writing Group. *Circulation* 1997;20:684–696.

Chapter 3

Cardiac Adaptation to Sport: The "Athlete's Heart"

Rory B. Weiner and Aaron L. Baggish

Cardiovascular Performance Program
Massachusetts General Hospital
Boston, MA, USA

Introduction

During exercise, the cardiovascular system is exposed to hemodynamic stress in the forms of pressure and volume. The magnitude of exercise-induced cardiovascular stress and relative contributions of pressure and volume are highly variable and are determined by numerous factors. When exercise is performed with sufficient intensity, duration, and frequency, the cardiovascular system remodels in response to these cardinal forms of stress. In aggregate, the changes in cardiac morphology and function that occur in response to exercise serve to minimize the energy cost of continued exercise exposure and may simultaneously serve to enhance athletic performance. This chapter is designed to provide a contemporary overview of exercise-induced cardiac remodeling with an emphasis on its relevance in clinical practice.

Historical Prespective

Cardiac enlargement in athletes was first described by Henschen and Darling in 1899.[1,2] Using rudimentary yet elegant physical examination techniques, these two pioneering investigators independently reported marked global cardiac enlargement among endurance-trained athletes. Over the ensuing century, much has been learned about the physiology of exercise-induced cardiac remodeling. Advances in our understanding of how the cardiovascular system responds to exercise have largely paralleled advances in diagnostic testing. In the early 1900s, Dr. Paul Dudley White used the "Mackenzie ink polygraph" to examine the rate and contour of the radial artery pulse among finishers of the Boston Marathon in an attempt to determine if prolonged exercise lead to cardiac fatigue and the ominous sign of *pulsus alternans*.[3] The subsequent development of chest radiography, a technique that permitted direct measurement of cardiac silhouette size, set the stage for numerous studies that confirmed Henschen's and Darling's original work.[4-6] The use of 12-lead electrocardiography and vectorcardiography provided further insights into exercise-induced cardiac adaptation by demonstrating distinct attributes of the athlete's heart, including marked sinus bradycardia[7,8] and abnormal but benign conduction patterns including the Wenckebach phenomenon.[9,10]

Studies examining cardiac adaptations to exercise have most recently relied on non-invasive cardiac imaging. Pioneering work using transthoracic echocardiography to assess cardiac dimensions among trained athletes reported mild left ventricular wall thickening,[11,12] biventricular chamber dilation,[13] and sport-specific remodeling patterns.[14] As summarized in detail below, a large body of literature now characterizes the structural and functional attributes of exercise-induced cardiac adaptation.

Overview of Revelant Exercise Physiology

A comprehensive understanding of exercise-induced cardiac remodeling requires consideration of basic exercise physiology. There is a direct relationship between exercise intensity (external work) and the body's demand for oxygen. Increasing oxygen demand is met by increasing oxygen uptake (VO_2). Peak oxygen consumption (Peak VO_2), a metric commonly measured in clinical practice, is defined as the amount of oxygen uptake/utilization that occurs at an individual athlete's maximal intensity of exercise. The cardiovascular system is responsible for transporting oxygen-rich blood from the lungs to the skeletal muscles, a process that is quantified as cardiac output (L/min). The Fick equation [VO_2 = cardiac output × (Δ arterial–venous O_2)] can be used to quantify the relationship between cardiac output and VO_2. In the healthy human, there is a direct and inviolate relationship between VO_2 and cardiac output, with every liter increase in VO_2 associated with a 5–6 liter increase in blood flow.

Cardiac output, the product of stroke volume and heart rate, may increase 5- to 6-fold during maximal exercise effort. Coordinated autonomic nervous system function, characterized by rapid and sustained parasympathetic withdrawal coupled with sympathetic activation, is required for this to occur. Heart rates may range from <40 bmp at rest to >200 bmp in a young, maximally exercising athlete. Heart rate increase is responsible for the majority of cardiac output augmentation during exercise. Maximal heart rate varies innately among individuals, decreases with age,[15] and may decrease slightly with chronic exercise training.[16]

In contrast, stroke volume both at rest and during exercise may increase significantly with prolonged exercise training. Stroke volume is defined as the quantity of blood ejected from the heart during each contraction. Stroke volume augmentation during exercise occurs as a result of increases in ventricular end-diastolic volume and, to a lesser degree, sympathetically medicated reduction in end-systolic volume. Cardiac chamber enlargement and the accompanying ability to generate a large stroke volume are direct results of exercise training and are the cardiovascular hallmarks of the endurance-trained athlete.

Hemodynamic conditions, specifically changes in cardiac output and peripheral vascular resistance, vary widely across sporting disciplines.[17] Although there is considerable overlap, exercise activity can be subdivided into two distinct physiologic categories each with defining hemodynamic differences. Isotonic exercise involves sustained elevations in cardiac output, with normal or reduced peripheral vascular resistance. This form of exercise underlies activities such as long-distance running, cycling, rowing, and swimming. Such activity represents a primary volume challenge for the heart and stimulates remodeling characterized by dilation of all four cardiac chambers. In contrast, isometric exercise involves activity characterized by increased peripheral vascular resistance and normal or only slightly elevated cardiac output. Isometric exercise leads to transient but potentially marked increases in systolic hypertension and left ventricular afterload that may lead to mild thickening of the left ventricular walls without chamber dilation. Strength training is the dominant form of exercise physiology in activities such as weightlifting, track and field throwing events, and American-style football. Popular team-based activities such as soccer, lacrosse, basketball, hockey and field hockey, and some endurance sporting disciplines such as rowing and cycling involve significant elements of both isotonic and isometric physiology and are consequently characterized by concomitant chamber dilation and wall thickening. The fundamental relationships between exercise hemodynamics and cardiac remodeling are summarized in Figure 1.

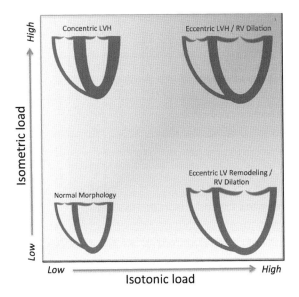

Figure 1.   Graphic representation of the relationship between the inherent physiologic demands of sporting activity and typical accompanying myocardial adaptations.

Structural and Functional Cardiac Adaptations

The left ventricle

Left ventricular chamber size

Dilation of the LV is common among athletes who engage in sports characterized by isotonic physiology and should be regarded as a normal finding among endurance athletes. Pelliccia *et al.* reported echocardiographic LV end-diastolic dimensions in a large group (*n* = 1,309) of Italian elite athletes (73% men) representing 38 different sports.[18] LV end-diastolic diameters varied widely from 38 to 66 mm in women (mean = 48 mm) and from 43 to 70 mm in men (mean = 55 mm). LV end-diastolic diameter was ≥55 mm in 45% and ≥60 mm in 14% of this combined male and female cohort. Markedly dilated LV chambers (defined as >60 mm) were associated with increased body mass and were most common among those participating in endurance sports (cross-country skiing, cycling, etc.). In clinical practice, 55–58 mm is commonly used to define the upper limits of normal for LV end-diastolic dimension,[19] meaning approximately 40% of male athletes in this study were above the normal reference point. More recently, in a US-based study of 500 university athletes, approximately 25% exceeded the gender recommended limit for LV end-diastolic diameter.[20] Taken together, these studies demonstrate that "cut-off" values for LV end-diastolic diameter are of limited value for differentiating the athlete's heart from pathologic cardiomyopathies.

Studies examining resting LV systolic function in athletes have consistently shown that LV ejection fraction, despite considerable LV dilation, is generally in the normal range.[21-24] However, it is important to note that trained athletes at rest may be found to have LV ejection fractions at or even slightly below the lower limits of normal. Among 147 Tour de France cyclists, 11% had an LV ejection fraction of ≤52%.[25] Similarly, in a study of National Football League players, 39% had LV ejection fractions in the range of 50–55%. Athletes with low-normal or mildly reduced LV ejection fractions are typically those with physiologic LV dilation who are capable of generating adequate stroke volumes to meet resting metabolic demands with minimal fractional ventricular emptying. Recent studies utilizing functional myocardial imaging, including tissue Doppler and speckle tracking echocardiography, suggest that endurance exercise training may lead to changes in regional LV systolic function that are not detected by assessment of a global indices such as LV ejection fraction.[26,27] Cross-sectional studies have observed differences in LV rotation and twist when comparing cyclists[27] and soccer players to sedentary controls,[28] and augmentation of LV apical rotation and LV twist has been documented in a short-term (90 days) longitudinal study of competitive rowers.[29] To what degree these changes in myocardial mechanics facilitate athletic performance remains speculative.

LV diastolic function has also been studied in endurance athletes with dilated LVs. Most studies have utilized pulsed-Doppler (transmitral and pulmonary venous flow) and tissue Doppler echocardiography to show that endurance exercise training leads to enhanced early diastolic LV filling.[30-32] These changes are due to a combination of enhanced intrinsic lusitropy and training-induced increases in plasma volume and thus LV pre-load. Speckle tracking echocardiography has provided further insight into diastolic function, with enhanced peak early diastolic untwisting rate observed in rowers after 90 days of endurance exercise training.[29] This ability of the LV to relax briskly during early diastole is an essential mechanism of stroke volume preservation during exercise at high heart rates.[33] A representative example of structural and functional echocardiographic data obtained from an international caliber endurance athlete with LV dilation (rower, combined high isotonic/high isometric physiology) is shown in Figure 2.

Exercise-induced LV dilation is often accompanied by mild increases in LV wall thickness. The resultant LV geometry, balanced LV chamber dilation and wall thickening, is known as eccentric LV hypertrophy (LVH) and occurs among athletes participating in sports with concomitant high isotonic and high isometric loads such as rowing and cycling.[30] Endurance disciplines with high isotonic but low isometric loads appear to lead to eccentric remodeling, an LV morphology characterized by dilation in the absence of significant wall thickening.[34]

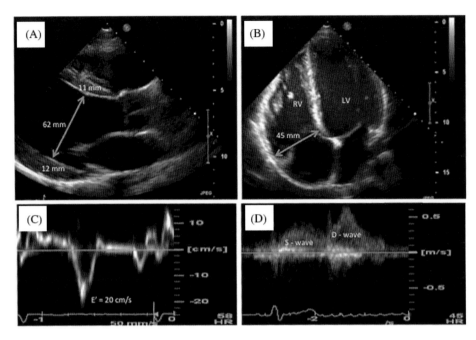

Figure 2.   Representative echocardiographic data derived from an elite level rower (combined high isotonic/high isometric physiology). (A) Parasternal long axis view demonstrating eccentric hypertrophy as defined by the presence of LV chamber dilation (62 mm end-diastolic internal dimension) and mild LV wall thickening (11–12 mm). (B) Apical four chamber view demonstrating concomitant RV dilation (basal end-diastolic dimension of 45 mm). (C) Pulse-wave tissue Doppler demonstrating supra-normal early LV relaxation velocity (20 cm/s) of the lateral mitral annulus. (D) Pulse-wave Doppler of pulmonary vein flow showing D-wave predominance due to rapid LV diastolic filling. LV = left ventricular, RV = right ventricular.

Left ventricular wall thickness

Thickening of the LV walls without associated LV chamber dilation, (i.e. concentric LVH) may develop among athletes who participate in strength-based activities such as weight lifting and American style football.[14,35,36] These sporting disciplines are characterized by repetitive bursts of high isometric loading which translate into pulsatile LV hypertension. Concentric LVH among strength-trained athletes is classically considered an adaptive remodeling process designed to normalize wall stress and cardiac work in the context of repetitive bouts of increasing afterload.

The concentric LVH phenotype appears to be far less common than the eccentric form of LVH discussed above and when present, is typically mild. In a longitudinal study of collegiate American-style football players ($n = 113$), 34% of those that played lineman position developed concentric LVH.[37]

It is noteworthy that the development of concentric LVH was associated with several key factors including resting systolic blood pressure, intraseason weight gain, and a family history of hypertension. Thus, it appears that concentric LVH among athletes may not only be due to the isometric loading inherent in actual sporting activity, but also a function of factors like the development of resting hypertension.

The finding of concentric LVH in an athlete may present a diagnostic challenge given the potential for overlap with mild forms of hypertrophic cardiomyopathy (HCM). Wall thickness "cut-off" values may be helpful in this scenario. Pelliccia *et al.* reported echocardiographic measurements of LV wall thicknesses among 947 elite Italian athletes and showed that only a small number (1.7%) had LV wall thicknesses ≥13 mm.[38] Sharma *et al.* similarly reported a low incidence (0.4%) of LV wall thickness >12 mm in 720 elite junior athletes.[39] In a recent study of nearly 500 collegiate athletes, not a single healthy university athlete had LV wall thickness >14 mm.[20] In summary, LV wall thickness in the range of 13–15 mm is a rare finding in healthy athletes and is often confined to individuals with large body size and those of Afro-Caribbean descent.[40] The finding of an LV wall thickness >15 mm should be considered pathologic until proven otherwise. In these situations, the pattern of LVH and a careful assessment of diastolic function may provide useful information.

The functional implication of concentric LVH among athletes remains incompletely understood. In one longitudinal study of male American-style football players, those that developed concentric LVH also demonstrated a relative impairment of LV early diastolic relaxation velocity by echocardiographic tissue Doppler imaging.[35] More recently, D'Andrea compared echocardiographic indices of LV diastolic function among a group of elite level strength athletes (n = 280) to those from a cohort of endurance athletes (n = 370) and showed that the strength-trained athletes had significantly lower values.[31] At present, it remains unclear whether strength training leads to decrements in diastolic function or whether strength training simply fails to produce the augmentation in diastolic function that is typical of endurance athletes.

The right ventricle

Exercise-induced cardiac remodeling is not confined to the LV. Endurance exercise training requires both the LV and right ventricle (RV) to accept and eject relatively large quantities of blood. Therefore, the cardiovascular response to repetitive endurance training includes biventricular remodeling. For the comparatively thin-walled RV, this remodeling typically takes the form of mild to moderate RV dilation without significant concomitant hypertrophy. Importantly, RV dilation in the endurance-trained athlete should always be associated with LV remodeling (eccentric LVH or remodeling) and the finding of isolated RV enlargement should raise suspicion of a pathologic process. Furthermore, RV dilation in endurance athletes tends to be a global process, without sacculation, aneurysmal dilation, or segmental dysfunction. Similar to LV dilation, in general strict "cut-off" values for RV end-diastolic diameter are not helpful in distinguishing exercise-related adaptation and pathologic cardiomyopathy.

Biventricular remodeling was documented in an early M-mode echocardiographic study which demonstrated symmetric RV and LV enlargement in a small cohort of highly trained endurance athletes.[41] In a larger M-mode and 2D echocardiorgaphy study of 127 male elite endurance athletes, the athletes demonstrated significantly larger RV cavities when compared to historical control subjects.[42] In a recent echocardiographic study of 102 endurance athletes, RV chamber dimensions were larger than "normal" values in over one-half of the athletes and 28% had RV outflow tract dimension that met the proposed major criteria for the diagnosis of arrhythmogenic RV cardiomyopathy (ARVC).[43] Cardiac MRI studies have also shown that RV enlargement is common among endurance athletes.[44,45] Differentiating exercise-induced RV changes from the diagnosis of ARVC is one of the most important clinical challenges that can arise, and awareness of the diagnostic criteria for ARVC which integrates family history, electrocardiography, and cardiac imaging is essential.[46]

The impact of strength training on the RV has not been as well studied. A recent echocardiographic study of endurance and strength athletes found that endurance athletes had greater internal RV dimensions, although RV function (systolic strain and diastolic function) were similar between the two groups.[47] A longitudinal study of RV structure in collegiate athletes before and after 90 days of team-based exercise training showed significant RV dilation in endurance athletes, but no changes in RV architecture in strength athletes.[35] Further characterization of how the RV responds to different forms of exercise and its contribution to exercise capacity is an important area for future investigation.

In similar fashion to the LV, mild reductions in RV systolic function are often observed in trained endurance athletes. A cardiac MRI study of over 300 subjects showed that RV ejection fraction was lower compared with non-athletic controls.[48] However, in a recent 3D echocardiography study, RV systolic indices were comparable between athletes and controls.[49] The finding of lower RV systolic function can be considered a physiological phenomenon since adequate resting stroke volumes at higher end-diastolic volumes will consequently be achieved at a lower ejection fraction. Therefore, preserved or mildly reduced RV systolic function can be expected in endurance athletes, although severe reductions in global function should be considered abnormal in any athlete. Regional systolic function of the

RV has also been assessed in athletes. In endurance athletes, both tissue Doppler and 2D strain studies have shown reduced systolic deformation in athletes compared to controls.[50,51] However, segments with reduced regional function showed complete normalization at peak exercise, indicating normal contractile reserve.[51]

Atria

An early echocardiograpghic study showed that endurance athletes had larger left atria (LA) than sedentary controls,[41] and that overt LA dilatation, particularly among older endurance athletes, is common.[52] Pelliccia *et al.* studied a large number of athletes ($n = 1,777$) and demonstrated that LA enlargement (≥ 40 mm anterior–posterior dimension by echocardiography) was present in 20%.[53] Interestingly, atrial fibrillation and other supraventricular tachyarrhythmias proved to be uncommon (prevalence < 1%) and similar to that in the general population in this cohort of relatively youthful athletes, despite the high frequency of LA enlargement. More recently, in a study of over 600 athletes, LA volume index determined by echocardiography confirmed a high prevalence of LA enlargement in trained athletes, particularly endurance athletes.[54] A recent meta-analysis of LA structure among more than 7,000 athletes and 1,000 controls provided clinically useful quantitative data about the magnitude of LA dilation in athletes.[55] Compared with sedentary controls, LA diameter was found to be 4.6 mm greater among endurance athletes, 3.5 mm greater among combined strength and endurance trained athletes, and 2.9 mm greater among purely strength-trained athletes. Recent studies have also begun to examine the right atrium (RA) in athletes and have documented similar increases in RA size among endurance athletes.[47,56]

Atrial function in athletes, assessed with speckle tracking echocardiography, has become an area of active investigation. A longitudinal study of elite female athletes before and after 16 weeks of training showed that LA global peak longitudinal strain and peak atrial contraction strain significantly decreased after training in athletes.[57] In contrast, other studies have not shown differences in atrial strain when comparing athletes and sedentary controls.[47,58] More studies in various groups of athletes are needed before conclusions can be drawn regarding atrial function in athletes' heart. This information will be needed to help determine if there is a mechanistic relationship between atrial size/function and the potential for increased incidence of atrial arrhythmias in certain athletic populations.[59]

Aorta

The aorta experiences a significant hemodynamic load during exercise and the nature of this load is dependent on sport type. It has been hypothesized that the pressure overload during strength training may lead to aortic remodeling and a study comparing elite strength-trained athletes and matched controls showed significantly larger aortic dimensions (annulus, sinuses of Valsalva, and proximal ascending aorta) in athletes.[60] Another study compared strength and endurance trained athletes and found that the aortic root diameter was significantly larger in strength-trained athletes.[61] In contrast, a study of over 2,000 Italian athletes found that the largest aortic root dimensions were observed in endurance-trained athletes, specifically swimmers and cyclists.[62] To help resolve this conflicting data regarding aortic size in athletes, a recent meta-analysis was conducted to determine whether endurance or strength training is associated with increased aortic dimensions. This analysis found that the weighted mean aortic root diameter measured at the sinuses of Valsalva was 3.2 mm larger in athletes compared to non-athletic controls, whereas aortic root size at the aortic valve annulus was 1.6 mm greater in athletes than in controls.[63] In sum, the available data indicate that athletes may have a small yet clinically insignificant increase in aortic root diameter compared to matched sedentary controls. Clinicians evaluating athletes should be aware that age and gender influence aortic dimensions, and that marked aortic root dilatation likely represents a pathological process not physiological adaptation.

Differentiating Athlete's Heart from Pathology

The above discussion of exercise-induced cardiac remodeling holds relevance to the clinician charged with the care of athletic patients since differentiating the athlete's heart from occult cardiac pathology is a common clinical challenge. While a comprehensive discussion of this topic is beyond the scope of this chapter, several considerations deserve mention. The need to differentiate adaptive cardiac remodeling from cardiomyopathy typically arises following documentation of one of three cardinal findings: (1) thick LV walls, (2) dilated LV chamber, and (3) dilated RV chamber. The approach to this problem requires a comprehensive understanding of what constitutes normality in the trained athlete and thus begins with consideration of training history, family history, and the presence or absence of subjective symptoms and exercise intolerance. A clinical algorithm for the approach to the patient with cardiac abnormalities of uncertain etiology is provided in Figure 3.

Determinants of Myocardial Adaptation

Cardiovascular adaptations to exercise vary considerably across individual athletes. Explanatory factors including gender, ethnicity, sporting discipline,

Thick LV Walls	Dilated LV Chamber	Dilated RV Chamber
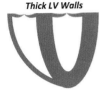		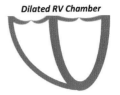

Thick LV Walls

Key Differential Diagnosis
Hypertrophic cardiomyopathy
Hypertensive heart disease
Infiltrative heart disease
Valvular heart disease

Clinical Factors c/w of Athlete's Heart
Strength training background
No subjective symptoms
Benign family history
Normal subjective exercise capacity

Echo Findings c/w Athlete's Heart
Mild symmetric LVH (walls <15 mm)
Normal RV dimensions
Normal / mildly enlarged LA
Normal aortic valve function
Normal mitral valve anatomy

Additional Diagnostic Considerations
Exercise testing (VO₂ assessment)
24h ambulatory BP monitor
Cardiac MRI
? Prescribed detraining

Dilated LV Chamber

Key Differential Diagnosis
Idiopathic dilated cardiomyopathy
Toxic (ETOH, drugs) cardiomyopathy
Infectious cardiomyopathy
Cardiomyopathy 2° tachyarrhythmia

Clinical Factors c/w of Athlete's Heart
Endurance training background
No subjective symptoms
Benign family history
No history of prior illness / substance abuse
Normal subjective exercise capacity

Echo Findings c/w Athlete's Heart
Concomitant RV dilation
Mild LV wall thickening
Supra-normal LV diastolic indices
Normal / mildly enlarged LA & RA

Additional Diagnostic Considerations
Exercise testing (VO₂ assessment)
Ambulatory rhythm monitoring
Cardiac MRI

Dilated RV Chamber

Differential Diagnosis
Arrhythmogenic RV cardiomyopathy
Idiopathic dilated cardiomyopathy
Pulmonary HTN / congenital heart disease
Sarcoidosis
Cardiomyopathy 2° tachyarrhythmia

Clinical Factors c/w of Athlete's Heart
Endurance training background
No subjective symptoms
Benign family history
Normal subjective exercise capacity

Echo Findings c/w Athlete's Heart
Concomitant LV dilation
Normal RV morphology
Supra-normal LV diastolic indices
Normal / mildly enlarged LA & RA
Normal RV systolic pressure

Additional Diagnostic Considerations
Signal averaged ECG
Exercise testing (VO₂ assessment)
Ambulatory rhythm monitoring
Cardiac MRI

Figure 3. Clinical considerations for the three most common cardiac structural scenarios (thick LV walls, dilated LV chamber, and dilated RV chamber) encountered in the clinical assessment of athletes. For each structural scenario, a differential diagnosis of the most common forms of overlap pathology, clinical/imaging attributes consistent with athlete's heart vs. occult pathology, and suggestions for adjunct diagnostic testing are provided. LV = left ventricular, RV = right ventricular, LA = left atrium, RA = right atrium.

underlying genetics, and duration of prior exercise exposure explain most but not all of this variability. Available data indicate that female athletes exhibit quantitatively less physiologic remodeling than their male counterparts. In an important early study, Pelliccia and colleagues presented cross-sectional echocardiographic data on 600 elite female Italian athletes and small group of sedentary controls.[64] Athletes in this study demonstrated larger left ventricular end-diastolic cavity dimension (49 ± 4 mm) and greater maximal wall thickness (8.2 ± 0.9 mm) than controls (46 ± 3 mm and 7.2 ± 0.6 mm; $p < 0.001$). Compared with data from previously studied male athletes ($n = 738$), female athletes showed significantly smaller left ventricular cavity dimension (11% less; $p < 0.001$) and wall thickness (23% less; $p < 0.001$) and were far less likely to have absolute measurements that exceeded normal cut-points. Similar findings have been reproduced by numerous investigators.[54,65–69] Although there are conflicting data in the literature, not all of the difference in absolute cardiac dimensions between men and women is eliminated when cardiac dimensions are corrected for the typically smaller female body size. Definitive mechanistic explanations for the gender-specific magnitude of exercise-induced cardiac adaptation remain elusive.

Ethnicity is also an important determinant of exercise-induced cardiac remodeling. Most notably, athletes of Afro-Caribbean descent, often termed Black athletes, tend to have thicker LV walls than Caucasian athletes. Basavarajaiah and colleagues studied a group of Caucasian and black male athletes utilizing echocardiographic imaging and found that nearly 20% of the black athletes had an LV wall thickness of at least 12 mm as compared to 4% of white athletes.[70] Importantly, 3% of black athletes in this cohort were found to have wall thickness of >15 mm. Similarly, Rawlins and colleagues studied ethnic/race related differences in a group of 440 black and white female athletes using echocardiography.[40] Black female athletes demonstrated significantly higher left ventricular wall thickness and mass compared to the white women (LV wall thickness = 9.2 ± 1.2 mm, LV mass = 187.2 ± 42 g in black athletes vs. LV wall thickness = 8.6 ± 1.2 mm, LV mass = 172.3 ± 42 g in the white athletes). At present, there are many ethnic populations that participate in athletics that have not been studied.

As discussed in detail above, exercise physiology differs markedly across sporting disciplines. In a landmark early paper, Morganroth and colleagues presented cross-sectional echocardiographic data which demonstrated strong associations between sport-type and left ventricular morphology.[14] Specifically, athletes participating in sports with predominantly isotonic physiology, swimmers and runners, were found to have larger left ventricular chamber diameters than athletes practicing wrestling, a sport with a largely isomteric physiology. Although the notion that cardiac dimensions vary as a function of sporting physiology has been challenged,[71] findings similar to those presented by Morganroth *et al.* have been reproduced by other investigators.[35,36,72] It must be emphasized that physiologic dichotomization of sporting disciplines into isometric and isotonic activities is a simplistic and inherently limited way of defining the cardiac stressors of exercise. Contemporary descriptions of exercise physiology acknowledge the fact that all athletic disciplines involve some element of each form of stress.[17] This is best illustrated by considering the broad category of endurance sports, which all share in common substantial amounts of isotonic stress, but which involve variable amounts of concomitant isometric stress. To what degree cardiac adaptations differ across the specific endurance disciplines has been largely unexplored and represents an area of important future work.

The genetics of exercise adaptation are an area of active investigation. Initial insights were gained from studies examining polymorphisms within gene coding for proteins of the renin-angiotensin-aldosterone axis. Among military recruits, the angiotensin-converting enzyme-DD polymorphism was associated with more

LVH than the II polymorphism during 10 weeks of exercise training.[73] Specific polymorphisms of the angiotensinogen gene have been similarly associated with LV remodeling.[74] Further work is required to examine alternative gene candidates in similar fashion. It has been shown that familial hypertension, a complex polygenic trait, is associated with both the magnitude and geometry of exercise-induced LV remodeling among endurance-trained athletes.[75] Further work will be required to determine the genetic and hemodynamic mechanisms underlying this observation.

Most recently, animal models of exercise have begun to clarify the molecular pathways that are responsible for cardiac adaptations to exercise. Several molecular mechanisms including the CCAAT/enhancer-binding protein β (C/EBPβ)/ (CITED)4 CBP/p300-Interacting Transactivators with E (glutamic acid)/D (aspartic acid) rich-carboxylterminal domain pathway and the IGF-1/neuregulin-1 (NRG-1) activated PI3K-AKT1 signaling pathway appear to be central to the process of exercise-induced cardiac remodeling.[76–79] Translational work documenting the role of such pathways in the human response to exercise will be required.

Finally, the influence of exercise exposure duration has recently been shown to play a role in the process of cardiac adaptation. Arbab-Zadeh *et al.* utilized a progressive exercise protocol to prepare 12 sedentary subjects (men, $n = 7$; age = 29 ± 6 years) for a marathon run (42 km) in which participants advanced through an incremental training protocol that began with light aerobic work characteristic of a clinical cardiac rehab program (1.5–3 h/week) and progressed to a more intense, recreational endurance athlete regimen (7–9 h/week).[80] In this setting, the authors observed a biphasic increase in LV mass with initial hypertrophy caused by LV wall thickening (0–6 months) and subsequent hypertrophy attributable to LV dilation (6–12 months). More recently, elite male rowers were followed with serial echocardiography over the 39-month period of high-intensity team-based training that spanned from college matriculation to graduation. In this study, there was a phasic remodeling response with distinct acute adaptations, including increases in LV chamber size, early diastolic function, and systolic twist, followed by a chronic phase of adaptation characterized by increasing wall thickness and regression in LV twist.[81] Although many questions about the role of exercise dose remain unanswered, it is increasingly clear that training duration is an important determinant of myocardial structure and function in athletes.

Uncertainties/Areas of Future Work

Although the last century of scientific investigation has lead to numerous advances in our understanding of how the heart and vascular system respond to exercise, key areas of uncertainty persist. The dose-response relationship between exercise and cardiac adaptation represents one such area. While it is well established that routine moderate intensity exercise promotes optimal cardiovascular health, several recent studies suggest that increasing "doses" of exercise may come with diminishing returns.[82,83] While this remains a controversial topic and is not the focus of this chapter, it serves to emphasize that we know relatively little about how varying levels of exercise volume and intensity dictate cardiac adaptation. There are several lines of evidence that suggest at least some association between the amount of exercise and the degree of cardiac remodeling. Large descriptive studies of elite athletes routinely report indices of cardiac chamber volume and mass that exceed those seen in less competitive athletic cohorts. One small prior study addressed this question directly by comparing cardiac parameters in international caliber rowers (22 ± 6 h of weekly training) to those in subelite rowers (11 ± 4 h of weekly training, $p < 0.001$).[30] In this study, metrics of both left and right ventricular size were significantly larger in the international caliber athletes. While some of the observed differences were accounted for by the significantly larger body sizes of the elite competitors, left ventricular volume, right ventricular volume, and left ventricular mass remained significantly larger after body size correction among the international level competitors. Due to the cross-sectional nature of the study design, this effort does not establish a cause and effect link between exercise dose and cardiac size, but serves as a hypothesis generating impetus for more definitive longitudinal studies.

The majority of data describing cardiac adaptation to sport have been derived from studies, such as the one above, that examine high-level competitors leaving questions about whether remodeling occurs in athletes of lower caliber who perform less exercise. Zilinski and colleagues recently conducted a prospective study in which approximately 50 recreational runners were studied with echocardiography before and after an 18-week marathon training plan that consisted of a relatively modest exercise dose of approximately 25 mi/week.[84] Interestingly, many of the adaptations that have been well described among high-level competitive athletes including mild eccentric LVH, left atrial dilation, and improvements in left ventricular diastolic function were observed. While more work will be required to characterize the myocardial response to moderate levels of exercise, it does appear that the process of exercise-induced cardiac remodeling is relevant to more that just elite athletes.

A final point about the exercise dose and cardiac remodeling relationship deserves mention. There are two principal components that define the magnitude of the exercise exposure: dose and intensity. The relative contribution of these two distinct factors to the process of cardiac remodeling remains completely unknown. The vast majority of studies examining exercise-induced cardiac remodeling provide quantitation of the exercise exposure as a sole function of duration, usually measured as hours per unit time. This fact is largely one of convenience as exercise duration is far simpler to measure and report with accuracy than exercise intensity. As such, we know very little about the role of exercise intensity as a determinant of the remodeling process. While methods that integrate both duration and intensity have been developed and applied in a limited capacity, we are unaware of any studies that have been completed with a primary goal of addressing this important issue. Although speculative, we suspect that both components of the exercise stimulus have independent and perhaps mechanistically discrete effects on cardiac remodeling.

Cardiac remodeling in response to exercise has traditionally been viewed as a benign and even health promoting phenomenon. However, recent preliminary data suggest that the most extreme degrees of remodeling may be accompanied by some maladaptive attributes. Two complementary studies of high level masters athletes, men and women with decades of intense, high-volume exercise exposure, have documented the presence of patchy myocardial fibrosis and associated ventricular arrhythmias.[85,86] When considered in tandem, these provocative cross-sectional studies raise the possibility that extreme amounts of exercise may lead to an ultimately maladaptive form of cardiac remodeling with potentially adverse clinical implications. At present, we view these data as hypothesis generating and as compelling grounds for longitudinal work in extreme performers with careful control for other factors that may cause cardiac muscle damage such as occult myocardial infection. While we await such work, it remains uncertain whether high levels of exercise should be discouraged, but it must be emphasized that moderate exercise exposure remains a key element of clinical disease prevention and should be encouraged in all patient populations.

Finally, to what degree exercise-induced cardiac remodeling is reversible in the contexts of both short- and long-term exercise abstinence remains uncertain. As described above, concentric LVH (LV wall thickening without chamber dilation) may develop in response to strength training. This form of athlete's heart may pose the greatest challenge when a clinician is asked to distinguish physiological adaptation (exercise-induced cardiac remodeling) from pathology (hypertrophic cardiomyopathy). At present, there is no single diagnostic test with adequate accuracy for making this distinction. Consequently, an integrated approach with consideration of personal and family history, 12-lead electrocardiography, imaging (echocardiography and/or cardiac MRI) and exercise testing is recommended.[87] Despite use of a systematic approach, "gray-zone" hypertrophy (13–15 mm) may remain ambiguous and prescribed detraining and follow-up cardiac imaging to assess for LVH regression may be required.

Despite the theoretical role of prescribed detraining, the time course and degree of expected LVH regression have not been well described. Most prior studies examining the LV response to exercise cessation have focused on eccentric LVH and have not standardized the duration of detraining. Maron *et al.* documented regression of eccentric LVH among Olympic athletes over 6–34 weeks (mean 13 weeks).[88] The largest detraining report to date included 40 elite Italian male athletes with eccentric LVH (LV dimension = 61.2 ± 2.9 mm, LV wall thickness = 12.0 ± 1.3 mm).[89] These athletes demonstrated complete normalization of wall thickness and significant but incomplete reduction in cavity dilation after 5.8 ± 3.6 years of detraining. The response of concentric LVH in strength athletes, the true mimicker of HCM, to prescribed detraining has not been well studied. A recent small study of five strength-trained athletes with concentric LVH showed significant regression of LV mass and LV wall thickness during a 6-month period of detraining.[90] Although a clinical profile of athletes with hypertrophic cardiomyopathy has recently been published,[91] there are currently no data defining the impact of exercise abstinence on cardiac parameters in patients with established cardiomyopathic conditions. It therefore remains unknown whether individuals with hypertrophic cardiomyopathy may demonstrate some regression of LVH following restriction from competitive sports. Further investigation is needed to address this important area of uncertainty and delineate the expected structural and functional changes in athletes with LVH and patients with cardiomyopathy undergoing a period of exercise cessation (prescribed detraining).

Personal Perspectives

Rory B. Weiner

I have always been interested in sports and physical activity, stemming from my earlier days as a cross-country runner and tennis player. In the latter, I was the right-handed member of a mirror-image identical twin doubles team which enjoyed success. Although we both became cardiologists, and not professional athletes, my interest in sports has persisted. At Massachusetts General Hospital, I have combined my passion for sports and also echocardiography to examine the cardiac remodeling that occurs in response to exercise training. As an investigator in the Harvard Athlete Initiative, I utilize echocardiography, including advanced techniques, such as speckle tracking, to study cardiac structure and function in athletes in longitudinal study designs. This work led to my first independent research funding, a Career Development Award from the American Society of Echocardiography, and subsequently a Scientist Development Grant from the

American Heart Association. A significant portion of my time is spent in the research investigation and clinical care of physically active individuals.

Aaron L. Baggish

My interest in the athletic heart began early in life and stemmed from my background as a competitive runner. The notion that the heart and vascular system are the primary determinants of endurance capacity and that with sustained training the cardiovascular system can adapt to enhanced performance has intrigued me since my days as a high school cross-country runner. Early in my medical training, it became clear to me that there was much to learn about the adaptive potential of the heart and that, as importantly, there was a growing need for cardiologists with interest and expertise in the care of athletes with heart disease. My career commitment to the study of athlete's heart and to the care of the athletic patient lead to the creation of the Cardiovascular Performance Program (CPP) at the Massachusetts General Hospital. Our productive and well-funded research program, our high volume clinical referral service, and our newly created sports cardiology fellowship continue to inspire me on a daily basis. It has and continues to be a privilege and a pleasure to study and to care for athletes of all ages, ambitions, and passions.

References

1. Henschen S. Skidlauf und Skidwettlauf. Eine medizinische Sportstudie. *Mitt Med Klin Upsala* 1899;2.
2. Darling EA. The effects of training. A study of the harvard university crews. *Boston Med Surg J* 1899;CXLI:229–233.
3. White PD. The pulse after a marathon race. *J Am Med Assoc* 1918;71:1047.
4. Keys A, Friedell HL. Size and stroke of the heart in young men in relation to athletic activity. *Science* 1938;88:456–458.
5. Farrell JT, Langan PC, Gordon B. Roentgen ray study of group of long-distance runners, with special reference to effects of exercise on size of heart. *Am J M Sc* 1929; 177:394.
6. Roesler H. A roentgenological study of the heart size in athletes. *Am J Roentgenol* 1936;36:849.
7. Shamroth L, Jokl E. Marked sinus and A-V nodal bradycardia with interference-dissociation in an athlete. *J Sports Med Phys Fitness* 1969;9:128.
8. Klemola E. Electrocardiographic observations on 650 Finnish athletes. *Ann Med Fenn* 1951;40:121.
9. Cullen KJ, Collin R. Daily running causing Wenckebach heart-block. *Lancet* 1964;2:729–730.

10. Sargin O, Alp C, Tansi C, Karaca L. Electrocardiogram of the month. Wenckebach phenomenon with nodal and ventricular escape in marathon runner. *Chest* 1970;57:102–105.

11. Allen HD, Goldberg SJ, Sahn DJ, Schy N, Wojcik R. A quantitative echocardiographic study of champion childhood swimmers. *Circulation* 1977;55:142–145.

12. Raskoff WJ, Goldman S, Cohn K. The "athletic heart". Prevalence and physiological significance of left ventricular enlargement in distance runners. *J Am Med Assoc* 1976;236:158–162.

13. Gilbert CA, Nutter DO, Felner JM, Perkins JV, Heymsfield SB, Schlant RC. Echocardiographic study of cardiac dimensions and function in the endurance-trained athlete. *Am J Cardiol* 1977;40:528–533.

14. Morganroth J, Maron BJ, Henry WL, Epstein SE. Comparative left ventricular dimensions in trained athletes. *Ann Intern Med* 1975;82:521–524.

15. Tanaka H, Monahan KD, Seals DR. Age-predicted maximal heart rate revisited. *J Am Coll Cardiol* 2001;37:153–156.

16. Whyte GP, George K, Shave R, Middleton N, Nevill AM. Training induced changes in maximum heart rate. *Int J Sports Med* 2008;29:129–133.

17. Mitchell JH, Haskell W, Snell P, Van Camp SP. Task Force 8: classification of sports. *J Am Coll Cardiol* 2005;45:1364–1367.

18. Pelliccia A, Culasso F, Di Paolo FM, Maron BJ. Physiologic left ventricular cavity dilatation in elite athletes. *Ann Intern Med* 1999;130:23–31.

19. Lang RM, Badano LP, Mor-Avi V, Afilalo J, Armstrong A, Ernande L, Flachskampf FA, Foster E, Goldstein SA, Kuznetsova T, Lancellotti P, Muraru D, Picard MH, Rietzschel ER, Rudski L, Spencer KT, Tsang W, Voigt JU. Recommendations for cardiac chamber quantification by echocardiography in adults: An update from the american society of echocardiography and the European association of cardiovascular imaging. *Eur Heart J Cardiovasc Imaging* 2015;16:233–271.

20. Weiner RB, Wang F, Hutter AM, Jr., Wood MJ, Berkstresser B, McClanahan C, Neary J, Marshall JE, Picard MH, Baggish AL. The feasibility, diagnostic yield, and learning curve of portable echocardiography for out-of-hospital cardiovascular disease screening. *J Am Soc Echocardiogr* 2012;25:568–575.

21. Fagard R, Aubert A, Staessen J, Eynde EV, Vanhees L, Amery A. Cardiac structure and function in cyclists and runners. Comparative echocardiographic study. *Brit Heart J* 1984;52:124–129.

22. Bar-Shlomo BZ, Druck MN, Morch JE, Jablonsky G, Hilton JD, Feiglin DH, McLaughlin PR. Left ventricular function in trained and untrained healthy subjects. *Circulation* 1982;65:484–488.

23. Bekaert I, Pannier JL, Van de Weghe C, Van Durme JP, Clement DL, Pannier R. Non-invasive evaluation of cardiac function in professional cyclists. *Brit Heart J* 1981;45:213–218.

24. Douglas PS, O'Toole ML, Hiller WD, Reichek N. Left ventricular structure and function by echocardiography in ultraendurance athletes. *Am J Cardiol* 1986;58:805–809.

25. Abergel E, Chatellier G, Hagege AA, Oblak A, Linhart A, Ducardonnet A, Menard J. Serial left ventricular adaptations in world-class professional cyclists: Implications for disease screening and follow-up. *J Am Coll Cardiol* 2004;44:144–149.

26. Baggish AL, Yared K, Wang F, Weiner RB, Hutter AM, Jr., Picard MH, Wood MJ. The impact of endurance exercise training on left ventricular systolic mechanics. *Am J Physiol* 2008;295:H1109–H1116.

27. Nottin S, Doucende G, Schuster-Beck I, Dauzat M, Obert P. Alteration in left ventricular normal and shear strains evaluated by 2D-strain echocardiography in the athlete's heart. *J Physiol* 2008;586:4721–4733.

28. Zocalo Y, Bia D, Armentano RL, Arias L, Lopez C, Etchart C, Guevara E. Assessment of training-dependent changes in the left ventricle torsion dynamics of professional soccer players using speckle-tracking echocardiography. *Conf Proc IEEE Eng Med Biol Soc* 2007;2007:2709–2712.

29. Weiner RB, Hutter AM, Jr., Wang F, Kim J, Weyman AE, Wood MJ, Picard MH, Baggish AL. The impact of endurance exercise training on left ventricular torsion. *JACC Cardiovasc Imaging* 2010;3:1001–1009.

30. Baggish AL, Yared K, Weiner RB, Wang F, Demes R, Picard MH, Hagerman F, Wood MJ. Differences in cardiac parameters among elite rowers and subelite rowers. *Med Sci Sports Exerc* 2010;42:1215–1220.

31. D'Andrea A, Cocchia R, Riegler L, Scarafile R, Salerno G, Gravino R, Golia E, Pezzullo E, Citro R, Limongelli G, Pacileo G, Cuomo S, Caso P, Russo MG, Bossone E, Calabro R. Left ventricular myocardial velocities and deformation indexes in top-level athletes. *J Am Soc Echocardiog* 2010;23:1281–1288.

32. Caso P, D'Andrea A, Galderisi M, Liccardo B, Severino S, De Simone L, Izzo A, D'Andrea L, Mininni N. Pulsed Doppler tissue imaging in endurance athletes: relation between left ventricular preload and myocardial regional diastolic function. *Am J Cardiol* 2000;85:1131–1136.

33. Stohr EJ, Gonzalez-Alonso J, Shave R. Left ventricular mechanical limitations to stroke volume in healthy humans during incremental exercise. *Am J Physiol* 2011;301: H478–H487.

34. Wasfy M, Weiner RB, Wang F, Berkstresser B, Lewis GD, DeLuca J, Hutter *AM Jr.*, Picard MH, Baggish A. Endurance exercise-induced cardiac remodling: not all sports are created equal. *J Am Soc Echocardiogr* 2015;28(12):1434–1440.

35. Baggish AL, Wang F, Weiner RB, Elinoff JM, Tournoux F, Boland A, Picard MH, Hutter AM, Jr., Wood MJ. Training-specific changes in cardiac structure and function: a prospective and longitudinal assessment of competitive athletes. *J Appl Physiol* 2008;104:1121–1128.

36. D'Andrea A, Limongelli G, Caso P, Sarubbi B, Della Pietra A, Brancaccio P, Cice G, Scherillo M, Limongelli F, Calabro R. Association between left ventricular structure and cardiac performance during effort in two morphological forms of athlete's heart. *Int J Cardiol* 2002;86:177–184.

37. Weiner RB, Wang F, Isaacs SK, Malhotra R, Berkstresser B, Kim JH, Hutter AM, Jr., Picard MH, Wang TJ, Baggish AL. Blood pressure and left ventricular hypertrophy during American-style football participation. *Circulation* 2013;128:524–531.

38. Pelliccia A, Maron BJ, Spataro A, Proschan MA, Spirito P. The upper limit of physiologic cardiac hypertrophy in highly trained elite athletes. *N Engl J Med* 1991;324:295–301.

39. Sharma S, Maron BJ, Whyte G, Firoozi S, Elliott PM, McKenna WJ. Physiologic limits of left ventricular hypertrophy in elite junior athletes: Relevance to differential diagnosis of athlete's heart and hypertrophic cardiomyopathy. *J Am Coll Cardiol* 2002;40:1431–1436.

40. Rawlins J, Carre F, Kervio G, Papadakis M, Chandra N, Edwards C, Whyte GP, Sharma S. Ethnic differences in physiological cardiac adaptation to intense physical exercise in highly trained female athletes. *Circulation* 2010;121:1078–1085.

41. Hauser AM, Dressendorfer RH, Vos M, Hashimoto T, Gordon S, Timmis GC. Symmetric cardiac enlargement in highly trained endurance athletes: A two-dimensional echocardiographic study. *Am Heart J* 1985;109:1038–1044.

42. Henriksen E, Landelius J, Wesslen L, Arnell H, Nystrom-Rosander C, Kangro T, Jonason T, Rolf C, Lidell C, Hammarstrom E, Ringqvist I, Friman G. Echocardiographic right and left ventricular measurements in male elite endurance athletes. *Eur Heart J* 1996;17:1121–1128.

43. Oxborough D, Sharma S, Shave R, Whyte G, Birch K, Artis N, Batterham AM, George K. The right ventricle of the endurance athlete: The relationship between morphology and deformation. *J Am Soc Echocardiog* 2012;25:263–271.

44. Scharhag J, Schneider G, Urhausen A, Rochette V, Kramann B, Kindermann W. Athlete's heart: Right and left ventricular mass and function in male endurance athletes and untrained individuals determined by magnetic resonance imaging. *J Am Coll Cardiol* 2002;40:1856–1863.

45. Scharf M, Brem MH, Wilhelm M, Schoepf UJ, Uder M, Lell MM. Cardiac magnetic resonance assessment of left and right ventricular morphologic and functional adaptations in professional soccer players. *Am Heart J* 2010;159:911–918.

46. Marcus FI, McKenna WJ, Sherrill D, Basso C, Bauce B, Bluemke DA, Calkins H, Corrado D, Cox MG, Daubert JP, Fontaine G, Gear K, Hauer R, Nava A, Picard MH, Protonotarios N, Saffitz JE, Sanborn DM, Steinberg JS, Tandri H, Thiene G, Towbin JA, Tsatsopoulou A, Wichter T, Zareba W. Diagnosis of arrhythmogenic right ventricular cardiomyopathy/dysplasia: proposed modification of the task force criteria. *Eur Heart J* 2010;31:806–814.

47. Pagourelias ED, Kouidi E, Efthimiadis GK, Deligiannis A, Geleris P, Vassilikos V. Right atrial and ventricular adaptations to training in male Caucasian athletes: An echocardiographic study. *J Am Soc Echocardiog* 2013;26:1344–1352.

48. Prakken NH, Velthuis BK, Teske AJ, Mosterd A, Mali WP, Cramer MJ. Cardiac MRI reference values for athletes and nonathletes corrected for body surface area, training hours/week and sex. *Eur J Cardiovasc Prev Rehabil* 2010;17:198–203.

49. D'Andrea A, Riegler L, Morra S, Scarafile R, Salerno G, Cocchia R, Golia E, Martone F, Di Salvo G, Limongelli G, Pacileo G, Bossone E, Calabro R, Russo MG. Right ventricular morphology and function in top-level athletes: A three-dimensional echocardiographic study. *J Am Soc Echocardiog* 2012;25:1268–1276.

50. Teske AJ, Prakken NH, De Boeck BW, Velthuis BK, Doevendans PA, Cramer MJ. Effect of long term and intensive endurance training in athletes on the age related decline in left and right ventricular diastolic function as assessed by Doppler echocardiography. *Am J Cardiol* 2009;104:1145–1151.

51. La Gerche A, Burns AT, D'Hooge J, Macisaac AI, Heidbuchel H, Prior DL. Exercise strain rate imaging demonstrates normal right ventricular contractile reserve and clarifies ambiguous resting measures in endurance athletes. *J Am Soc Echocardiog* 2012;25:253–262.e1.

52. Hoglund C. Enlarged left atrial dimension in former endurance athletes: an echocardiographic study. *Int J Sports Med* 1986;7:133–136.

53. Pelliccia A, Maron BJ, Di Paolo FM, Biffi A, Quattrini FM, Pisicchio C, Roselli A, Caselli S, Culasso F. Prevalence and clinical significance of left atrial remodeling in competitive athletes. *J Am Coll Cardiol* 2005;46:690–696.

54. D'Andrea A, Riegler L, Cocchia R, Scarafile R, Salerno G, Gravino R, Golia E, Vriz O, Citro R, Limongelli G, Calabro P, Di Salvo G, Caso P, Russo MG, Bossone E, Calabro R. Left atrial volume index in highly trained athletes. *Am Heart J* 2010;159:1155–1161.

55. Iskandar A, Mujtaba MT, Thompson PD. Left atrium size in elite athletes. *JACC Cardiovasc Imaging* 2015;8(7):753–762.

56. Grunig E, Henn P, D'Andrea A, Claussen M, Ehlken N, Maier F, Naeije R, Nagel C, Prange F, Weidenhammer J, Fischer C, Bossone E. Reference values for and determinants of right atrial area in healthy adults by 2-dimensional echocardiography. *Circ Cardiovasc Imaging* 2013;6:117–124.

57. D'Ascenzi F, Pelliccia A, Natali BM, Zaca V, Cameli M, Alvino F, Malandrino A, Palmitesta P, Zorzi A, Corrado D, Bonifazi M, Mondillo S. Morphological and functional adaptation of left and right atria induced by training in highly trained female athletes. *Circ Cardiovasc Imaging* 2014;7:222–229.

58. McClean G, George K, Lord R, Utomi V, Jones N, Somauroo J, Fletcher S, Oxborough D. Chronic adaptation of atrial structure and function in elite male athletes. *Eur Heart J Cardiovasc Imaging* 2015;16(4):417–422.

59. Andersen K, Farahmand B, Ahlbom A, Held C, Ljunghall S, Michaelsson K, Sundstrom J. Risk of arrhythmias in 52 755 long-distance cross-country skiers: a cohort study. *Eur Heart J* 2013;34:3624–3631.

60. Babaee Bigi MA, Aslani A. Aortic root size and prevalence of aortic regurgitation in elite strength trained athletes. *Am J Cardiol* 2007;100:528–530.

61. D'Andrea A, Cocchia R, Riegler L, Scarafile R, Salerno G, Gravino R, Vriz O, Citro R, Limongelli G, Di Salvo G, Cuomo S, Caso P, Russo MG, Calabro R, Bossone E. Aortic root dimensions in elite athletes. *Am J Cardiol* 2010;105: 1629–1634.

62. Pelliccia A, Di Paolo FM, De Blasiis E, Quattrini FM, Pisicchio C, Guerra E, Culasso F, Maron BJ. Prevalence and clinical significance of aortic root dilation in highly trained competitive athletes. *Circulation* 2010;122:698–706.

63. Iskandar A, Thompson PD. A meta-analysis of aortic root size in elite athletes. *Circulation* 2013;127:791–798.

64. Pelliccia A, Maron BJ, Culasso F, Spataro A, Caselli G. Athlete's heart in women. Echocardiographic characterization of highly trained elite female athletes. *J Am Med Assoc* 1996;276:211–215.

65. George KP, Wolfe LA, Burggraf GW, Norman R. Electrocardiographic and echocardiographic characteristics of female athletes. *Med Sci Sports Exerc* 1995;27:1362–1370.

66. Sun B, Ma JZ, Yong YH, Lv YY. The upper limit of physiological cardiac hypertrophy in elite male and female athletes in China. *Eur J Appl Physiol* 2007;101:457–463.

67. Whyte GP, George K, Nevill A, Shave R, Sharma S, McKenna WJ. Left ventricular morphology and function in female athletes: A meta-analysis. *Int J Sports Med* 2004;25:380–383.

68. Haykowsky M, Chan S, Bhambhani Y, Syrotuik D, Quinney H, Bell G. Effects of combined endurance and strength training on left ventricular morphology in male and female rowers. *Can J Cardiol* 1998;14:387–391.

69. Rowland T, Roti M. Influence of sex on the "Athlete's Heart" in trained cyclists. *J Sci Med Sport* 2010;13:475–478.

70. Basavarajaiah S, Boraita A, Whyte G, Wilson M, Carby L, Shah A, Sharma S. Ethnic differences in left ventricular remodeling in highly-trained athletes relevance to differentiating physiologic left ventricular hypertrophy from hypertrophic cardiomyopathy. *J Am Coll Cardiol* 2008;51:2256–2262.

71. Naylor LH, George K, O'Driscoll G, Green DJ. The athlete's heart: A contemporary appraisal of the 'Morganroth hypothesis'. *Sports Med* 2008;38:69–90.

72. D'Andrea A, Riegler L, Golia E, Cocchia R, Scarafile R, Salerno G, Pezzullo E, Nunziata L, Citro R, Cuomo S, Caso P, Di Salvo G, Cittadini A, Russo MG, Calabro R, Bossone E. Range of right heart measurements in top-level athletes: the training impact. *Int J Cardiol* 2013;164:48–57.

73. Montgomery HE, Clarkson P, Dollery CM, Prasad K, Losi MA, Hemingway H, Statters D, Jubb M, Girvain M, Varnava A, World M, Deanfield J, Talmud P, McEwan JR, McKenna WJ, Humphries S. Association of angiotensin-converting enzyme gene I/D polymorphism with change in left ventricular mass in response to physical training. *Circulation* 1997;96:741–747.

74. Karjalainen J, Kujala UM, Stolt A, Mantysaari M, Viitasalo M, Kainulainen K, Kontula K. Angiotensinogen gene M235T polymorphism predicts left ventricular hypertrophy in endurance athletes. *J Am Coll Cardiol* 1999;34:494–499.

75. Baggish AL, Weiner RB, Yared K, Wang F, Kupperman E, Hutter AM, Jr., Picard MH, Wood MJ. Impact of family hypertension history on exercise-induced cardiac remodeling. *Am J Cardiol* 2009;104:101–106.

76. Buerke M, Murohara T, Skurk C, Nuss C, Tomaselli K, Lefer AM. Cardioprotective effect of insulin-like growth factor I in myocardial ischemia followed by reperfusion. *Proc Natl Acad Sci U S A* 1995;92:8031–8035.

77. McMullen JR, Shioi T, Zhang L, Tarnavski O, Sherwood MC, Kang PM, Izumo S. Phosphoinositide 3-kinase(p110alpha) plays a critical role for the induction of physiological, but not pathological, cardiac hypertrophy. *Proc Natl Acad Sci USA* 2003; 100:12355–12360.

78. DeBosch B, Treskov I, Lupu TS, Weinheimer C, Kovacs A, Courtois M, Muslin AJ. Akt1 is required for physiological cardiac growth. *Circulation* 2006;113:2097–2104.

79. Bostrom P, Mann N, Wu J, Quintero PA, Plovie ER, Panakova D, Gupta RK, Xiao C, MacRae CA, Rosenzweig A, Spiegelman BM. C/EBPbeta controls exercise-induced cardiac growth and protects against pathological cardiac remodeling. *Cell* 2010;143:1072–1083.

80. Arbab-Zadeh A, Perhonen M, Howden E, Peshock RM, Zhang R, Adams-Huet B, Haykowsky MJ, Levine BD. Cardiac remodeling in response to 1 year of intensive endurance training. *Circulation* 2014;130:2152–2161.

81. Weiner RB, Deluca JR, Wang FW, Lin JJ, Wasfy M, Berkstresser B, Stohr EJ, Shave R, Lewis GD, Hutter *AM Jr.*, Picard MH, Baggish A. Exercise induced left ventricular remodeling among competitive athletes: A phasic phenomenon. *Circ Cardiovasc Imaging* 2015;8(12):e003651.

82. Lee DC, Pate RR, Lavie CJ, Sui X, Church TS, Blair SN. Leisure-time running reduces all-cause and cardiovascular mortality risk. *J Am Coll Cardiol* 2014;64:472–481.

83. Schnohr P, O'Keefe JH, Marott JL, Lange P, Jensen GB. Dose of jogging and long-term mortality: The copenhagen city heart study. *J Am Coll Cardiol* 2015;65:411–419.

84. Zilinski JL, Contursi ME, Isaacs SK, Deluca JR, Lewis GD, Weiner RB, Hutter AM, Jr., d'Hemecourt PA, Troyanos C, Dyer KS, Baggish AL. Myocardial adaptations to recreational marathon training among middle-aged men. *Circ Cardiovasc Imaging* 2015;8(2):e002487.

85. Wilson M, O'Hanlon R, Prasad S, Deighan A, Macmillan P, Oxborough D, Godfrey R, Smith G, Maceira A, Sharma S, George K, Whyte G. Diverse patterns of myocardial fibrosis in lifelong, veteran endurance athletes. *J Appl Physiol* 2011;110:1622–1626.

86. La Gerche A, Burns AT, Mooney DJ, Inder WJ, Taylor AJ, Bogaert J, Macisaac AI, Heidbuchel H, Prior DL. Exercise-induced right ventricular dysfunction and structural remodelling in endurance athletes. *Eur Heart J* 2012;33:998–1006.

87. Maron BJ. Distinguishing hypertrophic cardiomyopathy from athlete's heart physiological remodelling: Clinical significance, diagnostic strategies and implications for preparticipation screening. *Br J Sports Med* 2009;43:649–656.

88. Maron BJ, Pelliccia A, Spataro A, Granata M. Reduction in left ventricular wall thickness after deconditioning in highly trained Olympic athletes. *Brit Heart J* 1993;69:125–128.

89. Pelliccia A, Maron BJ, De Luca R, Di Paolo FM, Spataro A, Culasso F. Remodeling of left ventricular hypertrophy in elite athletes after long-term deconditioning. *Circulation* 2002;105:944–949.

90. Weiner RB, Wang F, Berkstresser B, Kim J, Wang TJ, Lewis GD, Hutter AM, Jr., Picard MH, Baggish AL. Regression of "gray zone" exercise-induced concentric left ventricular hypertrophy during prescribed detraining. *J Am Coll Cardiol* 2012;59:1992–1994.

91. Sheikh N, Papadakis M, Schnell F, Panoulas V, Malhotra A, Wilson M, Carre F, Sharma S. Clinical profile of athletes with hypertrophic cardiomyopathy. *Circ Cardiovasc Imaging* 2015;8:e003454.

Chapter 4

Mechanisms of Adaptation of the Coronary Circulation to Exercise/Exercise Training

M. Harold Laughlin and T. Dylan Olver

*Departments of Biomedical Sciences, and Medical Pharmacology
and Physiology, and DCRC, University of Missouri
Columbia, MO 65211, USA*

Introduction

Atherosclerotic coronary artery disease (CAD) of large coronary arteries (i.e. right, left main, circumflex, and left anterior descending coronary arteries) is a progressive disease starting with fatty streak lesions and culminating in complicated lesions producing thrombosis and myocardial infarction and/or sudden cardiac death. The development of CAD involves complex changes in the phenotypes of coronary vascular cells as well as infiltration of the artery wall by white blood cells. The two primary cell types responsible for vasomotor function of coronary arteries are vascular smooth muscle (VSM) and endothelial cells (EC). VSM cells modulate the diameter of the coronary arteries and EC influence VSM contraction. EC dysfunction is present throughout the process of atherosclerosis and plays an important role in development of CAD.[1] Physical activity/exercise is an important lifestyle factor that is now well established for being effective in prevention[2-5] and treatment of CAD.[5-7] Consistent with the idea that physical activity/exercise training are effective in prevention of CAD, Katzmarzyk *et al.* reported that all-cause

mortality and mortality resulting from cardiovascular disease are inversely proportional to cardiorespiratory fitness.[8] Indeed, available information indicates that
increasing or maintaining a high level of cardiorespiratory fitness is important for
vascular health in patients with known CAD, as well as people with type 2 diabetes mellitus (T2D), obesity, and even in normal weight lean individuals.[5] Exercise
training has emerged as an intervention for primary and secondary prevention of
coronary artery disease and is a Class 1a therapeutic option for treatment of
CAD.[7,9–11] Because of this, nearly every cardiologist and primary care physician
knows that physical activity is important for a healthy lifestyle and powerful in
prevention and treatment of CAD, although it is also clear that exercise training
does not provide immunity from atherosclerosis.[12,13]

It is now well established that cardiac rehabilitation and exercise-training programs produce beneficial effects on traditional cardiovascular risk factors including: plasma lipid profiles and glucose, body weight/obesity, blood pressure,
systemic inflammation, autonomic cardiovascular control, and improved cardiorespiratory fitness. There are several excellent reviews of the effects of exercise
training in patients with CAD to which the reader is referred.[5,9–11,14] A key paper in
the field is the prospective study of 27,000 apparently healthy women conducted
by Mora *et al.*[15] As summarized in Figure 1, these authors measured hemoglobin
A1c, blood lipids, novel lipids, creatinine, homocysteine, and inflammatory/
hemostatic biomarkers, as well as self-reported physical activity, weight, height,

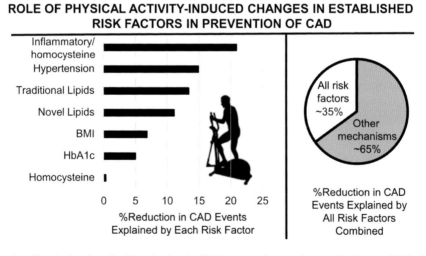

Figure 1.   Graph showing the % reduction in CAD events that can be ascribed to established risk
factors. Data are from Ref. 15. Data for each of the risk factors are presented in the bar graphs on
the left. On the right the pie chart shows that 35% of the protection provided by exercise can be
explained by the effects of exercise on all of these risk factors. Thus, the remaining protection must
be due to other mechanisms.

blood pressure, and indices of diabetes over a 10-year period. As shown on the right of Figure 1, their results indicated that 35.5% of the reduction in CAD events associated with physical activity could be attributed to exercise training-induced changes in established risk factors.[15] This key report raises the question: "What is the physiological basis for the 41–64.5% gap in our understanding of how physical activity attenuates atherosclerotic cardiovascular disease?" One hypothesis is that these additional beneficial effects of exercise training, not related to risk factors, result from changes in the biology of vascular cells and/or coronary blood vessels.[16] In a more recent review, Green *et al.* referred to these adaptations as "a vascular conditioning effect of exercise training."[17] Based on these observations, the primary purpose of this chapter is to summarize what is known about the effects of exercise on the coronary circulation and vascular cell mechanisms responsible for the beneficial effects of exercise. We first consider coronary vascular adaptations in normal subjects and then those demonstrated in CAD. As discussed below, although it is likely that mechanisms responsible for adaptations in the normal coronary circulation contribute to effectiveness of physical activity/exercise in the prevention and treatment of CAD, these adaptations do not appear to explain the entire benefit of exercise training in CAD patients. Understanding of the effects of exercise training on the coronary circulation in health and disease is important for those who prescribe exercise as part of the strategy to prevent CAD and for treatment of CAD as this is a key component of evidence-based medicine.

Although this chapter focuses on the effects of exercise on the coronary circulation, it is important to emphasize that, in a CAD patient, the ability of exercise training to increase maximal cardiac output through adaptations in left ventricular (LV) mass and diameter (i.e. eccentric hypertrophy) should not be overlooked. These adaptations are important for the training-induced increase in cardiorespiratory fitness. Further, coronary blood flow (CBF) per gram of myocardium is less in fit subjects at rest and during exercise because exercise training decreases myocardial oxygen demand by decreasing heart rate, contractility, and LV systolic wall stress and work.[18,19] These adaptations have a positive influence on the balance between oxygen supply and demand. Exercise training also induces adaptations in the coronary circulation and coronary vascular cells.

Exercise Training-induced Adaptations in the Normal Coronary Circulation

The coronary circulation provides about 100 mL/min/100 g of blood to the myocardium 24 h a day, every day of a person's life. Further, coronary blood flow can increase 4- to 6-fold during high-intensity exercise and other causes of cardiac stress. The coronary transport reserve capacity consists of an ability to increase CBF and capillary exchange above resting levels.[18,20] The transport reserve capacity of the normal coronary circulation is so large that it is not apparent why there is a need for an increase with exercise training.[18,20,21] Therefore, it is somewhat surprising that in normal mammals dynamic exercise training increases coronary transport capacity through increases in CBF capacity and capillary exchange capacity.[19] As we have described previously, exercise training-induced adaptations in the coronary circulation can be divided into functional (alterations in control of vascular resistance) and structural (angiogenesis and vascular remodeling).[16,19,21,22] Adaptations in control of coronary vascular resistance in normal subjects include changes in neurohumoral control and changes in vasomotor reactivity of coronary resistance arteries. These changes contribute to increased myocardial oxygen extraction following exercise training as exercise generally does not change the oxygen carrying capacity of blood.[19]

Structural vascular adaptations in the normal heart

In young rats exercise training increases myocardial capillary density, however, in older rats and larger mammals exercise training appears to match angiogenesis of capillaries to cardiac hypertrophy so that capillary density is maintained in the normal range.[19,23] Similarly, canine[24–26] and swine[27] show no change in coronary capillary/fiber ratio[24,27] or capillary density[24–27] following exercise training.[19,23] During exercise training in pigs, while capillary endothelial cell division and capillary sprouting were increased at 1, 3, and 8 weeks of training, there were no longer differences in capillary density after 16 weeks of exercise training.[28,29] Thus, in a fully-trained animal coronary capillary growth was matched to LV hypertrophy. This matching of capillary angiogenesis to cardiac hypertrophy is in contrast to pathologic forms of myocardial hypertrophy (due to hypertension or aortic stenosis) where capillary rarefaction often occurs.[30] The maintenance of capillary density in the hypertrophied myocardium reflects a prime difference between physiological and pathological cardiac remodeling and highlights the potential role of exercise training as a strategy to restore capillarity in pathological conditions.

Arteriolar density (number of coronary arterioles per mm^2) was also reported to be 40–60% greater in exercise trained than in sedentary swine.[27,28] Indeed, total cross-sectional area (μm^2 arterioles per mm^2 of myocardium) of arterioles is increased by exercise training, with a greater increase in total area of small (20–40 μm) than in larger (40–120 μm) arterioles.[29] In rats, exercise training may also influence compliance of coronary arterioles as it has been reported to reduce the collagen/elastin ratio within the vessel wall of coronary arterioles.[31] The increase in arteriolar cross-sectional area likely is central to increased total coronary blood flow capacity after exercise training.[19]

Exercise training also increases large epicardial coronary artery diameter. Increased coronary artery size has been reported in exercise-trained rodents, larger mammals, as well as humans.[19,32–35] Similar to changes in capillary density, increases in coronary artery size are proportional to increases in LV mass in elite athletes compared to healthy sedentary individuals.[34–36] Evidence suggests that outward remodeling of epicardial coronary arteries occurs to normalize the level of shear stress facing the arterial lumen wall. As discussed below, because shear stress upregulates eNOS expression it appears that there is a transient increase in eNOS expression early on in a training program that subsides as the epicardial arteries remodel, increase in diameter, and levels of shear stress normalize.

Haskell *et al.*[37] reported no differences in angiographicly measured, cross-sectional areas of the right, left main, and left anterior descending (LAD) coronary arteries of ultra-distance runners and sedentary subjects under basal resting conditions. But Haskell *et al.*[37] also reported that nitroglycerin-induced increases in coronary cross-sectional area were positively correlated with aerobic exercise capacity suggesting that the increased artery size was only apparent during nitroglycerin-induced dilation. Hildick-Smith[38] reported that nitroglycerin produced significantly greater dilation of the LAD in athletes than in sedentary men. Finally, Kozakova *et al.*[32] also reported a 2-fold greater dipyridamole-induced dilation of the left main coronary artery in athletes than in control subjects. Thus, results indicate that exercise training stimulates growth of epicardial arteries in proportion to the degree of cardiac hypertrophy and that conduit coronary artery vasodilator capacity is greater after exercise training.

Adaptations in coronary vascular control in the normal heart

Exercise training has been reported to increase parasympathetic and decrease sympathetic activity to the heart, but does not appear to alter autonomic control of CBF.[39–41] Thus, exercise training increases parasympathetic drive to the heart, but muscarinic receptor density/sensitivity in coronary vasculature is not altered and there is no evidence that exercise training alters parasympathetic control of coronary conduit and resistance vessel tone, and myocardial beta-adrenergic receptor density and sensitivity are also reported to be unchanged after exercise training (as reviewed in Ref. 19). Current literature suggests that, alpha-adrenergic tone is maintained or slightly increased in coronary resistance vessels after exercise training. This interpretation is supported by observations that coronary resistance vessels exhibit greater constriction in response to alpha$_1$-adrenergic stimulation after exercise training. During submaximal exercise it appears that there is maintained or slightly increased alpha-adrenergic and maintained beta-adrenergic tone in the coronary microcirculation of exercise trained subjects.[19]

Exercise training has also been reported to blunt the vasoconstrictor response of the proximal coronary arteries to $alpha_1$-adrenergic receptor stimulation in dogs[42,43] and swine.[44] Stehno-Bittel *et al.*[45,46] proposed the decreased vasoconstrictor reactivity is the result of exercise-induced decreases of intracellular calcium concentrations (Ca_i) in coronary VSM. Interestingly, exercise training did not alter vasoconstrictor responses of proximal coronary arteries to KCl or prostaglandin $F_2\alpha$.[43,44] Conversely, endothelium-dependent vasodilation produced by $alpha_2$-adrenergic receptor stimulation was not altered by exercise training in coronary arteries.[44]

Effects of exercise training on endothelium dependent dilator responses of coronary conduit arteries

In the early 1990s, Wang *et al.* reported that 7 days of exercise training, 2 h/day enhanced endothelium dependent dilation (EDD) to acetylcholine and reactive hyperemia in conduit coronary arteries and that the enhanced EDD was abolished by inhibition of nitric oxide synthase (NOS) with N-nitro-L-arginine while responses to nitroglycerine were not affected by training.[47] In contrast, longer exercise training programs (>10 weeks) reported that EDD of proximal arteries was not increased in dogs,[43] swine,[48] or rats.[49] It appears that during exercise training, progressive outward remodeling of the epicardial arteries occurs as summarized above. As a result of the increased diameter of the arteries, shear-stress levels during exercise are returned to normal and in response, eNOS expression is normalized,[50,51] thereby allowing EDD responses to return towards baseline levels.[43,48,50,52]

Effects of exercise training on vascular control in the coronary microcirculation

Coronary arterioles from exercise-trained pigs exhibit enhanced myogenic constriction compared to arterioles from sedentary pigs[53] and similar results were found in exercise-trained rats.[31] This enhanced tone may be due to altered calcium-dependent PKC signaling in the coronary VSM cells,[54] and increased voltage-gated calcium currents in VSM of large arterioles through L-type calcium channels.[55] The increased constriction in response to stretch (myogenic reactivity) is not accompanied by changes in receptor-mediated vasoconstriction (ET-1, acetylcholine,) or to direct stimulation of voltage-gated calcium channel activation with the L-type calcium channel agonist Bay K8644 or by K^+.[56] Exercise training may increase activity of K_v and K_{Ca} channels of coronary VSM and/or alter calcium control by the sarcoplasmic reticulum.[16,57,58]

Exercise training increases the maximal adenosine-induced increase in CBF per gram of myocardium in both dogs and miniature swine *in vivo*,[19] thus maximal CBF is increased. Although CBF capacity is increased by exercise training, CBF at rest and during submaximal exercise (same absolute intensities) is equal or slightly lower after exercise. At similar levels of cardiac work CBF is not changed by exercise training suggesting that exercise has a minimal effect on the coupling between myocardial metabolism and CBF.[18–20]

Exercise training has also been reported to increase coronary EDD in response to serotonin (increased CBF in anesthetized dogs)[42] and bradykinin in coronary arterioles (64–157 μm in diameter) isolated from exercise-trained swine.[53] The increased bradykinin-induced EDD appeared to be the result of increased NO release from eNOS because L-N^g-monomethyl arginine (L-NMMA) inhibited EDD to a greater extent in arterioles from exercise-trained pigs and eliminated the difference between trained and sedentary groups.[53] Consistent with this interpretation, subsequent work revealed increased endothelial NOS expression in coronary arterioles of exercise-trained swine.[51] It is interesting that in normal subjects, exercise training appears to produce sustained augmentation of EDD in the coronary microcirculation, but EDD is only transiently increased in conduit coronary arteries. In both cases, the enhanced EDD appears to be principally due to increased NO bioavailability.

Effects of exercise training on coronary transport capacity

Although current literature indicates that maximal CBF and coronary capillary diffusion capacity are both increased by exercise training there are reports of either no change[27,61–67] or an increase in maximal CBF.[18–20]

Our review of the literature indicates that in studies that rigorously assessed CBF capacity by assuring maximal vasodilation, controlling hemodynamic conditions, and documented the efficacy of the training program, CBF capacity was consistently reported to be increased following exercise training in swine,[29,68] dogs[24,69] and rats.[16,20,21,23,68–70] Importantly, clinical studies that assessed CBF capacity using echo-Doppler or positron emission tomography (PET) also provide a mixed view of the effects of exercise training on CBF capacity with some reporting increases[32,33,36,38,71] and others no change.[72–75] As is true for the animal studies, it is necessary to evaluate the quality of the CBF capacity measurements by determination of the assurance of maximal vasodilation, control of hemodynamic variables, and documentation of training effectiveness in these clinical studies. Importantly, the standard doses of adenosine used in most human studies measuring coronary reserve are not sufficient to cause maximal dilation so the measurements estimate coronary reserve, not CBF capacity.[76] These measures of coronary vasodilator reserve provide valuable prognostic information, but they may not rigorously estimate true coronary flow reserve. Therefore, the weight of current evidence suggests that exercise training increases maximal CBF per gram of myocardium.

Exercise training increases coronary capillary exchange capacity measured as coronary capillary permeability-surface area product in dogs and miniature swine.[18–20] Morphometric measurements of capillarization and capillary permeability-surface area product in the same hearts revealed that training increased coronary capillary permeability-surface area product with no change in capillary density.[18–20,28,77] It appears that exercise training induced changes in the distribution of coronary vascular resistance which resulted in increased effective capillary surface area and capillary permeability-surface area product without a change in coronary capillary numerical density.[19] These adaptations could be involved in the reported decrease in coronary sinus oxygen content and increase in oxygen extraction in exercise-trained dogs.[18–20]

In summary, available evidence indicates that both maximum CBF and coronary capillary permeability-surface area product are increased by exercise training and that this may improve the capacity and reserve to deliver oxygen to the myocardium. As summarized in Figure 2, these increases in coronary transport capacity are the result of increases in arteriolar and capillary density, enlargement of large coronary arteries, and changes in the vasomotor control of coronary epicardial arteries, resistance arteries, and arterioles.

Effects of exercise training on the coronary circulation in CAD

Suaya *et al.* reported results of a meta-analysis of 601,099 medicare beneficiaries who were hospitalized for CAD that demonstrate mortality rates were 21–34% lower in users of cardiac rehabilitation than in non-users.[78] As shown in Figure 3, from 1 to 5 years following discharge, rehabilitation provided substantial decreases in mortality rates. A key component of cardiac rehabilition is increased physical activity, i.e. exercise training. The mechanisms proposed to contribute to the beneficial effects of exercise training in CAD include regression of atherosclerosis, improvement of endothelial function, formation of collaterals (arteriogenesis), increases in circulating endothelial progenitor cells (EPCs), and development of new vessels (angiogenesis/vasculogenesis).[11,16,19] Below, we briefly summarize evidence concerning the effects of exercise training on coronary lesion

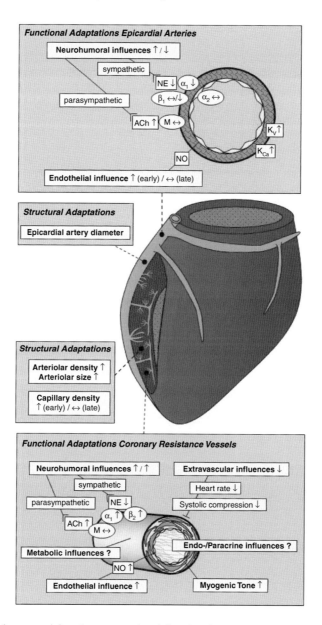

Figure 2.   Graph summarizing the structural and functional coronary adaptations to chronic exercise training in normal subjects. ACh = acetylcholine; M = muscarinic receptor; NE = norepinephrine; α_1 = alpha$_1$-adrenergic receptor; β_1 = beta$_1$-adrenergic receptor; β_2 = beta$_2$-adrenergic receptor; K_v = voltage-dependent K channel; K_{Ca} = Ca^{2+}-dependent K channel. Modified from Ref. 19 with permission of the American Physiological Society.

progression/regression, endothelial and coronary VSM cell function/phenotype in CAD, and on the collateral circulation and coronary microcirculation within collateral-dependent myocardium.

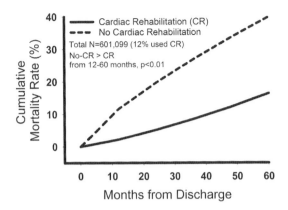

Figure 3.   Graph showing the relative mortality rate of subjects that participated in cardiac rehabilitation compared to those that did not. Results are taken from Ref. 78.

Exercise training effects on coronary plaque/lesion progression/regression

As summarized above, it is generally recognized that exercise training leads to enlargement of conduit coronary arteries in animals and humans.[20,26,32–35] There is also evidence that exercise training can reduce development of atherosclerotic lesions in coronary arteries of animal models of disease including Apo E-deficient mice,[79–81] rabbits,[82] and pigs[83] and/or may cause regression of atherosclerotic lesions in coronary arteries.

In contrast, our results indicate that exercise training did not retard progression or reverse coronary atherosclerosis in pigs in early stage disease,[1,84] but exercise training did seem to increase antioxidant protein content in coronary arterioles.[1] In primates, Kramsch *et al.*[85] reported that exercise training decreased CAD, but a more recent study by Williams *et al.*[86] found that wheel running in adult male monkeys did not retard progression or reverse CAD as measured with angiographic measures of lesion area even though exercise improved measures of cardiovascular health.[86] Although exercise training appears to have small effects on lesion size/progression, we and others have demonstrated that exercise training in CAD has beneficial effects on endothelial function/phenotype, as reflected in increased EDD and altered expression of endothelial genes toward a more atheroprotective phenotype.[87–89]

Randomized human trials that used angiography to evaluate the effects of exercise training on coronary lesion progression/regression provide important insight into whether or not exercise has a direct effect on lesion size in CAD.[10,90–93] The Lifestyle Heart Trial[92] included exercise in combination with low-fat diet as part of the lifestyle interventions and found that % stenosis decreased (regressed) in the coronary arteries of the treatment group but increased (progressed) in the control group. More recently, the Heidelberg Regression Study[90,93] reported that regular, leisure time exercise retarded progression of and/or reversed CAD. CAD patients were prospectively randomized either to an intervention exercise group ($n = 29$) (30 min of exercise/day recommended, plus 60 min of supervised exercise 2 times/week) or to a control group ($n = 33$) receiving usual care (including recommendation of 30 min/day of exercise) and no supervised exercise.[90] Leisure time physical activity from standardized questionnaires and participation in group exercise sessions was used to estimate energy expenditure. Repeat coronary angiography was performed after 1 year of participation and coronary lesions were measured by digital image processing. Oxygen uptake increased by 7% at ventilatory threshold and by 14% at peak exercise in the exercise intervention group, while oxygen uptake decreased under both conditions in the control group of patients. The exercise intervention group exhibited regression of CAD in 8 patients (28%), progression of disease in 3 patients (10%), and no change in coronary morphology in 18 patients (62%), whereas in the control group progression was observed in 45%, no change in 49%, and regression of disease in 6%. When the patient groups were combined into groups according to progression/no change/ regression of CAD, the lowest level of leisure time physical activity was noted in patients with progression of disease ($1,022 \pm 142$ kcal/week) as opposed to patients with no change ($1,533 \pm 122$ kcal/week) or regression of disease ($2,204 \pm 237$ kcal/week).[90] These seminal experiments suggested that leisure time exercise that consumes 2,204 kcal/week in a CAD patient for 1 year can induce regression of CAD lesions.[90] The Stanford Coronary Risk Intervention Project, which assigned patients to a risk-reduction group or usual care group, obtained similar results[91] as the risk-reduction group exhibited 47% less lesion progression after 1 year than the usual care group. Haskell *et al.* reported that the change in treadmill exercise performance was the best predictor of the change in coronary stenosis.[91] Because it does not appear that the ability of exercise training to cause regression or slow growth of coronary atherosclerotic lesions has been addressed since the studies mentioned above, the importance of this mechanism in the beneficial effects of exercise also remains unclear.[9]

Exercise training may have a greater effect on CAD lesion progression/regression following treatment with percutaneous transluminal coronary angiography and/or placement of intravascular stents. Belardinelli *et al.*[94] divided 118 patients who received percutaneous transluminal coronary angioplasty and/or stent treatments into an exercise training group (three supervised exercise bouts (at 60% peak oxygen consumption)/week) and a Control group (mild normal activity of life). After 6 months, results indicated improved functional capacity and quality of life of the exercise trained group relative to controls and that the exercise training group had fewer coronary events and hospital readmissions. The extent of restenosis was lower in the exercise trained patients in both the balloon-dilated and stented segments, but the number of patients exhibiting restenosis was not different between groups. Regression of CAD was seen in three exercise-trained patients, while none of the control subjects exhibited regression of CAD. Also, in the exercise trained group the number of new lesions in epicardial coronary arteries not undergoing angioplasty was lower than in the controls.[94] Fleenor and Bowles reported that exercise training can inhibit coronary artery lesion development and alter extracellular matrix composition of coronary neointima formed following percutaneous transluminal coronary angioplasty in Yucatan miniswine.[95] Although the circumflex branch was not affected by exercise training, exercise training significantly decreased lesion size and neointima proliferation in the LAD and attenuated type I collagen expression.

Also, total collagen was increased and fibronectin was decreased in the neointima of both LAD and left circumflex (LCx) coronary arteries of trained pigs. Similar results were obtained in the Ossabaw pig model of type 2 diabetes as exercise training reduced vascular disease in the peri-stent and non-stent regions of coronary arteries treated with percutaneous transluminal coronary angioplasty.[96] Importantly, similar results were obtained by Madssen *et al.*[102] who randomized 36 CAD patients, that received optimal treatment following intracoronary stent implantation, into either a moderate continuous (~70% peak heart rate) or an interval exercise (~90% peak heart rate) group (and evaluated plaque burden and vulnerability using intravascular ultrasound before and after training). Following the 12-week intervention, results suggest chronic exercise, regardless of the intensity, triggers a modest regression of plaque burden and necrotic core (distal to stent placement) in coronary lesions, resulting in a general shift of plaques classified as "vulnerable" to "less vulnerable." Thus, exercise training after percutaneous transluminal coronary angioplasty seems to decrease coronary lesion size and alter composition of the extracellular matrix of the wall of the coronary arteries which may result in less vulnerable plaques.[95] Importantly, exercise training in the context of cardiac rehabilitation has consistently been found to decrease mortality on CAD patients[78] and of CAD patients treated with percutaneous coronary intervention.[97] Indeed, cardiac rehabilitation results in substantial decreases in mortality rates[78] (Figure 3).

Overall the current literature paints a mixed picture concerning whether or not atherosclerotic lesion progression/regression is significantly altered by exercise training. In large mammals that have coronary arteries structurally more similar to human arteries, exercise training does not seem to alter lesion progression/regression. The most compelling evidence of a beneficial effect of exercise on lesion regression is from human subjects. However, there is evidence of beneficial effects of exercise in coronary arteries of humans and animals that have been treated with percutaneous transluminal coronary angioplasty and/or intravascular stents. It is not currently clear why exercise training would influence plaque formation/regression following interventional procedures but not limit lesion development and/or cause CAD plaque regression in the absence of such interventions. It seems possible that coronary hemodynamics are altered by interventional procedures and/or stenting such that exercise bouts generate more beneficial mechanical signals in the walls of these arteries, but this is speculation. Importantly, the reported changes in percent stenosis in these studies are quite small and therefore likely of little functional significance.[7,90–93] In this regard, Linke *et al.*[11] stated: "…the almost negligible amount of regression is unlikely to account for the tremendous relief in symptoms of CAD and the improvement of myocardial perfusion in patients undergoing exercise training" and Linke *et al.*[11] concluded that the beneficial effects of exercise training may be largely the result of training-induced improvement in EDD and/or overall endothelial function in the coronary circulation.

Exercise-induced alterations in atherosclerotic lesion composition may play an important role in reduced CAD mortality in physically active individuals even in the absence of any effects of exercise training on CAD lesion size. Acute coronary syndromes (ACS) and sudden death are most often associated with rupture of complex, vulnerable plaques that are otherwise clinically benign, i.e. <70% luminal stenosis, and asymptomatic.[98] There is evidence for an inverse relationship between chronic physical activity and incidence of first acute myocardial infarction, even in individuals with normal stress ECGs.[99] This observation is consistent with the concept that physical activity may shift a "vulnerable" thin-cap atheroma to a more stable lesion less prone to rupture. In support of this notion, exercise training in mice[100,101] reduces plaque rupture and increases cap thickness and collagen content perhaps due to lower matrix metalloproteinase (MPP-9) and increased tissue inhibitor of metalloproteinases (TIMP). Fleenor *et al.* report similar changes in lesion composition in post-angioplasty restenosis in swine.[95] More recently, Madssen *et al.* reported a reduction in the necrotic core area and a general shift from "vulnerable" to "less vulnerable" plaques in CAD patients with intracoronary stent implantation following 12 weeks of moderate continuous and interval exercise training.[102] More work is needed to determine the effects of exercise training on the composition of atherosclerotic lesions. In this regard, changes in the phenotype of coronary VSM may contribute to changes in lesion size and/or composition, and exercise training in CAD has beneficial effects on endothelial function/phenotype, as reflected in increased EDD and altered expression of endothelial genes toward a more atheroprotective phenotype.[87–89,103]

VSM interacts with endothelium thus playing an important role in both the initiation and progression of atherosclerotic lesions.[104,105] Exercise training may influence coronary VSM phenotypic modulation in atherosclerosis through altered ion channel regulation of intracellular calcium (Ca_i).[19,88] The same changes in intracellular calcium would also be expected to decrease the tendency for coronary vasospasm. It appears that exercise training interacts with proatherogenic factors resulting in decreased lesion progression and/or lesion regression through effects on shear stress stimulated release of NO by ECs, alterations in transmural pressure and/or altered circulating factors. It is clear that more work is needed to fully understand the effects or exercise training on coronary VSM phenotype and its role in atherogenesis.

As summarized above, there is substantial evidence that exercise training improves endothelial function in normal coronary and peripheral arteries due to increased NO production through eNOS and increased expression of superoxide dismutase (SOD).[18–20] Hambrecht *et al.*[106] reported that exercise training increased EDD of conduit and resistance coronary arteries of CAD patients.[106] Beck *et al.* also reported that endothelial function (i.e. EDD) in CAD patients was improved in peripheral arteries by exercise training and that this improvement correlated to serum levels of vascular endothelial growth factor (VEGF) and erythropoietin.[107] Exercise training also preserved EDD of coronary arteries of hypercholesterolemic pigs[87,103] in early stage CAD. Exercise training increased NO bioavailability (perhaps due to increased content of SOD enzyme) and decreased a prostanoid vasoconstrictor present in the hypercholesterolemic pig coronary arteries.[87,103] Exercise training did not alter the role of other endothelium-derived factors such as endothelium-derived hyperpolarizing factor.[87,103] Thus, exercise training increases EDD in coronary arteries and arterioles of animal models of CAD and in patients with CAD.[9,11,14,16,108] As outlined in several review articles, there is current debate about the relative role of endothelial progenitor cells (EPCs) in the beneficial effects of exercise training on the coronary endothelium.[4,7,11,109] Acute exercise bouts mobilize these cells from bone marrow and these cells in the circulation are believed to be attracted to damaged endothelium where they attach. These cells then either differentiate to mature ECs or secreted factors that modulate EC proliferation and vascular remodeling. Exercise training also increases the number of circulating EPCs and their function, and available evidence indicates that EPC number correlates with endothelial function.[4,7,11,109] We must look forward to results from ongoing research to fully appreciate the role of EPCs in the beneficial effects of exercise training in prevention and treatment of CAD.

In patients with long standing CAD, collateralization can be impressive and there is evidence that exercise training can increase collateral blood flow in CAD. This area remains a subject of controversy because measurements of collateral CBF using retrograde flow from a cannulated collateral-dependent coronary artery, and using radioactive microspheres, have consistently found that exercise training does not alter collateral CBF.[18–20] However, when collateral CBF was measured in chronically instrumented dogs before and after exercise training, results revealed that collateral CBF was increased by exercise training.[110,111] Cohen[111] found that the chronic instrumentation procedure stimulated the growth of coronary collaterals independent of exercise (similar increase in collateral CBF in sedentary animals). Thus, available literature indicates that exercise training does not increase collateral blood flow in the normal heart, and that increases in collateral CBF in chronically instrumented dogs after exercise training are likely due to the instrumentation and not to the exercise training.

Results indicate that exercise does increase collateral CBF in the presence of disease and in models of CAD. For example, exercise training in dogs with a chronic coronary artery stenosis does increase collateral formation.[112] Eckstein[112] measured retrograde blood flow from the cannulated collateral-dependent artery and found that exercise training produced the greatest increases in collateral CBF when the training started after formation of a mild coronary stenosis. These results were the first to suggest that if exercise bouts produce myocardial ischemia they are more effective in stimulating collateral vessel growth. Another model of CAD, ameroid constrictor which produces gradual coronary occlusion, has also provided mixed results as Heaton *et al.*[113] and Neill and Oxendine[114] reported no effect of exercise training on collateral CBF in dogs with ameroid constrictors while collateral CBF was reported to be increased (to 50% of normal) in the collateral-dependent region of pigs that were exercise trained, with an ameroid coronary occlude.[115,116]

Although several angiographic studies of collateralization in CAD patients have found no effect of exercise training on angiographicly detectable collateralization,[117,118] angiographic measures are limited to measurement of the size of relatively large coronary collaterals and do not assess collateral CBF. Belardinelli *et al.*[119] used thallium uptake to measure collateral-dependent CBF in patients with ischemic cardiomyopathy, and reported 8 weeks of moderate exercise training increased collateral CBF. Thus, exercise training does not appear to stimulate collateral formation in the coronary circulation of normal hearts, whereas if exercise bouts produce or aggravate myocardial ischemia in a region of myocardium distal to a coronary lesion (stenosis), then exercise training is effective in stimulating collateral vessel growth.

The literature consistently indicates that exercise training has beneficial effects on the vasomotor reactivity of collateral arteries and/or vasomotor control of resistance in collateral-dependent myocardium. Thus, exercise training was found to improve EDD in epicardial arteries isolated from the collateral-dependent region of the heart[120] and improve adenosine-induced vasodilation.[121] In coronary arterioles isolated from the collateral-dependent myocardium, exercise training improves bradykinin-induced EDD[122] and improves vascular endothelial growth factor (VEGF165)-induced EDD due to increased NO bioavailability.[123] Interestingly, exercise training did not improve bradykinin-induced EDD of arterioles isolated from the normally perfused region of collateralized hearts[122] in contrast to results from coronary arterioles isolated from normally trained pigs.[53] Griffin *et al.* proposed that the effects of exercise training on coronary arteriolar vasomotor reactivity are modified in the non-occluded arterial beds of chronically coronary occluded hearts.[122] Thus, the coronary arteries located in the non-occluded zones of hearts cannot be assumed to be "control" vessels.

Similar to what was reported for arterioles of normal pig hearts,[124] exercise training increased myogenic tone in arterioles isolated from collateral-dependent zones of the ameroid occlusion model of CAD.[125] Exercise training also resulted in enhanced endothelin-1 mediated contractile responses in collateral-dependent resistance arteries ($\sim$150 μm)[126] and vasodilator responses signaled through K_v channel activity.[125] As summarized in Figure 4, coronary resistance arteries isolated from the collateral-dependent region of hearts from exercise-trained pigs exhibit increased basal tone and increased vasodilator influences, increased EDD, increased NO production, and increased K^+ channel activity, whereas arterioles isolated from the remote (non-ischemic) myocardium exhibit some different adaptations to exercise training. Coronary resistance arteries isolated from the hearts of pigs with atherosclerotic CAD exhibit adaptations to exercise training that are similar to those of the arterioles from the collateral depend myocardium.[127] It seems reasonable to propose that these arteriolar adaptations to exercise training provide a greater capacity of the coronary microcirculation to sustain CBF to myocardium at risk of ischemia. Indeed, Linke *et al.*[11] proposed that the effects of exercise training on endothelium and EDD may be of greater importance than any other known effect of exercise training on the coronary circulation.

Conclusions

Physical activity/exercise training is beneficial in prevention and treatment of atherosclerotic CAD. As summarized in Figure 5, it is clear that this is partially the result of decreased risk factors, but some of the remaining benefits result from exercise-induced coronary vascular adaptation including structural remodeling and altered phenotype/function of VSM and EC. In the normal heart, exercise training produces a variety of structural adaptations in the coronary circulation, including: (i) increased conduit artery diameters, (ii) increased arteriolar densities and diameters, and (iii) maintained coronary capillary numerical density commensurate with the degree of cardiac hypertrophy. These changes likely underlie the increased CBF per gram of myocardium and increased diffusion capacity in exercise-trained hearts. It appears that the coronary circulation is not

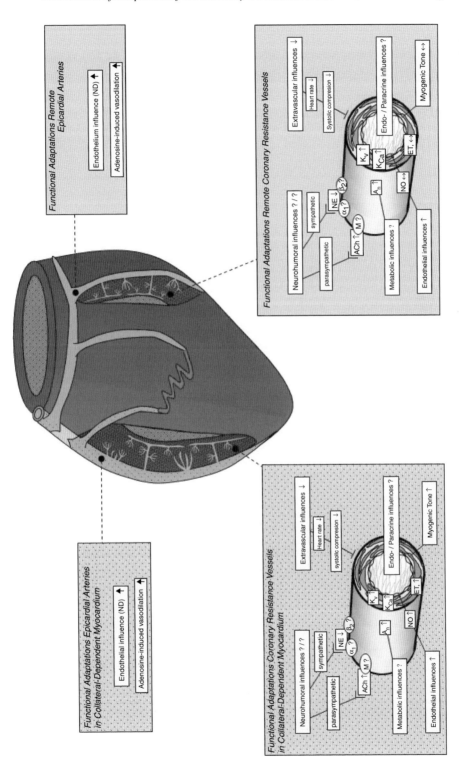

Figure 4.   Graph summarizing the structural and functional coronary adaptations to chronic exercise training in the collateral circulation. Abbreviations the same as in Figure 2. A = adenosine receptor; ET = Endothelin receptor. Modified from Ref. 19 with permission of the American Physiological Society.

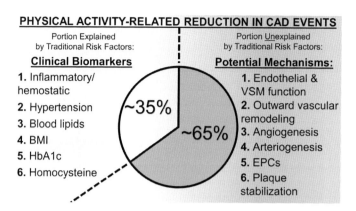

Figure 5.   Model summarizing the mechanisms responsible for the beneficial effects of physical activity/exercise training in prevention and treatment of coronary artery disease (CAD).

structurally static. Rather, the structure of the coronary vascular tree appears to be undergoing fine-tuning all the time, presenting non-linear, non-uniform adaptations throughout the course of an exercise training program. In the normal heart these effects appear to be relatively small. Conversely, CAD causes structural changes in the large coronary arteries that lead to decreased coronary transport function. As a result, in CAD, exercise-induced structural adaptations appear to be of greater importance. In both the normal and diseased coronary circulation, exercise-induced adaptation leads to sustained/enhanced coronary transport function. The effects of exercise training on coronary structure in the presence of atherosclerotic disease involves some of the phenomena described above for normal adaptations, but may also have additional beneficial effects on lesion volume/composition and the amount of the lesions that represent vulnerable plaque. There is evidence that exercise training modifies progression/regression of atherosclerosis, but the magnitude of these effects seems small relative to the overall clinical benefits provided by exercise training. This fact has led many to propose that the major benefit of exercise training may be on the phenotype/function of coronary vascular cells.

The functional adaptations induced by exercise in the coronary circulation include (i) an increased EDD (transient in conduit arteries; sustained in resistance vessels) that is principally NO-mediated, (ii) altered alpha-adrenergic influence (reduced in conduit vessels and increased in resistance vessels), and (iii) a change in local control of the diameter of resistance vessels. Coronary arterioles exhibit increased myogenic tone after exercise training. In models of disease and in CAD patients, if exercise bouts produce or increase ischemia, there is evidence that collateral growth can be enhanced. In CAD patients and animal models of CAD, evidence indicates that exercise training also increases EDD in conduit arteries and in the arterial tree in the areas of myocardium at risk.

Thus, while there have been major advances in our understanding of coronary vascular adaptation to exercise training in health and CAD, several research questions remain outstanding. For example, the molecular mechanisms underlying the structural and functional adaptations to exercise training in the coronary vascular tree of the normal heart remain incompletely understood. Hemodynamic signals (shear and stretch[128]) and chemical signals (i.e. myokines, adipokines, insulin, and glucagon) generated by exercise bouts are likely what initiate changes in gene expression of vascular cells.[129] Hemodynamic signals may also be involved in the mechanism by which exercise training induces/enhances collateral formation in hearts with a coronary artery stenosis. Another puzzling set of observations is that evidence indicates that exercise training has beneficial effects on endothelial function/phenotype, yet does not influence atherosclerosis progression/regression in animal models of CAD.

Although we do not fully understand the mechanisms underlying the clinical benefit of exercise training in patients with CAD, there is no doubt about the benefits both in prevention and treatment.[4,5] What is perhaps of greatest concern is that cardiac rehabilitation programs (that include exercise training) are underutilized[5] and further, compliance to prescribed exercise is also poor. For example, the HF-ACTION trial reported 84% initial compliance of patients, 65% compliance at 1 year, and 40% compliance at 3 years.[130] Schuler *et al.*[4] indicated that the Heart Failure Association of the European Society of Cardiology concluded that low adherence of patients to prescribed exercise training is the "Achilles heel" of the use of exercise training in treating patients. Clearly it is important for each cardiologist to spend time convincing their patients of the importance of physical activity and exercise training programs in cardiovascular and coronary health at the time they recommend exercise to their patients.

Personal Perspectives

M. Harold Laughlin

I became interested in the effects of exercise on the coronary circulation when I was a graduate student in 1970 at the University of Iowa. My advisor John Diana studied microcirculation and Dr. Charles Tipton was a renouned exercise physiologist. Under their leadership, I combined their approaches to my interests. At the time I was intrigued by the lack of understanding of the coronary circulation and the effects of acute and chronic exercise on this circulatory bed. In 1981, this became the focus of my NIH grant entitled: "Exercise: Coronary Reserve,

Coronary Heart Disease" which funded my work in this area until my focus shifted to CAD in 1993 after my coronary event. This lead to the funding of our program project grant in 1995; "Vascular Cell Biology: Exercise Training and Coronary Disease." While we have learned a lot about CAD and the mechanisms responsible for the beneficial effects of exercise in prevention and treatment of CAD, much remains to be established. As summarized above, there is no doubt about the fact that a physically active lifestyle is central to cardiovascular health and a lack of this lifestyle in Western culture causes substantial mortality and morbidity. I believe that we will be better equipped to prescribe exercise to patients and encourage humans to be physically active when we understand the mechansims responsible for these beneficial effects on the circulation in general and specifically the coronary circulation.

T. Dylan Olver

As a Physiologist, I enjoy investigating the mechanisms that regulate physiological function from a systems perspective down to the molecular level. My love for integrative physiology developed as a result of my ongoing interest and involvement in physical activity and nutritional strategies to improve physical performance. Over the years, as I experienced the health of loved ones deteriorate and was exposed to more and more research, I became fascinated by the relationship between physical activity and vascular disease; from both a contemporary and evolutionary standpoint. My chief thrust is to identify major gaps in our knowledge of vascular disease throughout the lifespan and differentiate the physiological vs. pathological vascular adaptations that accelerate disease progression. Further, given the benefits of routine physical activity, my goal is to develop strategies for catalyzing progress towards the formation and implementation of targeted, customized exercise prescriptions to improve vascular health outcomes. Understanding the nature of, and identifying the underlying mechanisms of, specific physical activity-induced vascular adaptations holds extraordinary promise in the development of personalized exercise medicine.

Acknowledgments

The authors' work was supported by grants from the National Heart, Lung, and Blood Institute Grant #'s HL-52490, HL-35088, and HL112998.

References

1. Arce-Esquivel AA, Kreutzer KV, Rush JW, Turk JR, Laughlin MH. Exercise does not attenuate early cad progression in a pig model. *Med Sci Sports Exer* 2012; 44:27–38.

2. Blair SN, Church TS. The fitness, obesity, and health equation: Is physical activity the common denominator? *J Am Med Assoc* 2004;292:1232–1234.

3. Dhaliwal SS, Welborn TA, Howat PA. Recreational physical activityh as an independent predictor of multivariable cardiovascular disease risk. *PloS One* 2013;8: e83435.

4. Schuler G, Adams V, Goto Y. Role of exercise in the prevention of cardiovascular disease: Results, mechanisms, and new perspectives. *Eur Heart J* 2013;34: 1790–1799.

5. Swift DL, Lavie CJ, Johannsen NM, Arena R, Earnest CP, P'Keefe JH, Milani RV, Blair SN. Physical activity, cardiorespiratory fitness, and exercise training in primary and secondary coronary prevention. *Circ J* 2013;77:281–292.

6. Gielen S, Laughlin MH, O'Conner C, Duncker DJ. Exercise training in patients with heart disease: Review of beneficial effects and clinical recommendations. *Prog Cardiovasc Dis* 2015;57:347–355.

7. Wienbergen H, Hambrecht R. Physical exercise and its effects on coronary artery disease. *Curr Opin Pharmacol* 2013;13:218–225.

8. Katzmarzyk PT, Church TS, Blair SN. Cardiorespiratory fitness attenuates the effects of the metabolic syndrome on all-cause and cardiovascular disease mortality in men. *Arch Intern Med* 2004;164:1092–1097.

9. Gielen S, Schuler G, Adams V. Cardiovascular effects of exercise training: Molecular mechanisms. *Circulation* 2010;122:1221–1238.

10. Gielen S, Schuler G, Hambrecht R. Exercise training in coronary artery disease and coronary vasomotion. *Circulation* 2001;103:e1–e6.

11. Linke A, Erbs S, Hambrecht R. Exercise and the coronary circulation — alterations and adaptations in coronary artery disease. *Prog Cardiovasc Dis* 2006;48:270–284.

12. Mohlenkamp S, Bose D, Mahabadi AA, Heusch G, Erbel R. On the paradox of exercise: Coronary atherosclerosis in an apparently healthy marathon runner. *Nat Clin Pract Cardiovasc Med* 2007;4:396–401.

13. Currens JH, White PD. Half a century of running. Clinical, physiologic and autopsy findings in the case of clarence demar ("Mr. Marathon"). *N Engl J Med* 1961;265: 988–993.

14. Ribeiro F, Alves AJ, Duarte JA, Oliveira J. Is exercise training an effective therapy targeting endothelial dysfunction and vascular wall inflammation? *Int J Cardiol* 2010;141:214–221.

15. Mora S, Cook N, Buring JE, Ridker PM, Lee I-M. Physical activity and reduced risk of cardiovascular events: Potential mediating mechanisms. *Circulation* 2007;116: 2110–2118.

16. Laughlin MH, Joseph B. Wolfe memorial lecture. Physical activity in prevention and treatment of coronary disease: The battle line is in exercise vascular cell biology. *Med Sci Sports Exer* 2004;36:352–362.

17. Green DJ, O'Driscoll G, Joyner MJ, Cable NT. Exercise and cardiovascular risk reduction: Time to update the rationale for exercise? *J Appl Physiol* 2008; 150(2):766–768.

18. Laughlin MH, Davis MJ, Secher NH, van Lieshout JJ, Arce-Esquivel AA, Simmons GH, Bender SB, Padilla J, Bache RJ, Merkus D, Duncker DJ. Peripheral circulation. *Compr Physiol* 2012;2:321–447.

19. Laughlin MH, Bowles DK, Duncker DJ. The coronary circulation in exercise training. *Am J Physiol Heart Circ Physiol* 2012;302:H10–H23.

20. Laughlin MH, Korthuis RJ, Duncker DJ, Bache RJ. *Control of Blood Flow to Cardiac and Skeletal Muscle During Exercise. Chapter 16.* New York: American Physiological Society and Oxford University Press, 1996.

21. Laughlin MH. Coronary transport reserve in normal dogs. *J Appl Physiol* 1984;57:551–561.

22. Brown MD. Exercise and coronary vascular remodelling in the healthy heart. *Exp Physiol* 2003;88:645–658.

23. Duncker DJ, Bache RJ. Regulation of coronary blood flow during exercise. *Physiol Rev* 2008;88:1009–1086.

24. Laughlin MH, Tomanek RJ. Myocardial capillarity and maximal capillary diffusion capacity in exercise-trained dogs. *J Appl Physiol* 1987;63:1481–1486.

25. Wyatt HL, Mitchell JH. Influences of physical training on the heart of dogs. *Cir Res* 1974;35:883–889.

26. Wyatt HL, Mitchell JH. Influences of physical conditioning and deconditioning on coronary vasculature of dogs. *J Appl Physiol* 1978;45:619–625.

27. Breisch EA, White FC, Nimmo LE, McKirnan MD, Bloor CM. Exercise-induced cardiac hypertrophy: A correlation of blood flow and microvasculature. *J Appl Physiol* 1986;60:1259–1267.

28. White FC, McKirnan MD, Breisch EA, Guth BD, Liu YM, Bloor CM. Adaptation of the left ventricle to exercise-induced hypertrophy. *J Appl Physiol* 1987;62:1097–1110.

29. White FC, Bloor CM, McKirnan MD, Carroll SM. Exercise training in swine promotes growth of arteriolar bed and capillary angiogenesis in heart. *J Appl Physiol* 1998;85:1160–1168.

30. Bache RJ. Effects of hypertrophy on the cornary circulation. *Prog Cardiovasc Disease* 1988;30:403–440.

31. Hanna MA, Taylor CR, Chen B, La HS, Maraj JJ, Kilar CR, Behnke BJ, Delp MD, Muller-Delp JM. Structural remodeling of coronary resistance arteries: Effects of age and exercise training. *J Appl Physiol* 2014;117:616–623.

32. Kozakova M, Galetta F, Gregorini L, Bigalli G, Franzoni F, Giusti C, Palombo C. Coronary vasodilator capacity and epicardial vessel remodeling in physiological and hypertensive hypertrophy. *Hypertension* 2000;36:343–349.

33. Kozakova M, Paterni M, Bartolomucci F, Morizzo C, Rossi G, Galetta F, Palombo C. Epicardial coronary artery size in hypertensive and physiologic left ventricular hypertrophy. *Am J Hypertens* 2007;20:279–284.

34. Pelliccia A, Spataro A, Granata M, Biffi A, Caselli G, Alabiso A. Coronary arteries in physiological hypertrophy: Echocardiographic evidence of increased proximal size in elite athletes. *Int J Sports Med* 1990;11:120–126.

35. Zandrino F, Molinari G, Smeraldi A, Odaglia G, Masperone MA, Sardanelli F. Magnetic resonance imaging of athlete's heart: Myocardial mass, left ventricular function, and cross-sectional area of the coronary arteries. *Eur Radiol* 2000;10: 319–325.

36. Windecker S, Allemann Y, Billinger M, Pohl T, Hutter D, Orsucci T, Blaga L, Meier B, Seiler C. Effect of endurance training on coronary artery size and function in healthy men: An invasive followup study. *Am J Physiol Heart Circ Physiol* 2002;282:H2216–H2223.

37. Haskell WL, Sims C, Myll J, Bortz WM, St Goar FG, Alderman EL. Coronary artery size and dilating capacity in ultradistance runners. *Circulation* 1993;87:1076–1082.

38. Hildick-Smith DJ, Johnson PJ, Wisbey CR, Winter EM, Shapiro LM. Coronary flow reserve is supranormal in endurance athletes: An adenosine transthoracic echocardiographic study. *Heart* 2000;84:383–389.

39. Blomqvist CG, Saltin B. Cardiovascular adaptations to physical training. *Ann Rev Physiol* 1983;45:169–189.

40. Raven PB, Rohm-Young D, Blomqvist CG. Physical fitness and cardiovascular response to lower body negative pressure. *J Appl Physiol* 1984;56:138–144.

41. Scheuer J, Tipton CM. Cardiovascular adaptations to physical training. *Ann Rev Physiol* 1977;39:221–251.

42. Bove AA, Dewey JD. Proximal coronary vasomotor reactivity after exercise training in dogs. *Circulation* 1985;71:620–625.

43. Rogers PJ, Miller TD, Bauer BA, Brum JM, Bove AA, Vanhoutte PM. Exercise training and responsiveness of isolated coronary arteries. *J Appl Physiol* 1991;71: 2346–2351.

44. Oltman CL, Parker JL, Adams HR, Laughlin MH. Effects of exercise training on vasomotor reactivity of porcine coronary arteries. *Am J Physiol* 1992;263:372–382.

45. Stehno-Bittel L, Laughlin MH, Sturek M. Exercise training alters ca release from coronary smooth muscle sarcoplasmic reticulum. *Am J Physiol* 1990;259: H643–H647.

46. Stehno-Bittel L, Laughlin MH, Sturek M. Exercise training depletes sarcoplasmic reticulum calcium in coronary smooth muscle. *J Appl Physiol* 1991;71:1764–1773.

47. Wang J, Wolin MS, Hintze TH. Chronic exercise enhances endothelium-mediated dilation of epicardial coronary artery in conscious dogs. *Circ Res* 1993;73: 829–838.

48. Oltman CL, Parker JL, Laughlin MH. Endothelium-dependent vasodilation of proximal coronary arteries from exercise-trained pigs. *J Appl Physiol* 1995;79:33–40.

49. Parker JL, Mattox ML, Laughlin MH. Contractile responsiveness of coronary arteries from exercise-trained rats. *J Appl Physiol* 1997;83:434–443.

50. Laughlin MH. Endothelium-mediated control of coronary vascular tone after chronic exercise training. *Med Sci Sports Exerc* 1995;27:1135–1144.

51. Laughlin MH, Pollock JS, Amann JF, Hollis ML, Woodman CR, Price EM. Training induces nonuniform increases in enos content along the coronary arterial tree. *J Appl Physiol* 2001;90:501–510.

52. Laughlin MH, Turk JR, Schrage WG, Woodman CR, M. PE. Influence of coronary artery diameter on enos protein content. *Am J Physiol* 2003;284:H1307–H1312.

53. Muller JM, Myers PR, Laughlin MH. Vasodilator responses of coronary resistance arteries of exercise-trained pigs. *Circulation* 1994;89:2308–2314.

54. Korzick DH, Laughlin MH, Bowles DK. Alterations in pkc signaling underlie enhanced myogenic tone in exercise-trained porcine coronary resistance arteries. *J Appl Physiol* 2004;96:1425–1432.

55. Bowles DK, Hu Q, Laughlin MH, Sturek M. Exercise training increases l-type calcium current density in coronary smooth muscle. *Am J Physiol* 1998;275: H2159–H2169.

56. Laughlin MH, Muller JM. Vasoconstrictor responses of coronary resistance arteries in exercise- trained pigs. *J Appl Physiol* 1998;84:884–889.

57. Heaps C, Bowles DK, Sturek M, Laughlin MH, Parker JL. Enhanced l-type Ca2+ channel current density in coronary smooth muscle of exercise-trained pigs is compensated to limit myoplasmic free ca2+ accumulation. *J Physiol* 2000;528: 435–445.

58. Bowles DK, Wamhoff BR. Coronary smooth muscle adaptation to exercise: Does it play a role in cardioprotection? *Acta Physiol Scand* 2003;178:117–121.

59. Heiss HW, Barmeyer J, Wink J, Hell G, Cerny FJ, Keul J, Reindell H. Studies on the regulation of myocardial blood flow in man I: Training effects on blood flow and metabolism of the healthy heart at rest and during standardized heavy exercise. *Basic Res Cardiol* 1976;71:658–675.

60. von Restorff W, Holtz J, Bassenge E. Exercise induced augmentation of myocardial oxygen extraction in spite of normal coronary dilatory capacity in dogs. *Pflug Arch* 1977;372:181–185.

61. Barnard RJ, Duncan HW, Baldwin KM, Grimditch G, Buckberg DD. Effects of intensive exercise training on myocardial performance and coronary blood flow. *J Appl Physiol* 1980;49:444–449.

62. Bove AA, Hultgren PB, Ritzer TF, Carey RA. Myocardial blood flow and hemodynamic responses to exercise training in dogs. *J Appl Physiol* 1979;46: 571–578.

63. Carey RA, Santamore WP, Michele JJ, Bove AA. Effects of endurance training on coronary resistance in dogs. *Med Sci Sports Exerc* 1983;15:355–359.

64. Cohen MV. Coronary vascular reserve in the greyhound with left ventricular hypertrophy. *Cardiovasc Res* 1986;20:182–194.

65. Liang IY, Hamra M, Stone HL. Maximum coronary blood flow and minimum coronary resistance in exercise-trained dogs. *J Appl Physiol* 1984;56:641–647.

66. Scheel KW, Ingram LA, Wilson JL. Effects of exercise on the coronary and collateral vasculature of beagles with and without coronary occlusion. *Circ Res* 1981;48: 523–530.

67. Stone HL. Coronary flow, myocardial oxygen consumption, and exercise training in dogs. *J Appl Physiol* 1980;49:759–768.

68. Laughlin MH, Overholser KA, Bhatte MJ. Exercise training increases coronary transport reserve in miniature swine. *J Appl Physiol* 1989;67:1140–1149.

69. Laughlin MH. Effects of exercise training on coronary transport capacity. *J Appl Physiol* 1985;58:468–476.

70. Buttrick PM, Levite HA, Schaible TF, Ciambrone G, Scheuer J. Early increases in coronary vascular reserve in exercised rats are independent of cardiac hypertrophy. *J Appl Physiol* 1985;59:1861–1865.

71. Hagg U, Wandt B, Bergstrom G, Volkmann R, Gan L-M. Physical exercise capacity is associated with coronary and peripheral vascular function in healthy young adults. *Am J Physiol Heart Circ Physiol* 2005;289:H1627–H1634.

72. Radvan J, Choudhury L, Sheridan DJ, Camici PG. Comparison of coronary vasodilator reserve in elite rowing athletes versus hypertrophic cardiomyopathy. *Am J Cardiol* 1997;80:1621–1623.

73. Hannukainen JC, Janatuinen T, Toikka JO, Jarvisalo MJ, Heinonen OJ, Kapanen J, Nagren K, Nuutila P, Kujala UM, Kaprio J, Knuuti J, Kalliokoski KK. Myocardial and peripheral vascular functional adapation to exercise training. *Scand J Med Sci Spor* 2007;17:139–147.

74. Kjaer A, Meyer C, Wachtell K, Olsen MH, Ibsen H, Opie L, Holm S, Hesse B. Positron emission tomographic evaluation of regulation of myocardial perfusion in physiological (elite athletes) and pathological (systemic hypertension) left ventricular hypertrophy. *Am J Cardiol* 2005;96:1692–1698.

75. Heinonen I, Nesterov SV, Liukko K, Kemppainen J, Någren K, Luotolahti M, Virsu P, Oikonen V, Nuutila P, Kujala UM, Kainulainen H, Boushel R, Knuuti J, Kalliokoski KK. Myocardial blood flow and adenosine a2a receptor density in endurance athletes and untrained men. *J Physiol* 2008;586:5193–5202.

76. Heusch G. Adenosine and maximum coronary vasodilation in humans: Myth and misconceptions in the assessment of coronary reserve. *Basic Res Cardiol* 2010; 105:1–5.

77. Overholser KA, Bhatte MJ, Laughlin MH. Modeling the effect of flow heterogeneity on coronary permeability-surface area. *J Appl Physiol* 1991;71:758–769.

78. Suaya JA, Stason WB, Ades PA, Normand ST, Shepard DS. Cardiac rehabilitation and survival in older coronary patients. *J Am Coll Cardiol* 2009;54:25–33.

79. Okabe T, Kishimoto C, Murayama T, Yokode M, Kita T. Effects of exercise on the development of atherosclerosis in apolipoprotein e-deficient mice. *Exp Clin Cardiol* 2006;11:4276–4279.

80. Okabe TA, Shimada K, Hattori M, Murayama T, Yokode M, Kita T, Kishimoto C. Swimming reduces the severity of atherosclerosis in apolipoprotein e deficient mice by antioxidant effects. *Cardiovasc Res* 2007;74:537–545.

81. Shimada K, Kishimoto C, Okabe T, Hattori M, Murayama T, Yokode M, I, Kita T. Exercise training reduces severity of atherosclerosis in apolipoprotein e knockout mice via nitric oxide. *Circulation* 2007;71:1147–1151.

82. Yang AL, Jen CJ, Chen HI. Effects of high-cholesterol diet and parallel exercise training on the vascular function of rabbit aortas: A time course study. *J Appl Physiol* 2003;95:1194–1200.

83. Link RP, Pedersoli WM, Safanie AH. Effect of exercise on development of atherosclerosis in swine. *Atherosclerosis* 1972;15:107–122.

84. Turk JR, Laughlin MH. Physical activity and atherosclerosis: Which animal model? *Can J Appl Physiol* 2004;29:657–683.

85. Kramsch DM, Aspen AJ, Abramowitz BM, Kreimendahl T, Hood WB, Jr. Reduction of coronary atherosclerosis by moderate conditioning exercise in monkeys on an atherogenic diet. *N Engl J Med* 1981;305:1483–1489.

86. Williams JK, Kaplan JR, Suparto IH, Fox JL, Manuck SB. Effects of exercise on cardiovascular outcomes in monkeys with risk factors for coronary heart disease. *Arterioscler Thromb Vasc Biol* 2003;23:864–871.

87. Woodman CR, Turk JR, Rush JWE, Laughlin MH. Exercise attenuates the effects of hypercholesterolemia on endothelium-dependent relaxation in female porcine coronary arteries. *J Appl Physiol* 2004;96:1105–1113.

88. Wamhoff BR, Bowles DK, Dietz NJ, Hu Q, Sturek M. Exercise training attenuates coronary smooth muscle phenotypic modulation and nuclear ca2+ signaling. *Am J Physiol Heart Circ Physiol* 2002;283:H2397–H2410.

89. Simmons GH, Padilla J, Jenkins NT, Laughlin MH. Exercise training and vascular cell phenotype in a swine model of familial hypercholesterolaemia: Conduit arteries and veins. *Exp Physiol* 2014;99:454–465.

90. Hambrecht R, Niebauer J, Marburger C, Grunze M, Kalberer B, Hauer K, Schlierf G, Kubler W, Schuler G. Various intensities of leisure time physical activity in patients with coronary artery disease: Effects on cardiorespiratory fitness and progression of coronary atherosclerotic lesions. *J Am College Cardiol* 1993;22:468–477.

91. Haskell W, Alderman E, Fair J, Maron D, Mackey S, Superko H, Williams P, Johnstone I, Champagne M, Krauss R. Effects of intensive multiple risk factor reduction on coronary atherosclerosis and clinical cardiac events in men and women with coronary artery disease. The stanford coronary risk intervention project (scrip). *Circulation* 1994;89:975–990.

92. Ornish D, Brown SE, Scherwitz LW, Billings JH, Armstrong WT, Ports TA, McLanahan SM, Kirkeeide RL, Brand RJ, Gould KL. Can lifestyle changes reverse coronary heart disease? The lifestyle heart trial. *Lancet* 1990;336:129–133.

93. Schuler G, Hambrecht R, Schlierf G, Neibauer J, Hauer K, Neumann J, Hoberg E, Drinkmann A, Bacher F, Grunze M. Regular physical exercise and low-fat diet. Effects on progression of coronary artery disease. *Circulation* 1992; 86:1–11.

94. Belardinelli R, Paolini I, Cianci G, Piva R, Georgiou D, Purcaro A. Exercise training intervention after coronary angioplasty: The etica trial. *J Am Coll Cardiol* 2001;37: 1891–1900.

95. Fleenor BS, Bowles DK. Exercise training decreases the size and alters the composition of the neointima in a porcine model of percutaneous transluminal coronary angioplasty (ptca). *J Appl Physiol* 2009;107:937–945.

96. Edwards JM, Neeb ZP, Alloosh MA, Long X, Bratz IN, Peller CR, Byrd JP, Kumar S, Obukhov AG, Sturek M. Exercise training decreases store-operated Ca2+ entry associated with metabolic syndrome and coronary atherosclerosis. *Cardiovasc Res* 2010;85:631–640.

97. Goel K, Lennon RJ, Tilbury RT, Squires RW, Thomas RJ. Impact of cardiac rehabilitation on mortality and cardiovascular events after percutaneous coronary intervention in the community. *Circulation* 2011;123:2344–2352.
98. Casscells W, Naghavi M, Willerson JT. Vulnerable atherosclerotic plaque: A multifocal disease. *Circulation* 2003;107:2072–2075.
99. Lakka TA, Venalainen JM, Rauramaa R, Salonen R, Tuomilehto J, Salonen JT. Relation of leisure-time physical activity and cardiorespiratory fitness to the risk of acute myocardial infarction. *N Engl J Med* 1994;330:1549–1554.
100. Kadoglou NPE, Kostomitsopoulos N, Kapelouzou A, Moustardas P, Katsimpoulas M, Giagini A, Dede E, Boudoulas H, Konstantinides S, Karayannacos PE, Liapis CD. Effects of exercise training on the severity and composition of atherosclerotic plaque in apoe-deficient mice. *J Vasc Res* 2011;48:347–356.
101. Napoli C, Williams-Ignarro S, de Nigris F, Lerman LO, D'Armiento FP, Crimi E, Byrns RE, Casamassimi A, Lanza A, Gombos F, Sica V, Ignarro LJ. Physical training and metabolic supplementation reduce spontaneous atherosclerotic plaque rupture and prolong survival in hypercholesterolemic mice. *Proc Natl Acad Sci USA* 2006;103:10479–10484.
102. Madssen E, Moholdt T, Videm V, Wisloff U, Hegbom K, Wiseth R. Coronary atheroma regression and plaque characteristics assessed by grayscale and radiofrequency intravascular ultrasound after aerobic exercise. *Am J Cardiol* 2014;114:1504–1511.
103. Thompson MA, Henderson KK, Woodman CR, Turk JR, Rush JWE, Price E, Laughlin MH. Exercise preserves endothelium-dependent relaxation in coronary arteries of hypercholesterolemic male pigs. *J Appl Physiol* 2004;96:1114–1126.
104. Schwartz SM. Smooth muscle migration in atherosclerosis and restenosis. *J Clin Invest* 1997;100:S87–S89.
105. Schwartz SM, deBlois D, O'Brien ERM. The intima: Soil for atherosclerosis and restenosis. *Circ Res* 1995;77:445–465.
106. Hambrecht R, Wolf A, Gielen S, Linke A, Hofer J, Erbs S, Schoene N, Schuler G. Effect of exercise on coronary endothelial function in patients with coronary artery disease. *N Engl J Med* 2000;342:454–460.
107. Beck EB, Erbs S, Mogius-Winkler S, Adams V, Woitek FJ, Walther T, Hambrecht R, Mohr FW, Strumvoll M, Bluher M, Schuler G, Linke A. Exercise training restores the endothelial response to vascular growth factors in patients with stable coronary artery disease. *Eur J Prev Cardiol* 2012;19:412–418.
108. Linke A, Adams V, Schulze PC, Erbs S, Gielen S, Fiehn E, Mobius-Winkler S, Schubert A, Schuler G, Hambrecht R. Antioxidative effects of exercise training in patients with chronic heart failure: Increase in radical scavenger enzyme activity in skeletal muscle. *Circulation* 2005;111:1763–1770.
109. Lenk K, Uhlemann M, Schuler G, Adams V. Role of endothelial progenitor cells in the beneficial effects of physical exercise on atherosclerosis and coronary artery disease. *J Appl Physiol* 2011;111:321–328.

110. Knight DR, Stone HL. Alteration of ischemic cardiac function in normal heart by daily exercise. *J Appl Physiol* 1983;55:52–60.

111. Cohen MV. Training in dogs with normal coronary arteries: Lack of effect on collateral development. *Cardiovasc Res* 1990;24:121–128.

112. Eckstein RW. Effect of exercise and coronary artery narrowing on coronary collateral circulation. *Circ Res* 1957;5:230–235.

113. Heaton WH, Marr KC, Capurro NL, Goldstein RE, Epstein SE. Beneficial effect of physical training on blood flow to myocardium perfused by chronic collaterals in the exercising dog. *Circulation* 1978;27:575–581.

114. Neill WA, Oxendine JM. Exercise can promote coronary collateral development without improving perfusion of ischemic myocardium. *Circulation* 1979;60: 1513–1519.

115. Bloor CM, White FC, Sanders TM. Effects of exercise on collateral development in myocardial ischemia in pigs. *J Appl Physiol* 1984;56:656–665.

116. Roth DM, White FC, Nichols ML, Dobbs SL, Longhurst JC, Bloor CM. Effect of long-term exercise on regional myocardial function and coronary collateral development after gradual coronary artery occlusion in pigs. *Circulation* 1990;82:1778–1789.

117. Franklin BA. Exercise training and coronary collateral circulation. *Med Sci Sports Exerc* 1991;23:648–653.

118. Niebaurer J, Hambrecht R, Marburger C, Hauer K, Velich T, von Hodenberg E, Schlierf G, Kubler W, Schuler G. Impact of intensive physical exercise and low-fat diet on collateral vessel formation in stable angina pectoris and angiographically confirmed coronary artery disease. *Am J Cardiol* 1995;76:771–775.

119. Belardinelli R, Georgiou D, Ginzton L, Cianci G, Purcaro A. Effects of moderate exercise training on thallium uptake and contractile response to low-dose dobutamine of dysfunctional myocardium in patients with ischemic cardiomyopathy. *Circulation* 1998;97:553–561.

120. Griffin KL, Laughlin MH, Parker JL. Exercise training improves endothelium-mediated vasorelaxation after chronic coronary occlusion. *J Appl Physiol* 1999;87: 1948–1956.

121. Heaps CL, Sturek M, Rapps JA, Laughlin MH, Parker JL. Exercise training restores adenosine induced relaxation in coronary arteries distal to chronic occlusion. *Am J Physiol Heart Circ Physiol* 2000;278:H1984–H1992.

122. Griffin KL, Woodman CR, Price EM, Laughlin MH, Parker JL. Endothelium-mediated relaxation of porcine collateral-dependent arterioles is improved by exercise training. *Circulation* 2001;104:1393–1398.

123. Fogarty JA, Muller-Delp JM, Delp MD, Mattox ML, Laughlin MH, Parker JL. Exercise training enhances vasodilation responses to vascular endothelial growth factor in porcine coronary arterioles exposed to chronic coronary occlusion. *Circulation* 2004;109:664–670.

124. Muller JM, Myers PR, Laughlin MH. Exercise training alters myogenic responses in porcine coronary resistance arteries. *J Appl Physiol* 1993;75:2677–2682.

125. Heaps CL, Mattox ML, Kelly KA, Meininger CJ, Parker JL. Exercise training increases basal tone in arterioles distal to chronic coronary occlusion. *Am J Physiol Heart Circ Physiol* 2006;290:H1128–H1135.

126. Robles JC, Sturek M, Parker JL, Heaps CL. Ca2+ sensitization and pkc contribute to exercise training-enhanced contractility in porcine collateral-dependent coronary arteries. *Am J Physiol Heart* 2011;300:H1201–H1209.

127. Henderson KK, Turk JR, Rush JWE, Laughlin MH. Endothelial function in coronary arterioles from pigs with early-stage coronary disease induced by high-fat, high-cholesterol diet: Effect of exercise. *J Appl Physiol* 2004;97:1159–1168.

128. Laughlin MH, Roseguini B. Mechanisms for exercise training-induced increases in skeletal muscle blood flow capacity: Differences with interval sprint training versus aerobic endurance training. *J Physiol Pharmacol* 2008;59:71–88.

129. Padilla J, Simmons GH, Bender SB, Arce-Esquivel AA, Whyte JJ, Laughlin MH. Vascular effects of exercise: Endothelial adaptations beyond active muscle beds. *Physiology* 2011;26:132–145.

130. O'Connor CM, Whellan DJ, Lee KL, Keteyian SJ, Cooper LS, Ellis SJ, Leifer ES, Kraus WE, Kitzman DW, Blumenthal JA, Rendall DS, Miller NH, Fleg JL, Schulman KA, McKelvie RS, Zannad F, Piña IL. Efficacy and safety of exercise training in patients with chronic heart failure: Hf-action randomized controlled trial. *J Am Med Assoc* 2009;301:1439–1450.

Chapter 5

Electrophysiologic Adaptation to Exercise and Management of Arrhythmias in the Athlete

**Flavio D'Ascenzi*, Alessandro Zorzi[†],
and Domenico Corrado[†]**

*Department of Medical Biotecnologies
Division of Cardiology, University of Siena
Siena, Italy
[†]Department of Cardiac, Thoracic, and Vascular Sciences
University of Padua, Padua, Italy

Introduction

During the last decades, data obtained by studying large populations of trained athletes has provided insight into our understanding of adaptive changes of the cardiovascular system to sustained physical training and has helped to differentiate physiologic cardiac remodeling from the pathologic changes produced by diseases that increase the risk for sudden cardiac death (SCD) during sports.[1] Adolescent and young adults, both males and females, who practice competitive sports activity have a three times greater risk to die suddenly compared to non-athletes of same age and gender.[2] Sport is not itself the cause of the increased mortality, but acts as a trigger for cardiac arrest in the presence of cardiovascular diseases that predispose life-threatening ventricular arrhythmias. Such conditions include arrhythmogenic right ventricular cardiomyopathy (ARVC), premature coronary artery disease, hypertrophic cardiomyopathy (HCM), and coronary artery anomalies.[2]

Because of the neuroautonomic remodeling with increased vagal tone that occurs in the athlete's heart, trained athletes commonly develop benign rhythm and conduction disturbances including sinus bradyarrhythmia, junctional rhythm, and 1st degree and Wenckebach atrioventricular (AV) block (Mobitz type I).[3–6] In addition, athletes may develop an increased ectopic ventricular automaticity resulting in isolated premature ventricular beats (PVBs), that are generally innocent in the absence of an underlying structural heart disease.[7,8]

This chapter reviews the electrophysiologic adaptive changes of the athlete's heart and focuses on the prevalence, mechanisms, and clinical significance of arrhythmias in the athletic population.

Structural and Neuroautonomic Remodeling of the Athlete's Heart

The heart of the athlete has intrigued clinicians and scientists for more than a century. Early investigations in the late 1800s and early 1900s documented cardiac enlargement and bradyarrhythmias in individuals with above-normal exercise capacity. Since that time, scientific understanding of the association between sport participation and specific cardiac adaptations has paralleled advances in cardiovascular diagnostic techniques. Now, it is well known that participation in high-volume, high-intensity training programs results in significant neuroautonomic, morphological, and functional remodeling (Figure 1). These central and peripheral cardiovascular adaptations facilitate the generation of a large and sustained cardiac output and enhance the extraction of oxygen from exercising muscles.[9]

The development and rapid dissemination of echocardiography led to further advances in our understanding of the athlete's heart.[10] Identification of ventricular chamber enlargement, myocardial hypertrophy, and atrial dilatation in trained athletes has led to a more comprehensive understanding of cardiac adaptation to exercise conditioning. Moreover, physiologic adaptation of the cardiac autonomic nervous system, including increased vagal tone and/or withdrawal of sympathetic activity, results in sinus bradycardia, AV conduction impairment, and early repolarization.[11] The extent of cardiac morphological and electrical changes in trained athletes varies with the athlete's gender, race, level of fitness, and type of sport.[12–14] Adaptive changes are more prevalent and significant in male athletes and in those of Afro-Caribbean descent.[13–16] This most likely reflects the role of genetic/ethnic predisposing factors, which account for a more prominent cardiovascular remodeling, either structural or neuro-autonomic, in response to physical training and

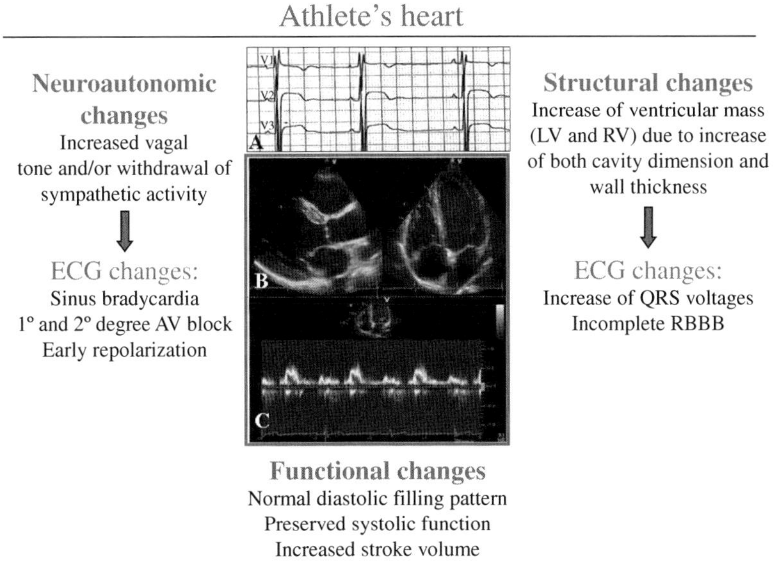

Athlete's heart

Neuroautonomic changes
Increased vagal tone and/or withdrawal of sympathetic activity

↓

ECG changes:
Sinus bradycardia
1° and 2° degree AV block
Early repolarization

Structural changes
Increase of ventricular mass (LV and RV) due to increase of both cavity dimension and wall thickness

↓

ECG changes:
Increase of QRS voltages
Incomplete RBBB

Functional changes
Normal diastolic filling pattern
Preserved systolic function
Increased stroke volume

Figure 1. Neuroautonomic, functional, and structural adaptations of the heart to sustained exercise (athlete's heart). Reproduced with permission from Ref. 96.

competition. Although short-term sports conditioning does not induce changes of cardiac dimensions, prolonged training is commonly associated with structural left ventricular (LV) remodeling. The morphological changes depend on the type of exercise undertaken.[14] High dynamic (isotonic) forms of exercise, which characterize endurance sports, such as long-distance running and cycling, are more likely to result in an increase in absolute ventricular chamber dimensions with a proportional increase in wall thickness (eccentric hypertrophy). Such ventricular changes are required to adapt to the volume overload associated with the increase in cardiac output during activity. In contrast, high static (isometric) exercise, such as weight lifting and wrestling, tends to increase LV mass without increasing chamber size (concentric hypertrophy), in response to the pure pressure overload produced by the very high systemic arterial pressures generated by this sporting activity. Athletes who participate in sports combining high dynamic and high static demands, such as rowing and canoeing, exhibit intermediate morpho-functional changes. Adaptive LV hypertrophy is typically symmetric (i.e. hypertrophy of the septum and LV free wall is equal), occurs early in conditioning, and rapidly reverses to baseline within weeks of detraining. The ECG of highly trained athletes characteristically shows sinus bradycardia/arrhythmia, increased QRS voltages, and early repolarization changes.[11,17] Experimental studies demonstrated that acetylcholine depresses the action potential plateau in right ventricular epicardium but not endocardium, by suppressing the calcium current and/or augmenting the potassium current. This leads to an 'up-sloping' ST segment elevation that is readily reversed with atropine. Although acetylcholine alone is capable of causing loss of the action potential dome in isolated right ventricular epicardial tissues, acetylcholine or vagotonia alone are unlikely to lead to loss of the action potential dome *in vivo* or to provoke phase 2 reentry. This may explain why the right precordial early repolarization pattern in the normal athlete is not associated with the risk of sudden arrhythmic death.[18]

Participation in endurance sport disciplines, such as cycling, cross-country skiing, and rowing/canoeing, provokes greater cardiac remodeling, and is associated with a higher rate and greater extent of physiologic ECG changes such as sinus bradycardia and increase of QRS voltages.

Arrhythmias depend on triggers, substrates, and modulators, and these factors may be present in relation to physical activity.[19,20] Unfortunately, the pathophysiological mechanisms responsible for the development of arrhythmias in athletes without structural heart disease are unclear, although an increased automaticity is the most likely explanation. Atrial fibrillation (AF) is rarely seen in young athletes, but may be increased in older athletes. The mechanisms responsible for this supraventricular arrhythmia remain speculative and mostly rely on experimental data. Atrial enlargement and fibrosis, atrial ectopy, increased vagal tone, and changes in electrolytes, among others, have been proposed as mechanisms. However, recent data in humans do not support pathological remodeling of the atria as a substrate for AF in young healthy athletes.[21–23]

Physiological Electrical Changes of the Athlete's Heart: The Athlete's Electrocardiogram

ECG abnormalities occur frequently in trained athletes as a consequence of electrical/structural adaptive changes of the heart to sustained physical exercise ('athlete's heart') but may also represent the sign of an underlying cardiovascular disease. Figure 2 reports "physiologic vs. pathologic ECG abnormalities" of the athlete's ECG.[24] Abnormalities are divided into two groups according to their prevalence, relation to exercise training, association with an increased cardiovascular risk, and need for further clinical investigation to confirm (or exclude) an underlying cardiovascular disease. Athlete's heart is commonly (up to 80%) associated with ECG changes such as sinus bradycardia, 1st degree AV block, and early repolarization (Group 1) resulting from physiologic adaptation of the cardiac autonomic nervous system to training. Moreover, the ECG of trained athletes often exhibits pure voltage criteria for LV hypertrophy that reflect the physiological LV remodeling, consisting of increased LV wall thickness and chamber size (Figure 3). These ECG changes should be clearly separated from uncommon ECG

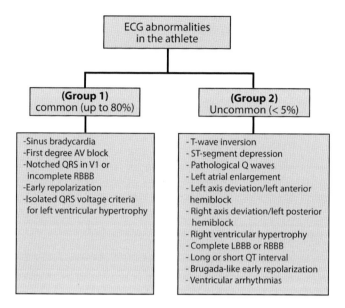

Figure 2.   Classification of ECG abnormalities in the athlete. Common ECG abnormalities: up to 80% of trained athletes exhibit ECG changes such as sinus bradycardia, 1st degree AV block, early repolarization, incomplete right bundle branch block, and pure increase of QRS voltages (Group 1). Such common ECG changes are the consequence of the physiologic cardiovascular adaptation to sustained physical exertion and do not reflect the presence of an underlying cardiovascular disease. Therefore, they are not associated with an increase of cardiovascular risk and allow eligibility to competitive sports without additional evaluation.

Uncommon ECG abnormalities: this subset includes uncommon ECG patterns (<5%) such as ST-segment and T-wave repolarization abnormalities, pathological Q-waves, intraventricular conduction defects, and ventricular arrhythmias (Group 2). These ECG abnormalities are unrelated to athletic conditioning and should be regarded as an expression of a possible underlying cardiovascular disorders, notably cardiomyopathies, and cardiac ion channel diseases, and, thus, associated with an inherent increased risk of sudden arrhythmic death. Adapted with permission from Ref. 24.

patterns (<5%) such as ST-segment and T-wave repolarization abnormalities, pathologic Q-waves, intraventricular conduction defects, ventricular pre-excitation, long and short QT interval, and ventricular arrhythmias (Group 2), which are unrelated to athletic training and may be an expression of cardiovascular disorders, notably cardiomyopathies, and cardiac ion channel diseases, which increase the risk of SCD during sports.

Appropriate interpretation of ECG abnormalities by qualified physicians is essential for proper cardiovascular evaluation and management of young competitive athletes. Misinterpretation of the ECG by inexperienced physicians may lead to serious consequences. Athletes may undergo expensive diagnostic work-ups or be unnecessarily disqualified from competition for abnormalities that fall

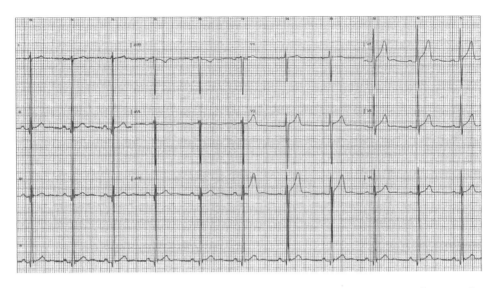

Figure 3. Typical electrocardiogram of an endurance athlete. 12-lead electrocardiogram of a 21-year-old runner showing pure voltage criteria (Sokolow–Lion) for left ventricular hypertrophy and diffuse early repolarization (J-point elevation).

within the normal range for athletes. ECG abnormalities in HCM are a good example since they overlap marginally with ECG findings in healthy trained athletes. Isolated QRS voltage criteria for LV hypertrophy (Socolow–Lyon or Cornell criteria) are unusual in patients with HCM in whom pathologic hypertrophy is characteristically associated with additional non-voltage criteria such as left atrial enlargement, left QRS axis deviation, a 'strain' pattern of repolarization, and delayed intrinsicoid deflection, T-wave inversion, and pathologic Q-waves (Figure 4).[25] Such ECG abnormalities of HCM need to be clearly distinguished from the ECG patterns of healthy trained athletes in whom physiologic hypertrophy manifests as an isolated increase of QRS amplitude, with right QRS axis deviation, normal atrial and ventricular activation patterns, and normal ST–T repolarization. A corollary is that further investigation by echocardiography is not recommended in athletes showing an isolated increase of QRS voltages at preparticipation screening, unless such subjects have other ECG changes suggesting pathologic LV hypertrophy, relevant symptoms, an abnormal physical examination, or a positive family history for cardiovascular diseases and/or SCD.[24]

On the other hand, signs of potentially lethal organic heart disease may be misinterpreted as normal variants of the athlete ECG. Particularly, T-wave inversion in right precordial leads (V1–V3) is often dismissed in young competitive athletes as non-specific or as persistence of the juvenile T-wave pattern. Migliore

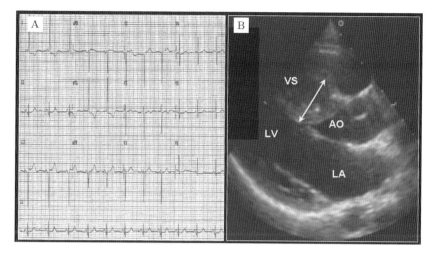

Figure 4. Electrocardiographic and echocardiographic finding of an athlete with hypertrophic cardiomyopathy. (A) The ECG shows T-wave inversion in lateral leads (I and aVL) and pathological Q-wave in inferior leads (III and aVF). (B) The echocardiogram shows an asymmetrical left ventricular hypertrophy with a maximal septal thickness of 31 mm. VS = ventricular septum; LV = left ventricle; LA = left atrium; AO = aorta. Reproduced with permission from Ref. 26.

et al. found a 4.7% prevalence of T-wave inversion in V1–V2/V3 among young Caucasian athletes (aged 9–19 years) and demonstrated a decreasing prevalence of T-wave inversion with increasing age (8.4% in athletes younger than 14 years old vs. 1.7% in those older than 14 years). Moreover, at multivariate analysis, pubertal development rather than age was independently associated with right-precordial T-wave inversion and the clinical meaning of this ECG feature also depended on the development stage: no cardiac disease was found among pre-pubertal children with right-precordial T-wave inversions whereas 11% of post-pubertal individuals with persistent negative T-waves in V1–V2/V3 were diagnosed with definite or borderline ARVC (Figure 5).[26] According to this study, right-precordial T-wave inversion should be regarded in the context of age and pubertal development and further investigation should be performed only if the ECG abnormality persists beyond puberty. Black athletes demonstrate a higher prevalence of T-wave inversion in precordial leads V1–V4 than Caucasian athletes, but most anterior inverted T-waves in Afro-Caribbean athletes are preceded by J-point elevation and convex ST-segment elevation.[27] It has been recently shown that in both post-pubertal black and white athletes, anterior T-wave inversion confined to leads V1–V4 and preceded by J-point elevation represents an "early repolarization variant" and can be considered a normal finding in the athlete. Instead, T-wave inversion not preceded by J-point elevation or extending beyond V4 or involving the limb leads should

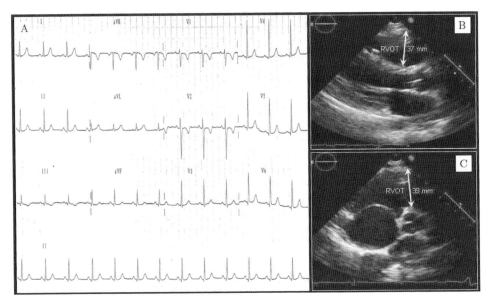

Figure 5.   Electrocardiographic and echocardiographic findings in a 14-year-old male soccer player with complete pubertal development and right-precordial negative T-waves. (A) The ECG shows T-wave inversion in right precordial leads (V1–V2) and (B) the echocardiogram reveals right ventricular dilation and dysfunction. (C) At the end of the clinical work-up a diagnosis of Arrhythmogenic cardiomyopathy was made. RVOT = right ventricular outflow tract. Reproduced with permission from Ref. 26.

be seen as the sign of an underlying cardiomyopathy and should prompt further investigation (Figure 6).[28]

Bradyarrhythmias and Conduction Disturbances

Athletic bradycardia is a non-pathologic condition commonly associated with aerobic exercise, in well-conditioned endurance athletes.[29] Sinus bradycardia is by far the most common bradyarrhythmia in the athlete. It is correlated with the training level and can result in heart rates at rest as low as 30–40 bpm.[29–33] Sinus pauses >2 seconds are quite common, with a reported prevalence of 37% in the study by Viitasalo *et al.*[34] Sinus arrhythmia and wandering atrial pacemaker are also more prevalent in athletes compared with the general population. Sinus bradycardia is usually correlated to type and intensity of training.[33] Its incidence varies widely among the populations oscillating from 4% to 8% in general, to 40% to 90% in selected athletic populations. Sinus rates at rest in the 30 to 40 bpm range are fairly common in the highly conditioned athlete.[29–34] With significant sinus bradycardia, a junctional or ventricular escape rhythm can compete with sinus

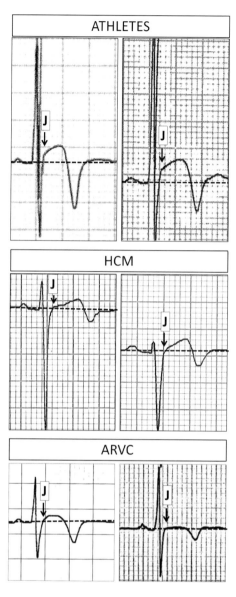

Figure 6.   Patterns of anterior T-wave inversion in healthy athletes and athletes with cardiomyopathy. Note that athletes typically demonstrate J-point elevation preceding the negative T-wave so that this J-point elevation/T-wave inversion pattern can be considered an early repolarization variant and further investigations can be avoided if T-wave inversion is confined to leads V1–V4. On the other hand, in patients with hypertrophic cardiomyopathy (HCM) or arrhythmogenic right ventricular cardiomyopathy (ARVC) and anterior T-wave inversion, there is no J-point elevation. Anterior T-wave inversion with no J-point elevation or extending beyond V4 or to the limb leads should prompt additional investigations to exclude an underlying structural heart disease. Reproduced with permission from Ref. 28.

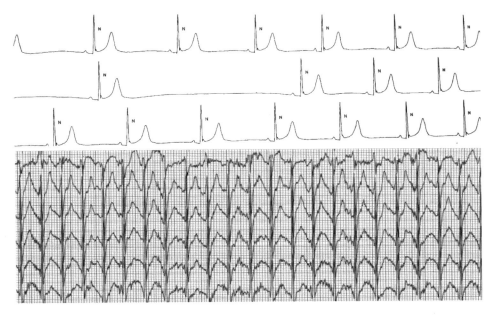

Figure 7.   Sinus bradycardia in an endurance athlete. Top: Marked sinus bradycardia with pauses >3 s during sleeping in a 19-year-old competitive rower. Bottom: Maximal exercise testing demonstrating preserved chronotropic reserve and confirming the benign (neuroauthonomic) nature of nocturnal sinus bradycardia.

rhythm. Sports eligibility can be granted in athletes without heart disease and without bradycardia-related symptoms (syncope, presyncope, asthenia, dyspnea, etc.).[35] In dubious cases, maximal stress test electrocardiogram must show a normal chronotropic response and 24-h Holter ECG monitoring must show the absence of daytime sinus pauses longer than 3 s (Figure 7). In athletes practicing aerobic sports, sinus pauses more than 3 s may also be accepted, as long as they are not associated with symptoms or arrhythmias that correlate with bradycardia. In selected cases, 3–6 months of detraining can be very useful in documenting a reduction of the sinus arrhythmia.

The incidence of 1st- and Mobitz type I 2nd degree AV block (AVB) is very high in endurance athletes while Mobitz type II 2nd degree AVB and 3rd degree AVB are very rare.[36–40] With exercise all of these individuals show normalization of the PR interval (Figure 8). 1st degree AVB that normalizes during hyperpnoea and/or exercise does not contraindicate sports activity. In 2nd degree AVB with narrow QRS and Luciani–Wenckebach periodism (Mobitz type 1), sports is permitted in the absence of heart disease or symptoms and if AV conduction normalizes with the increase in HR during maximal exercise stress testing.[35] Athletes practicing aerobic sports may be eligible even in the presence of sinus pauses

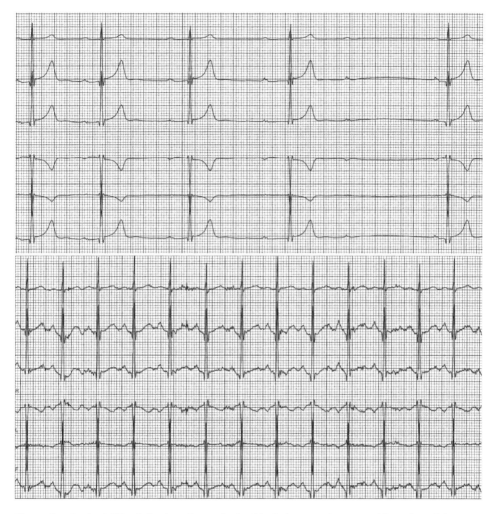

Figure 8. Luciani–Wenckeback atrioventricular block in an endurance athlete. Top: 2nd degree Mobitz I (Luciani–Wenckebach) AV block during sleeping in a 28-year-old runner. Note that sinus bradycardia is also present at the time of the block, suggesting the role of increased vagal tone in the etiopathogenesis of impaired atrioventricular conduction (rather than structural disease of the atrioventricular node). Bottom: during moderate exercise atrioventricular conduction completely normalizes, confirming the benign (neuroauthonomic) nature of the atrioventricular block.

more than 3 s, provided these are not associated with symptoms. 2nd degree AVB Mobitz type 2, advanced and complete AVB require investigation of the conduction system. These forms, when sporadic and related to hypervagotonia, may be compatible with sports if AV conduction normalizes during maximal stress testing and in the absence of ventricular pauses more than 3 s during 24-h Holter ECG monitoring. Persistent forms and those unrelated to hypervagotonia contraindicate sports activity. Similarly, according to European Society of Cardiology recommendations for the interpretation of 12-lead ECGs in the athlete,[24] sinus bradycardia, prolonged PR interval, and Wenckebach phenomenon are common in athletes as a result of the high resting vagal tone and significantly lower intrinsic heart rates. Prolonged PR intervals of up to 300 milliseconds should not prompt further work-up, but longer intervals should be investigated with an exercise test (the PR interval should shorten as vagal tone is withdrawn). Similarly, Wenckebach phenomenon in isolation need not prompt further work-up, but an exercise test could resolve any concern.

Thus, taken together, these considerations suggest that, unless associated with symptoms, an abnormal response to exercise, or other arrhythmias, sinus bradycardia and AV blocks are benign findings in the athlete.

Atrial Fibrillation

Reports from epidemiological studies evaluating AF in athletes have provided different results depending on the age, years of training, and type of sport of the study population. Karjalainen *et al.* in 1998[41] demonstrated an increased risk of AF in healthy middle-aged men practicing sport. The authors studied 300 top-ranking orienteering veterans compared to 495 controls and observed AF in 5.3% of athletes and 0.9% of controls. In 2002, Mont *et al.* published a retrospective analysis of lone AF patients seen at the outpatient arrhythmia clinic, showing that the proportion of regular sport practice among men with lone AF was higher than among men from the general population (63% vs. 15%).[42] The same population was analyzed in a case-control study with two age-matched controls for each case from the general population.[43] The analysis showed that sports practice increased the risk of developing lone AF more than five times. The association between sport practice and lone AF became significant at over 1,500 cumulative hours of sport practice. The same research group investigated 183 individuals who ran the Barcelona Marathon in 1992 and 290 sedentary healthy subjects.[44,45] After 10 years of follow-up, the annual incidence of lone AF among marathon runners and sedentary men was 0.43/100 and 0.11/100, respectively. Vigorous physical activity was also associated with an increased risk of AF in a prospective study that enrolled 107 consecutive patients with AF recruited at the emergency room.[46] Myrstad *et al.*[47] demonstrated a 6.0% higher incidence of AF in 509 elderly Norwegian men who had a long history of cross-country skiing compared with 1,768 elderly men in the general population. Interestingly, light and moderate leisure-time physical activity during the previous years reduced the risk for AF. The authors hypothesized that exercise intensity was associated with a risk for AF in a U-shaped pattern: while moderate intensity was associated with a lower incidence of AF, people reporting the highest intensity had the same incidence as people not exercising. Finally, among middle-aged patients undergoing cavo-tricuspid isthmus ablation for common atrial flutter, those engaged in endurance sport more frequently developed AF during the follow-up as compared with non-endurance athletes (81% vs. 48%, $p = 0.02$, respectively).[48] This study suggests that endurance sport may increase the recurrence of AF after ablation for atrial flutter.

While these studies have demonstrated a possible association between exercise and AF, this relationship is controversial.[49] In 2005, Pelliccia *et al.*[50] found a prevalence of AF of 0.3% among 1,777 healthy athletes (age: 24 ± 6 years), thus similar to that observed in the general population, but it must be underlined that, at variance with other investigations, this study was conducted in a relatively young population of athletes engaged in different sporting disciplines. More recently, Woodward *et al.* demonstrated that during 6 years of follow-up the rate of hospital admission for AF was not increased above the national rate in 2,590 non-elite cyclists, suggesting that the level of activity practiced by this cohort of cyclists was not sufficient to increase the risk of hospitalization for AF.[51] A systematic review and meta-analysis found no significant increase in AF with a higher level of physical activity.[52] Furthermore, although a direct relationship between AF and exercise has to be definitively confirmed, lone AF in athletes is not necessarily associated with increased risk of death, maybe because other factors like the lower prevalence of coronary artery disease may reduce the overall risk of mortality and also because persistent AF develops in only a minority of male endurance athletes.[53]

The pathophysiological mechanisms responsible for the development of AF in athletes remain speculative and mostly dependent on experimental data. Atrial enlargement and fibrosis, atrial ectopy, increased vagal tone, and changes in electrolytes have been proposed as mechanisms (Figure 9). However, as previously reported, recent data on humans do not support the interpretation of a pathological remodeling of the atria as a substrate for AF in young healthy athletes.[21–23]

Wolff–Parkinson–White Syndrome

Wolff–Parkinson–White (WPW) syndrome is a congenital heart disease characterized by the abnormal persistence of a muscular bundle (accessory AV pathway) which provides an alternative way of electrical connection between atrial and ventricular myocardium, other than the normal AV node-His bundle axis. Typical ECG features of ventricular pre-excitation in the WPW syndrome

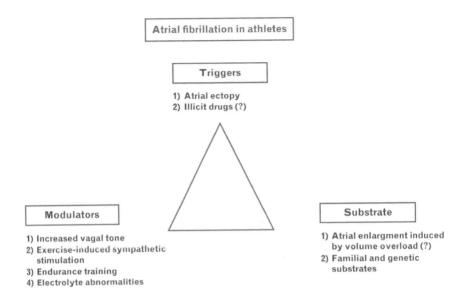

Figure 9.   Possible etiopathogenic factors contributing to atrial fibrillation in athletes. This figure reports the possible triggers, modulators, and substrates involved in the development of atrial fibrillation in athletes. Note that atrial fibrosis and atrial dilatation induced by pressure overload have not been included, according to the scant data available in humans. The term atrial 'dilatation' has been replaced by atrial 'enlargement' in order to underline the physiological benign meaning of atrial remodeling in athletes. Reproduced with permission from Ref. 49.

include: (1) a PR interval less than 0.12 s (2) with a slurring of the initial segment of the QRS complex, known as a delta wave, and (3) a QRS complex widening with a total duration greater than 0.12 s. The delta wave may be particularly evident in highly trained athletes who exhibit an increase in vagal tone and prolonged atrioventricular conduction time. It may be complicated by different types of arrhythmia, in particular: (1) orthodromic atrioventricular reentrant tachycardia (AVRT); (2) antidromic AVRT; (3) pre-excited AF that can degenerate into ventricular fibrillation, leading to sudden death. Physical activity may increase the occurrence of arrhythmias in WPW syndrome.[54]

Cardiac Ion Channel Disorders

The cardiac ion channel disorders are genetically determined diseases that are associated with a structurally normal heart and a propensity to develop polymorphic ventricular tachycardia or ventricular fibrillation that may lead to syncope or SCD. These diseases include long QT syndrome, short QT syndrome, Brugada syndrome, and catecholaminergic polymorphic ventricular tachycardia.

Short QT syndrome

Short QT (SQT) syndrome is a recently identified genetic disorder and characterized by SQT (QTc < 320 ms) often associated with tall and peaked T-wave. SQT has been associated with paroxysmal AF and ventricular fibrillation, leading to sudden death. The effect of physical effort on such arrhythmic complications is not known. Data are still limited, but adrenergic stress has been linked to the development of life-threatening arrhythmias.[55] Eligibility for competitive sport should be denied in both symptomatic and asymptomatic individuals according to European and Italian recommendations.[35,56] Conversely, the recent recommendations from the American Heart Association/American College of Cardiology (AHA/ACC) suggest that participation in competitive sports may be considered in patients with SQT syndrome if precautionary measures and disease-specific treatment are in place and if the athlete has been asymptomatic on treatment for at least 3 months.[57]

Brugada syndrome

The Brugada syndrome is characterized by a distinctive ECG pattern of J-point and ST-segment elevations in the right precordial leads and increased vulnerability to ventricular fibrillation, in the absence of clinical evidence of structural heart disease. In about one-third of patients, the origin of the syndrome can be linked to a genetically-induced cardiac sodium channel dysfunction due to a mutation in the SCN5A gene. Distinctive clinical manifestations consist of dynamic changes of the ECG over time, polymorphic ventricular tachycardia, and exercise-unrelated syncope or sudden death. Three different types of repolarization abnormalities have been described, of which only the most prominent form (type 1) is diagnostic.[58] In others, provocation by class-1antiarrhythmic drugs such as procainamide, flecanide, or ajmaline may unmask a diagnostic type 1 ECG. Also a febrile state, electrolyte disturbances, and autonomic changes may increase the ECG manifestation and even trigger ventricular arrhythmias.[58] Although SCD in patients with Brugada syndrome typically occurs at rest, the increased vagal tone as a consequence of chronic athletic conditioning may increase the risk of SCD at rest. Increased body temperature is also a risk factor for SCD in Brugada syndrome, and hyperthermia during exercise could trigger SCD during strenuous activity. Differentiating right precordial early repolarization (which may be present in about 4% of athletes) from Brugada syndrome can be difficult. Recently, the ratio of the ST-segment elevation at J-point (STJ) and at 80 milliseconds after the J-point (ST80), the STJ/ST80 ratio, is a highly accurate electrocardiographic parameter for differentiating anterior early repolarization of the athlete from that of Brugada syndrome (Figure 10).[59]

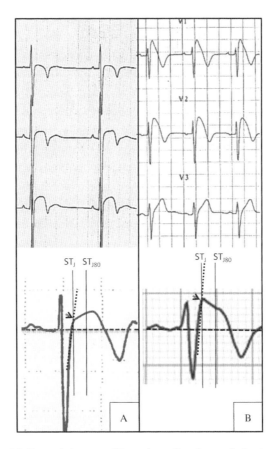

Figure 10.   Differential diagnosis between "domed-type" early repolarization of athlete's heart and coved-type Brugada electrocardiogram. Electrocardiographic leads V1–V3 of a healthy Afro-Caribbean soccer player showing "domed type" anterior repolarization abnormalities (A) and of a patient with Brugada syndrome and a spontaneous "coved type" electrocardiogram (B). The athlete's ECG is characterized by an upsloping ST-segment elevation ($ST_j/ST_{j+80ms} < 1$) while the patient with Brugada syndrome shows a downsloping ST-segment ($ST_j/ST_{j+80ms} > 1$). Modified with permission from Ref. 59.

Patients with Brugada syndrome (i.e. with a distinctive spontaneous or drug-induced type 1 ECG, symptoms of cardiac arrest or syncope, or ventricular tachycardia inducibility at electrophysiological study) are usually treated with an internal cardioverter defibrillator (ICD). According to the current European recommendations, patients with Brugada syndrome should be restricted from all competitive sports except those with low cardiovascular demand.[56] In contrast, and similar to other ion channel diseases, the recent recommendations from the AHA/ACC[57] suggest that genotype positive/phenotype negative individuals and patients with Brugada syndrome may engage in competitive sports if hyperthermia and potassium depletion are avoided, an automatic external defibrillator is available, the athlete has had appropriate treatment, and been asymptomatic on treatment for at least 3 months.

Catecholaminergic polymorphic ventricular tachycardia

Mutations in the ryanodine receptor (RyR2; the calcium release channel of the sarcoplasmic reticulum), calsequestrin (CASQ2; another protein involved in intra-cellular calcium handling), or the structural protein ankyrin-B (also referred to as LQT4-syndrome) have been identified as the underlying molecular causes of cat-echolaminergic polymorphic ventricular tachycardia.[60] The baseline ECG is not diagnostic, but the exercise ECG shows multi-focal premature ventricular beats (PVBs) or ventricular tachycardia (VT) with alternating QRS-axis, known as 'bi-directional VT', that may degenerate into polymorphic VT or ventricular fibril-lation. No structural changes are present. Maximal stress testing usually repro-duces the arrhythmia at heart rates >120 bpm. This inherited form of adrenergically-dependent arrhythmia leads to syncope or SCD at a young age. About one-third of individuals with catecholaminergic polymorphic VT have a family history of syncope and/or SCD, occurring before the age of 30 years. This clinical entity may comprise 5–10% of patients with familial arrhythmias but without QTc prolongation or Brugada type ECG abnormalities.[60]

Competitive and even moderate leisure-time sports are contraindicated.[35,56,57] Beta-blockers are the first choice therapy. If stress testing during beta-blocker treatment shows the absence of arrhythmias, low to moderate leisure-time sports can be performed, but patients should be immediately re-evaluated if symptoms recur.

Ventricular Arrhythmias

Prevalence and significance of premature ventricular beats in athletes

Ventricular arrhythmias are common in the general, non-athletic population, occurring in 40–75% of healthy individuals undergoing a 24-h ambulatory ECG monitoring, and frequent (>60/h) or complex (repetitive, polymorphic, R-on-T) PVBs occur in 1–4% of healthy subjects.[61] In the general athletic population, PVBs occur with the same frequency as they do in the sedentary population,[62,63] although some authors reported a higher prevalence of PVBs and complex ectopy in endurance athletes compared with controls.[36] In a study on athletes with ven-tricular arrhythmias discovered on an ECG, obtained at preparticipation screening, subsequent 24-h ambulatory ECG monitoring demonstrated that PVBs were frequent but usually isolated and monomorphic. Couplets were present in 30% of these athletes and were usually rare and monomorphic, with wide coupling intervals.[64]

The discovery of frequent PVBs in otherwise healthy subjects raises the question as to whether non-invasive examinations, such as ECG, stress test, and echocardiography, are sufficient to exclude heart diseases or whether, in the absence of prominent cardiac abnormalities, PVBs are benign or are an early manifestation of a concealed heart disease.[65] Biffi *et al.* reported that even a high prevalence of complex ventricular arrhythmias on 24-h ECG monitoring in trained athletes without cardiovascular abnormalities were benign over a 8-year follow-up.[7] Furthermore, athletic deconditioning can abolish frequent and complex ventricular arrhythmias in most athletes.[8] In contrast to the apparently benign PVBs at rest, the occurrence of ventricular arrhythmias during exercise raises clinical concern, particularly in a population where SCD is frequently triggered by intense physical activity. Indeed, malignant ventricular arrhythmias induced or worsened by exercise in young patients are a recognized feature of ion channel disease, HCM, and ARVC, acute/subacute myocarditis, and dilated cardiomyopathy.[65,66–68] Thus, clinicians are faced with the dilemma of whether exercise-induced PVBs are benign or signal a potentially life-threatening condition.

Although the disappearance of PVBs with exercise is typical,[62,69] in some cases ventricular arrhythmias do occur during the exercise test and most athletes (up to 85%) are referred for cardiologic screening because of this finding.[64] It is unclear whether persistence/worsening of ventricular arrhythmias is independently associated with a poorer prognosis. Some authors suggest that exercise-induced PVBs indicate a poorer prognosis[70–73] and Sofi *et al.* found that exercise testing was able to identify pathological findings in athletes with innocent findings at physical examination and resting ECG.[74] Conflicting data have been reported also in the non-athletic population. Some authors demonstrated the benign nature of exercise-induced PVBs,[75,76] whereas others found an association with increased mortality.[76,77] More reassuring data come from long-term follow-up studies in subjects with outflow tract PVBs which showed a benign prognosis.[78,79] Recently Verdile *et al.* demonstrated that 367 (7.5%) of 5,011 top-level athletes demonstrated at least one PVB during exercise. Most (331 or 90%) had ≤10 PVBs and were not restricted from athletics, but of 36 with frequent or complex arrhythmias, 23 had a spontaneous reduction and 13 were evaluated for ablation which was successful in 6.[80] Furthermore, in the vast majority of athletes (64%) investigated by Verdile and colleagues, exercise-induced PVBs decreased with deconditioning, but this could simply represent regression to the mean. None of the athletes had cardiovascular events over 7.4 years of follow-up, even if athletes continued sport at a competitive level.[80]

An important variant when evaluating athletes with ventricular arrhythmias is the PVB morphology since determining the PVBs origin is important to determine the prognosis and whether to investigate the athletes with arrhythmias. Among the athletes reported by Verdile *et al.*[80] most (68%) PVBs had right ventricular outflow tract morphology, with inferior axis and left bundle branch block (LBBB) configuration, with R/S transition beyond lead V3. Around 15% had fascicular ventricular arrhythmias with right bundle branch block (RBBB) morphology and superior axis. Around 9% showed PVBs with LV outflow tract morphology, that is, inferior axis and LBBB configuration and R/S transition in lead V1/V2. Other morphologies (e.g. LBBB and superior axis or RBBB and inferior axis) were present in the remaining 26 athletes. These findings agree with those by Delise *et al.*, who found that PVBs in competitive athletes frequently demonstrate a LBBB morphology (72.8%), followed by fascicular morphology (21%), and RBBB (6.1%).[81] Steriotis *et al.* studied a cohort of 145 young athletes with ventricular arrhythmias discovered at baseline ECG who underwent 24-h ambulatory ECG monitoring and demonstrated that PVBs were usually isolated and monomorphic. They also found that the most frequent PVB morphologies were LBBB with inferior axis deviation (59 subjects, 50%), RBBB with left axis deviation (LAD) (21, 18%), LBBB with LAD (18, 15%), RBBB with right axis deviation (14, 12%), LBBB with normal axis (14, 12%), and RBBB with inferior axis deviation (8, 7%).[64] Effort-induced PVBs showed LBBB morphology with inferior axis deviation (7, 37%), RBBB with LAD (6, 31%), LBBB with LAD (3, 16%), LBBB with normal axis (1, 0.7%), and RBBB with right axis deviation (1, 0.7%). Thus, in athletes, the most frequent PVB morphology has a LBBB pattern and inferior axis, indicating origin in the right ventricular outflow tract, which is a recognized idiopathic and benign entity. Also, ventricular arrhythmias with a borderline width QRS (≤ 0.12 s) and a right bundle branch block/superior axis pattern, which is pathognomonic for origin in the left posterior fascicle, carry no adverse prognosis unless associated with heart disease or syncope during exercise. In contrast, arrhythmias with different configurations such as LBBB and intermediate/superior axis or RBBB with wide QRS are rare in healthy athletes and may be the sign of an underlying structural heart disease (Figure 11).[64, 65, 80–83]

Evaluation and management of athletes with ventricular arrhythmias

The first objective in evaluating an athlete with ventricular arrhythmias is to exclude life-threatening cardiovascular disease by echocardiography, 24-h Holter monitoring, and exercise testing. Holter recordings should be performed during intense physical activity and preferably when the athlete is performing his/her specific sports activity. Careful assessment of the morphology of the arrhythmic

QRS complex and coexistent ECG abnormalities may help to characterize the anatomic origin and the probability of an underlying disease. Exercise tests should mimic the exercise/sport responsible for the arrhythmic events, because a conventional exercise test may not replicate the specific clinical situation and the arrhythmogenic mechanisms produced by the sport. An increase in the arrhythmia at the beginning of exercise, disappearance at peak exercise, and reappearance during recovery usually suggest a benign process.[65,80–83] Triggering or worsening of the arrhythmia during exercise may indicate an underlying cardiomyopathy or ion channel disease.[84–86] A possible exception is the right ventricular outflow tract (RVOT) VT, which is characterized by repetitive monomorphic bouts of PVBs or paroxysmal sustained episodes, with the typical left bundle branch block/inferior axis pattern. RVOT tachycardia is usually triggered by exercise and can be interrupted by adenosine. It is an idiopathic and benign condition, provided that ARVC is excluded.[87] Another common ventricular arrhythmia is fascicular ventricular tachycardia, which has a borderline wide QRS (0.12 s) and a right bundle branch block/superior axis pattern, which is pathognomonic for origin in the left posterior hemifascicle (Figure 11). This entity also carries no adverse prognosis unless it is associated with syncope during exercise or heart disease.[88] The induction of polymorphic VT during exercise always carries a bad prognosis. Polymorphic VT with alternating complexes ("bidirectional" pattern), induced during exercise, suggests the inherited ion channel disorder, catecholaminergic polymorphic ventricular tachycardia, which causes exercise-induced arrhythmic cardiac arrest in the absence of structural heart disease as discussed above.

The analysis of concomitant repolarization/depolarization ECG abnormalities may help interpret the clinical significance of a documented ventricular arrhythmia. The association between a PVB with a left bundle branch block pattern and repolarization abnormalities, such as T-wave inversion in the right precordial leads, is highly suggestive of ARVC.[24] The coexistence of a right ventricular conduction defect in the form of a prolonged QRS duration or a delayed S-wave upstroke in V1–V3 further increases the likelihood of ARVC. On the other hand, PVBs with a right bundle branch block configuration in lead V1 indicate a left ventricular origin and suggest possible LV heart muscle diseases such as dilated/inflammatory cardiomyopathy, HCM, LV non-compaction, or a predominantly left-sided ARVC. In these patients, even if echocardiography is negative, contrast-enhanced cardiovascular magnetic resonance imaging may disclose concealed left-ventricular scar tissue that may be a substrate for life-threatening ventricular arrhythmias and SCD in the athlete.[89] In selected athletes in whom non-invasive clinical and instrumental findings are inconclusive, other invasive tests such as electrophysiological study, cardiac catheterization, and endomyocardial biopsy may be required to achieve a definite diagnosis. Molecular genetic

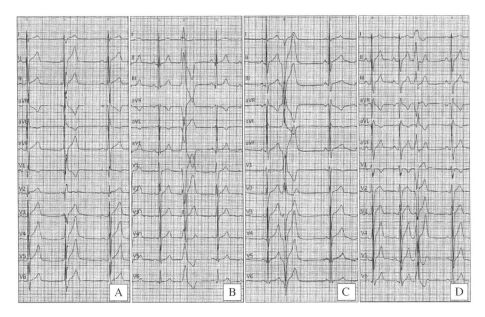

Figure 11. Common and uncommon morphologies of premature ventricular beats in athletes. (A) Premature ventricular beat (PVB) with a right bundle branch block (RBBB) morphology and relatively narrow QRS, suggesting a fascicular origin (common), (B) PVB with a left bundle branch block (LBBB) morphology, inferior axis, and QRS transition in V4, suggesting the origin from the right ventricular outflow tract (common), (C) PVB with a RBBB morphology, wide QRS and axis towards a VR, suggesting the origin from the infero-lateral wall of the left ventricle (rare), (D) PVB with a LBBB morphology and intermediate axis suggesting the origin from the RV free wall (rare).

studies are increasingly available for the diagnosis of inherited arrhythmogenic heart muscle diseases, including channelopathies. Work-up should also include a search for agents that may enhance electrical ventricular irritability, such as the use of excessive amount of alcohol, illicit drugs, or stimulants, particularly ephedrine and caffeine.

Current European recommendations[90] suggest that all sports are allowed in asymptomatic athletes, with no family history of SCD, <2,000 PVBs/24 h, no polymorphic PVBs or couplets, no increased PVBs by exercise, and exclusion of underlying structural or arrhythmogenic disease (with or without treatment). Deconditioning (3–6 months) is recommended in symptomatic athletes or with >2,000 PVBs/24 h or polymorphic PVBs or couplets, or PVBs increased by exercise. If an underlying cardiovascular disease is excluded and resolution of arrhythmias with detraining is demonstrated, all sports are allowed, but the athlete has to be revaluated every year. Conversely, in the presence of underlying disease, no competitive sports are allowed, possibly with the exception of light to moderate leisure-time sports. Similarly, the recent recommendations from the AHA/ACC suggest that athletes without structural heart disease who have PVBs can participate in all competitive sports.[91] However, when PVBs increase in frequency during exercise or exercise testing and convert to repetitive forms, further evaluation by appropriate imaging or monitoring strategies are recommended before clearance for participation in high-intensity sports. If uncontrollable, exercise-induced arrhythmias produce symptoms of lightheadedness or near-syncope, fatigue, or dyspnea, the athlete should be limited to competitive sports below the level at which marked frequency increased or symptoms appeared during testing. Conversely, athletes with defined structural heart disease should be limited to low-intensity competitive sports.

Syncope

Syncope is a sudden transient loss of consciousness and postural tone with spontaneous recovery after a brief period, which does not require electrical or medical therapy.[92] The athlete with syncope presents a unique challenge for the physician. The causes of syncope in athletes range from benign neurocardiogenic episodes to life-threatening conditions such as ventricular arrhythmias leading to SCD. Thus, it is mandatory to identify causes and mechanisms of syncope with the aim to exclude underlying heart disease.

The most common cause of syncope in athletes is neurally-mediated or vasovagal syncope.[93] Specific triggers are blood draws and prolonged standing. Classic prodromal symptoms such as warmth, nausea, or palpitations are present in most cases. Usually the syncopal episodes are brief (5–30 s) and patients awake nauseous. Orthostatic hypotension may also cause syncope during sports or immediately after exertion. Orthostatic hypotension can be asymptomatic or associated with symptoms such as lightheadedness, dizziness, blurred vision, weakness, palpitations, and syncope. Orthostatic hypotension is favored by volume depletion from recent exercise and reduced vasomotor tone caused by long periods of training. Approximately 1% of syncope in athletes is secondary to cardiac disease, so-called cardiogenic syncope.[94] While neurally-mediated syncope usually occurs at rest, cardiogenic syncope typically occurs during effort.[95] Syncope during exertion should be differentiated from syncope immediately after exercise. With the later, exercise-induced peripheral vasodilatation is no longer counteracted by the active "peripheral muscle pump" causing a fall in central circulation volume and syncope.

There are few available data on the epidemiology and causes of syncope in the athlete. Colivicchi *et al.* studied a large population of 7,568 athletes undergoing preparticipation screening.[94] A syncopal episode was reported by 474 (6.2%) in the previous 5 years. With regard to circumstances, it is noteworthy that syncope was not exercise related in 87.7%, and exercise related in 13.3%, i.e. post-exertional in 12.0%, and exertional in 1.3%. Over an average of 6.4 +/− 3.1 years of follow-up, the recurrence rate of syncope was 20/1,000 subject-years, whereas the rate of new syncopal episodes was 2.2/1,000 subject-years. In athletes with exercise-unrelated episodes, the diagnosis was either vasovagal or situational syncope. In athletes with post-exertional syncope, cardiac work-up was normal and no SCD occurred. Among those with syncope during exertion (n 46, or 1.3%), one HCM and one right ventricular tachycardia were diagnosed.

Clinical evaluation of syncope in the athlete remains a challenge. The major aim is to identify athletes at risk and to protect them from SCD. Although benign mechanisms predominate, syncope may be arrhythmic and precede SCD. Syncope during exercise should be regarded as an alarming symptom and carefully evaluated to exclude an underlying cardiac disease predisposing to arrhythmic cardiac arrest. All athletes with syncope should undergo a focused and detailed work-up for underlying cardiac causes, either structural or electrical. The work-up includes medical and family history, and a resting ECG. Often the assessment requires additional testing such as a echocardiography, stress testing, 24-h Holter monitoring and/or loop monitoring, and cardiac MRI; in selected cases may also require invasive studies such as coronary angiography, electrophysiological study, and endomyocardial biopsy. In athletes with neurocardiogenic syncope, the restriction from sports is dictated by the possibility that any transient loss of consciousness could produce danger for the athlete and the people nearby. In athletes with syncope of arrhythmic origin, with or without an underlying heart disease, recommendations depend on the type of arrhythmia and/or on the associated abnormal cardiovascular condition.

Personal Perspective

Domenico Corrado

I began studying the electrophysiologic changes of the athlete's heart and the arrhythmogenic conditions predisposing to sudden cardiac death during sports in 1982, the year of my graduation in Medicine at the University of Padua, Italy. At that time, I became curious and fascinated by the mystery of cardiac arrest occurring suddenly and unexpectedly in young people and athletes who were apparently healthy and achieved extraordinary exercise performance without complaining of any symptoms. In 1986, under the guidance of Dr. Gaetano Thiene who was professor of cardiovascular pathology at the University of Padua, I wrote my thesis for cardiology specialization in clinical-pathological correlations in young subjects who died suddenly from arrhythmogenic right ventricular cardiomyopathy, a previously unrecognized cause of fatality in the athlete; the thesis became an article that was published in the *New England Journal of Medicine* in 1988. Since then, I have been increasingly involved in the research field of sports cardiology. In 1998, together with Dr. Maurizio Schiavon who was chief of the Centre for Sports Medicine in Padua, I published an article in the *New England Journal of Medicine* that demonstrated the efficacy of the Italian preparticipation electrocardiographic screening in identifying athletes with hypertrophic cardiomyopathy, the leading cause of sudden death in US athletes. About one decade later, we reported in *JAMA* on a time-trend analysis of the incidence of sudden cardiovascular death in young competitive athletes between the ages of 12 and 35 years in the Veneto region between 1979 and 2004. The study demonstrated a sharp decline of ≈90% in death rates among athletes after the introduction of the Italian screening program in 1982, particularly because of fewer sudden deaths from cardiomyopathies. In a provocative article published in the Lancet in 2005, I used a quotation from the Greek dramatist Menander, "Those whom the gods love die young," in reference to sudden death among athletes. I wanted to highlight that, by virtue of the results of our long-running investigation in the Veneto region of Italy, fatalities occurring in the young should no longer be considered as predestined and beyond our control, but a consequence of an underlying heart disease that may be identified and treated during life. In 2005, I coordinated an ESC study group that recommended implementing a common European protocol of preparticipation screening for athletes along the lines of the electrocardiographic screening system in Italy. In 2010, I chaired a consensus document that provided recommendations for appropriate interpretation of the electrocardiogram of the athlete.

References

1. Maron BJ, Pelliccia A. The heart of trained athletes: Cardiac remodeling and the risks of sports, including sudden death. *Circulation* 2006;114:1633–1644.
2. Maron BJ. Sudden death in young athletes. *N Engl J Med* 2003;349:1064–1075.
3. Cavallaro V, Petretta M, Betocchi S, *et al*. Effects of sustained training on left ventricular structure and function in top level rowers. *Eur Heart J* 1993;14:898–903.
4. Choo JK, Abernethy WB III, Hutter AM Jr. Electrocardiographic observations in professional football players. *Am J Cardiol* 2002;90:198–200.

5. Balady GJ, Cadigan JB, Ryan TJ. Electrocardiogram of the athlete: An analysis of 289 professional football players. *Am J Cardiol* 1984;53:1339–1343.

6. Corrado D, Basso C, Rizzoli G, *et al.* Does sports activity enhance the risk of sudden death in adolescents and young adults? *J Am Coll Cardiol* 2003;42:1959–1963.

7. Biffi A, Pelliccia A, Verdile L, *et al.* Long-term clinical significance of frequent and complex ventricular tachyarrhythmias in trained athletes. *J Am Coll Cardiol* 2002;40: 446–452.

8. Biffi A, Maron BJ, Verdile L, *et al.* Impact of physical deconditioning on ventricular tachyarrhythmias in trained athletes. *J Am Coll Cardiol* 2004;44:1053–1058.

9. Pluim BM, Zwinderman AH, van der Laarse A, *et al.* The athlete's heart. A meta-analysis of cardiac structure and function. *Circulation* 2000;101:336–344.

10. Spirito P, Pelliccia A, Proschan MA, *et al.* Morphology of the "athlete's heart" assessed by echocardiography in 947 elite athletes representing 27 sports. *Am J Cardiol* 1994;71:802–806.

11. Pelliccia A, Maron BJ, Culasso F, *et al.* Clinical significance of abnormal electrocardiographic patterns in trained athletes. *Circulation* 2000;102:278–284.

12. Pelliccia A, Culasso F, Di Paolo F, *et al.* Physiologic left ventricular cavity dilatation in elite athletes. *Ann Intern Med* 1999;130:23–31.

13. Pelliccia A, Maron BJ, Culasso F, *et al.* Athlete's heart in women: Echocardiographic characterization of highly trained elite female athletes. *J Am Med Assoc* 1996;276:211–215.

14. Pluim BM, Zwinderman AH, van der Laarse A, *et al.* The athlete's heart: A meta-analysis of cardiac structure and function. *Circulation* 1999;100:336–344.

15. Magalski A, Maron BJ, Main ML, *et al.* Relation of race to electrocardiographic patterns in elite American football players. *J Am Coll Cardiol* 2008;51:2250–2255.

16. Basavarajaiah S, Boraita A, Whyte G, *et al.* Ethnic differences in left ventricular remodeling in highly-trained athletes: Relevance to differentiating physiologic left ventricular hypertrophy from hypertrophic cardiomyopathy. *J Am Coll Cardiol* 2008;51:2256–2262.

17. Corrado D, McKenna WJ. Appropriate interpretation of the athlete's electrocardiogram saves lives as well as money. *Eur Heart J* 2007;28:1920–1922.

18. Zorzi A, ElMaghawry M, Migliore F, *et al.* ST-segment elevation and sudden death in the athlete. *Card Electrophysiol Clin* 2013;5:73–84.

19. Mont L, Elosua R, Brugada J. Endurance sport practice as a risk factor for atrial fibrillation and atrial flutter. *Europace* 2009;11:11–17.

20. Mascia F, Perrotta L, Galanti G, *et al.* Atrial fibrillation in athletes. *Int J Sports Med* 2013;34:379–384.

21. D'Ascenzi F, Cameli M, Zacà V, *et al.* Supernormal diastolic function and role of left atrial myocardial deformation analysis by 2D speckle tracking echocardiography in elite soccer players. *Echocardiography* 2011;28:320–326.

22. D'Ascenzi F, Cameli M, Padeletti M, *et al.* Characterization of right atrial function and dimension in top-level athletes: A speckle tracking study. *Int J Cardiovasc Imaging* 2013;29:87–94.

23. D'Ascenzi F, Pelliccia A, Natali BM, *et al*. Increased left atrial size is associated with reduced atrial stiffness and preserved reservoir function in athlete's heart. *Int J Cardiovasc Imaging* 2015;31:669–705.
24. Corrado D, Pelliccia A, Heidbuchel H, *et al*. Recommendations for interpretation of 12-lead electrocardiogram in the athlete. *Eur Heart J* 2009;31:243–259.
25. Calore C, Melacini P, Pelliccia A, *et al*. Prevalence and clinical meaning of isolated increase of QRS voltages in hypertrophic cardiomyopathy versus athlete's heart: Relevance to athletic screening. *Int J Cardiol* 2013;168:4494–4497.
26. Migliore F, Zorzi A, Michieli P, *et al*. Prevalence of cardiomyopathy in Italian asymptomatic children with electrocardiographic T-wave inversion at preparticipation screening. *Circulation* 2012;125:529–538.
27. Papadakis M, Carre F, Kervio G, *et al*. The prevalence, distribution, and clinical outcomes of electrocardiographic repolarization patterns in male athletes of African/Afro-Caribbean origin. *Eur Heart J* 2011;32:2304–2313.
28. Calore C, Zorzi A, Sheikh N, *et al*. Electrocardiographic anterior T-wave inversion in athletes of different ethnicities: differential diagnosis between athlete's heart and cardiomyopathy. *Eur Heart J* 2016;37:2515–2527.
29. Blake JB, Larrabee RC. Observations upon long distance runners. *Boston Med Surg J* 1903;148:195.
30. Chapman JH. Profound sinus bradycardia in the athletic heart syndrome. *J Sports Med Phys Fitness* 1982;22:45–48.
31. Hanne-Paparo N, Kellermann JJ. Long-term Holter ECG monitoring of athletes. *Med Sci Sports Exerc* 1981;13:294–298.
32. Zehender M, Meinertz T, Keul J, *et al*. ECG variants and cardiac arrhythmia in athletes: Clinical relevance and prognostic importance. *Am Heart J* 1990;119:1378–1391.
33. Huston TP, Puffer JC, Rodney WM. The athletic heart syndrome. *N Engl J Med* 1985;313:24–32.
34. Viitasalo MT, Kala R, Eisalo A. Ambulatory electrocardiographic findings in young athletes between 14 and 16 years of age. *Eur Heart J* 1984;5:2–6.
35. Biffi A, Delise P, Zeppilli P, *et al*. Italian cardiological guidelines for sports eligibility in athletes with heart disease: part 1. *J Cardiovasc Med* 2013;14:477–499.
36. Palatini P, Maraglino G, Sperti G, *et al*. Prevalence and possible mechanisms of ventricular arrhythmias in athletes. *Am Heart J* 1985;110:560–567.
37. Talan DA, Bauernfeind RA, Ashley WW, *et al*. Twentyfour hour continuous ECG recordings in longdistance runners. *Chest* 1982;82:19–24.
38. Viitasalo M, Kala R, Eisalo A. Ambulatory electrocardiographic recording in endurance athletes. *Br Heart J* 1982;47:213–220.
39. Meytes I, Kaplinsky E, Yahini JH. Wenckebach A-V block: A frequent feature following heavy physical training. *Am Heart J* 1975;90:426–430.
40. Zeppilli P, Fenici R, Sassara M, *et al*. Wenckebach second-degree AV block in top-ranking athletes: An old problem revisited. *Am Heart J* 1980;100:291–294.

41. Karjalainen J, Kujala UM, Kaprio J, *et al*. Lone atrial fibrillation in vigorously exercising middle aged men: Case-control study. *Brit and J* 1998;316:1784–1785.

42. Mont L, Sambola A, Brugada J, *et al*. Long-lasting sport practice and lone atrial fibrillation. *Eur Heart J* 2002;23:477–482.

43. Elosua R, Arquer A, Mont L, *et al*. Sport practice and the risk of lone atrial fibrillation: A case-control study. *Int J Cardiol* 2006;108:332–337.

44. Molina L, Mont L, Marrugat J, *et al*. Long-term endurance sport practice increases the incidence of lone atrial fibrillation in men: A follow-up study. *Europace* 2008;10: 618–623.

45. Masia R, Pena A, Marrugat J, *et al*. High prevalence of cardiovascular risk factors in Gerona, Spain, a province with low myocardial infarction incidence. REGICOR Investigators. *J Epidemiol Commun Health* 1998;52:707–715.

46. Mont L, Tamborero D, Elosua R, *et al*. GIRAFA (Grup Integrat de Recerca en Fibril·lació Auricular) Investigators. Physical activity, height, and left atrial size are independent risk factors for lone atrial fibrillation in middle-aged healthy individuals. *Europace* 2008;10:15–20.

47. Myrstad M, Løchen ML, Graff-Iversen S, *et al*. Increased risk of atrial fibrillation among elderly Norwegian men with a history of long-term endurance sport practice. *Scand J Med Sci Sports* 2014;24:e238–e244.

48. Heidbuchel H, Anné W, Willems R, *et al*. Endurance sports is a risk factor for atrial fibrillation after ablation for atrial flutter. *Int J Cardiol* 2006;107:67–72.

49. D'Ascenzi F, Cameli M, Ciccone MM, *et al*. The controversial relationship between exercise and atrial fibrillation: Clinical studies and pathophysiological mechanisms. *J Cardiovasc Med* 2015;16:802–810.

50. Pelliccia A, Maron BJ, Di Paolo FM, *et al*. Prevalence and clinical significance of left atrial remodeling in competitive athletes. *J Am Coll Cardiol* 2005;46:690–695.

51. Woodward A, Tin Tin S, Doughty RN, Ameratunga S. Atrial fibrillation and cycling: Six year follow-up of the Taupo bicycle study. *BMC Public Health* 2015;15:23.

52. Kwok CS, Anderson SG, Myint PK, Mamas MA, Loke YK. Physical activity and incidence of atrial fibrillation: A systematic review and meta-analysis. *Int J Cardiol* 2014;177:467–476.

53. Hoogsteen J, Schep G, Van Hemel NM, *et al*. Paroxysmal atrial fibrillation in male endurance athletes. A 9-year follow up. *Europace* 2004;6:222–228.

54. Sarubbi B. The Wolff–Parkinson–White electrocardiogram pattern in athletes: How and when to evaluate the risk for dangerous arrhythmias. The opinion of the paediatric cardiologist. *J Cardiovasc Med* 2006;7:271–278.

55. Gaita F, Giustetto C, Bianchi F, *et al*. Short QT syndrome. A familial cause of sudden death. *Circulation* 2003;108:965–970.

56. Heidbüchel H, Corrado D, Biffi A, *et al*. Study Group on Sports Cardiology of the European Association for Cardiovascular Prevention and Rehabilitation. Recommendations for participation in leisure-time physical activity and competitive sports of patients with arrhythmias and potentially arrhythmogenic conditions.

Part II: Ventricular arrhythmias, channelopathies and implantable defibrillators. *Eur J Cardiovasc Prev Rehabil* 2006;13:676–686.

57. Ackerman MJ, Zipes DP, Kovacs RJ, Maron BJ. Eligibility and disqualification recommendations for competitive athletes with cardiovascular abnormalities: Task force 10: the cardiac channelopathies: A scientific statement from the American Heart Association and American College of Cardiology. *J Am Coll Cardiol* 2015;66:2424–2428.

58. Antzelevitch C, Brugada P, Borggrefe M, *et al.* Brugada syndrome: Report of the second consensus conference. *Heart Rhythm* 2005;2:429–440.

59. Zorzi A, Leoni L, Di Paolo FM, *et al.* Differential diagnosis between early repolarization of athlete's heart and coved-type brugada electrocardiogram. *Am J Cardiol* 2015;115:529–532.

60. Van der Werf C, Wilde AA. Catecholaminergic polymorphic ventricular tachycardia: From bench to bedside. *Heart* 2013;99:497–504.

61. Kennedy HL, Whitlock JA, Sprague MK, *et al.* Long-term follow-up of asymptomatic healthy subjects with frequent and complex ventricular ectopy. *N Engl J Med* 1985;312:193–197.

62. Selzman KA, Gettes LS. Exercise-induced premature ventricular beats: Should we do anything differently? *Circulation* 2004;109:2374–2375.

63. Fuchs T, Torjman A, Galitzkaya L, *et al.* The clinical significance of ventricular arrhythmias during an exercise test in non-competitive and competitive athletes. *Isr Med Assoc J* 2011;13:735–739.

64. Steriotis AK, Nava A, Rigato I, *et al.* Noninvasive cardiac screening in young athletes with ventricular arrhythmias. *Am J Cardiol* 2013;111:557–562.

65. Lampert R. Evaluation and management of arrhythmia in the athletic patient. *Progr Cardiovasc Dis* 2012;54:423–431.

66. Heidbuchel H, Hoogsteen J, Fagard R, *et al.* High prevalence of right ventricular involvement in endurance athletes with ventricular arrhythmias: Role of an electro-physiologic study in risk stratification. *Eur Heart J* 2003;24:1473–1480.

67. Gimeno JR, Tomé-Esteban M, Lofiego C, *et al.* Exercise-induced ventricular arrhythmias and risk of sudden cardiac death in patients with hypertrophic cardiomyopathy. *Eur Heart J* 2009;30:2599–2605.

68. Heidbuchel H, Prior DL, La Gerche A. Ventricular arrhythmias associated with long-term endurance sports: What is the evidence? *Brit J Sports Med* 2012;46:44–50.

69. Morshedi-Meibodi A, Evans JC, Levy D, *et al.* Clinical correlates and prognostic significance of exercise-induced ventricular premature beats in the community: The Framingham Heart Study. *Circulation* 2004;109:2417–2422.

70. Califf RM, McKinnis RA, Burks J, *et al.* Prognostic implications of ventricular arrhythmias during 24 hour ambulatory monitoring in patients undergoing cardiac catheterization for coronary artery disease. *Am J Cardiol* 1982;50:23–31.

71. Marieb MA, Beller GA, Gibson RS, *et al.* Clinical relevance of exercise-induced ventricular arrhythmias in suspected coronary artery disease. *Am J Cardiol* 1990;66:172–178.

72. Schweikert RA, Pashkow FJ, Snader CE, *et al*. Association of exercise-induced ventricular ectopic activity with thallium myocardial perfusion and angiographic coronary artery disease in stable, low-risk populations. *Am J Cardiol* 1999;83: 530–534.

73. Sami M, Chaitman B, Fisher L, *et al*. Significance of exercise-induced ventricular arrhythmia in stable coronary artery disease: A coronary artery surgery study project. *Am J Cardiol* 1984;54:1182–1188.

74. Sofi F, Capalbo A, Pucci N, *et al*. Cardiovascular evaluation, including resting and exercise electrocardiography, before participation in competitive sports: Cross sectional study. *Brit Med J* 2008;337:88–92.

75. Ventura R, Steven D, Klemm HU, *et al*. Decennial follow-up in patients with recurrent tachycardia originating from the right ventricular outflow tract: Electrophysiologic characteristics and response to treatment. *Eur Heart J* 2007;28:2338–2345.

76. Beckerman J, Mathur A, Stahr S, *et al*. Exercise-induced ventricular arrhythmias and cardiovascular death. *Ann Noninvasive Electrocardiol* 2005;10:47–52.

77. Jouven X, Zureik M, Desnos M, *et al*. Long-term outcome in asymptomatic men with exercise-induced premature ventricular depolarizations. *N Engl J Med* 2000;343: 826–833.

78. Gaita F, Giustetto C, Di Donna P, *et al*. Long-term follow-up of right ventricular monomorphic extrasystoles. *J Am Coll Cardiol* 2001;38:364–370.

79. Niwano S, Wakisaka Y, Niwano H, *et al*. Prognostic significance of frequent premature ventricular contractions originating from the ventricular outflow tract in patients with normal left ventricular function. *Heart* 2009;95:1230–1237.

80. Verdile L, Maron BJ, Pelliccia A, *et al*. Clinical significance of exercise-induced ventricular tachyarrhythmias in trained athletes without cardiovascular abnormalities. *Heart Rhythm* 2015;12:78–85.

81. Delise P, Sitta N, Lanari E, *et al*. Long-term effect of continuing sports activity in competitive athletes with frequent ventricular premature complexes and apparently normal heart. *Am J Cardiol* 2013;112:1396–1402.

82. Rahilly GT, Prystowsky EN, Zipes DP, *et al*. Clinical and electrophysiologic findings in patients with repetitive monomorphic ventricular tachycardia and otherwise normal electrocardiogram. *Am J Cardiol* 1982;50:459–468.

83. Buxton AE, Marchlinski FE, Doherty JU, *et al*. Repetitive, monomorphic ventricular tachycardia: Clinical and electrophysiologic characteristics in patients with and patients without organic heart disease. *Am J Cardiol* 1984;54:997–1002.

84. Partington S, Myers J, Cho S, *et al*. Prevalence and prognostic value of exercise-induced ventricular arrhythmias. *Am Heart J* 2003;145:139–146.

85. Udall JA, Ellestad MH. Predictive implications of ventricular premature contractions associated with treadmill stress testing. *Circulation* 1977;56:985–989.

86. Casella G, Pavesi PC, Sangiorgio P, *et al*. Exercise-induced ventricular arrhythmias in patients with healed myocardial infarction. *Int J Cardiol* 1993;40:229–235.

87. Lerman BB. Mechanism, diagnosis, and treatment of outflow tract tachycardia. *Nat Rev Cardiol* 2015;12:597–608.

88. Nogami A. Purkinje-related arrhythmias part I: Monomorphic ventricular tachycardias. *Pacing Clin Electrophysiol* 2011;34:624–650.
89. Schnell F, Claessen G, La Gerche A, *et al*. Subepicardial delayed gadolinium enhancement in asymptomatic athletes: Let sleeping dogs lie? *Br J Sports Med* 2016;50: 111–117.
90. Heidbüchel H, Panhuyzen-Goedkoop N, Corrado D, *et al*. Recommendations for participation in leisure-time physical activity and competitive sports in patients with arrhythmias and potentially arrhythmogenic conditions Part I: Supraventricular arrhythmias and pacemakers. *Eur J Cardiovasc Prev Rehabil* 2006;13:475–484.
91. Zipes DP, Link MS, Ackerman MJ, *et al*. Eligibility and disqualification recommendations for competitive athletes with cardiovascular abnormalities: Task force 9: Arrhythmias and conduction defects: A scientific statement from the American Heart Association and American College of Cardiology. *J Am Coll Cardiol* 2015;66: 2412–2423.
92. Brignole M, Hamdan MH. New concepts in the assessment of syncope. *J Am Coll Cardiol* 2012;59:1583–1591.
93. Vettor G, Zorzi A, Basso C, Thiene G, Corrado D. Syncope as a warning symptom of sudden cardiac death in athletes. *Cardiol Clin* 2015;33:423–432.
94. Colivicchi F, Ammirati F, Santini M. Epidemiology and prognostic implications of syncope in young competing athletes. *Eur Heart J* 2004;25:1749–1753.
95. Grubb BP. Neurocardiogenic syncope and related disorders of orthostatic intolerance. *Circulation* 2005;111:2997–3006.
96. Corrado D, Calore C, Zorzi A, Migliore F. Improving the interpretation of the athlete's electrocardiogram. *Eur Heart J* 2013;34:3606–3609.

Chapter 6

The Athlete's Electrocardiogram

Sanjay Sharma and Keerthi Prakash

St George's, University of London
Cranmer Terrace, London SW17 0RE, United Kingdom

Regular intense exercise is associated with alterations in cardiac structure and function which facilitate the generation of a large and sustained increase in cardiac output for prolonged periods. Such adaptations are commonly represented on the surface EKG of the athlete and influenced by a variety of demographic factors including age, gender, ethnicity, and the sporting discipline. Several studies in large populations of athletes have revealed a spectrum of EKG patterns that are considered benign. It is prudent to emphasize that in the presence of symptoms or abnormalities on cardiac examination, apparently normal EKG patterns warrant further investigation.

Occasionally some electrical patterns in athletes, specifically repolarization anomalies, may overlap with morphologically mild or incomplete phenotypic expression of both the cardiomyopathies and the ion channel diseases which are implicated in exercise-related sudden cardiac death. Marked repolarization changes overlapping with these disease processes are usually observed in male endurance athletes and athletes of African/Afro-Caribbean origin. The differentiation between benign physiological adaptation from electrical harbingers of diseases implicated in exercise-related sudden cardiac death is essential because erroneous interpretation has profound consequences that may lead to unnecessary disqualification from sport at one extreme, to jeopardizing a young life at the other.

The steady trickle of deaths among athletes and the high visibility afforded by these catastrophes has led several sporting bodies, including the International Olympic Committee, the National Basketball Association, and the Union of European Football Associations, to advocate cardiac screening for their athletes. Such practice frequently incorporates a 12-lead EKG hence the interpretation of the athlete's EKG is pivotal for the assessment of individuals engaged in competitive sport or high-intensity routine recreational exercise.

This chapter will provide an in-depth analysis of the normal physiological alterations in electrical patterns that are major components of the athlete's heart and will aim to highlight specific anomalies that should raise the possibility of underlying cardiac pathology.

Physiological EKG Patterns in Athletes

Normal athletes' EKG patterns can be divided broadly into those which reflect increased vagal tone and those which reflect an increase in cardiac chamber size and ventricular wall thickness. Sinus bradycardia, sinus arrhythmia, early repolarization consisting of J-point elevation, ST segment elevation with tall T-waves, 1st degree atrioventricular (AV) block, voltage criteria for left and right ventricular hypertrophy, and incomplete right bundle branch block are recognized manifestations of the athlete's EKG.[1,2]

Sinus bradycardia and sinus arrhythmia

Sinus bradycardia (Figure 1) and sinus arrhythmia are common. Over 80% of athletes exhibit a resting heart rate between 45 and 60 bpm. Approximately 5% show a heart rate <40 bpm, but a resting pulse <35 bpm is rare and usually confined to athletes engaging in endurance sports. Sinus arrhythmia is common particularly in young athletes and is present in up to 70% of cases. 1st degree AV block is detected in 5% of unselected athletes, but has been reported in over 30% of endurance athletes[3] whereas Mobitz type 1 AV block (Wenckebach block), sinus pauses, and junctional rhythms can be observed at rest or during sleep in a smaller proportion of athletes. An ectopic atrial rhythm or a wandering atrial pacemaker are also recognized and are due to increased vagal tone. All of these anomalies resolve with relatively gentle exercise which causes sympathetic tone to override vagal tone.

In contrast, Mobitz type 2nd or 3rd degree AV block are extremely rare and usually observed in a very small proportion (0.5%) of lifelong veteran endurance athletes.[2] In such instances, markers of cardiac conduction tissue disease include symptoms such as dizziness or syncope, persistence of the heart block or chronotropic incompetence during exercise, or failure of the 2nd or 3rd degree AV block to resolve after a 6-week trial of detraining.

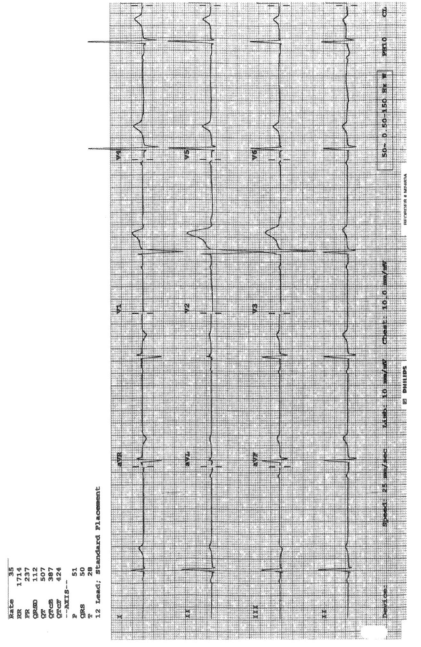

Figure 1.   EKG of an endurance athlete showing sinus bradycardia.

Voltage criteria for left ventricular hypertrophy

Isolated large QRS voltage fulfilling the criteria for left ventricular hypertrophy (LVH) is common in young, slim male athletes[4] and does not warrant further investigation in the absence of symptoms or an abnormal physical examination unless there is a family history of hypertrophic cardiomyopathy. Almost 70% of thin, young male athletes fulfil the Sokolow–Lyon voltage criteria for LVH (S-wave in V1 + largest R-wave in V5 or V6 > 3.5 mV [0.1 mV = 1 small square on standard EKG] or R-wave in AVL ≥ 1.1 mV).[5] Although there is poor correlation between electrical voltage criteria for LVH and structural LVH at echocardiography, we suspect that the increase in QRS voltage represents a relative increase in left ventricular size and mass since the magnitude of the QRS complexes regress with detraining. Among athletes with physiological increases in left ventricular size, large QRS complexes represent the only electrical manifestation of LVH. The co-existence of ST segment depression, T-wave inversion (TWI), pathological Q-waves, or delayed intrinsicoid deflection in the left ventricular leads is highly suggestive of diseases associated with pathological LVH.[6–9]

Partial right bundle branch block

Incomplete right bundle branch block (RBBB) (rSR' in V1; QRS <120 ms) may be detected in almost one-third of athletes[1,4,10,11] and is probably representative of an increased conduction time from physiological right ventricular dilation rather than disease of the His–Purkinje fibres. Incomplete RBBB is not a typical feature of arrhythmogenic right ventricular cardiomyopathy (ARVC)[12] and further investigation of this specific pattern is not warranted in the absence of symptoms or physical signs suggestive of an intracardiac shunt. Complete RBBB is observed in 1% of the general population and one report suggests a slightly higher frequency in endurance athletes.[13]

Early repolarization

Early repolarization changes consisting of J-point elevation, ascending ST segments, and tall T-waves are present in over 60% of athletes[1,4,10,11,13,14] and are most prevalent in male endurance athletes and in athletes of African/Afro-Caribbean origin.[15] Classically, there is elevation of the QRS–ST junction (J-point) >0.1 mV, accompanied by a concave ST segment and a tall T-wave. This is most pronounced in the anterior precordial leads (V1–V4) (Figure 2), but can also commonly affect the inferior and lateral leads. The J-point may also manifest as a notched deflection

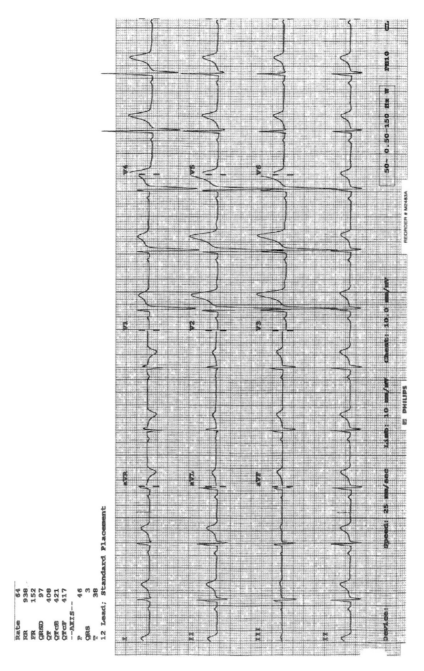

Figure 2.   Early repolarization in a Caucasian athlete demonstrating J-point elevation with concave ST segment elevation and peaked upright T-waves.

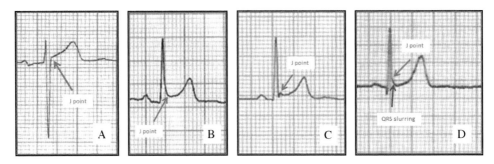

Figure 3.   Early repolarization changes in athletes: (A) J-point elevation with concave ST segment elevation; (B) a discrete J-point; (C) a notched J-point after the S-wave; (D) a J-point embedded in the terminal portion of the S-wave.

after the S-wave or as terminal slurring of the QRS complex in the inferior and/or lateral leads (Figure 3). In athletes of African/Afro-Caribbean origin there is frequently ST segment elevation after the J-point in the anterior leads (V1–V4) that may be accompanied by asymmetrical TWI[15–17] (Figure 4). Such repolarization changes are thought to be due to increased vagal tone and resolve at higher heart rates during exercise testing or after a period of detraining. A longitudinal study of 148 athletes noted that a higher proportion of athletes demonstrated early repolarization changes post-training (52.7%) compared to pre-training (37.2%).[14]

Early repolarization has always been considered a benign manifestation of athletic training, but over the past 7–8 years there have been reports linking early repolarization in the inferior and/or lateral leads to idiopathic ventricular fibrillation (VF).[18,19] However, J-point elevation in the inferior and lateral leads is present in 25% of Caucasian athletes and 40% of African/Afro-Caribbean athletes and is almost always associated with ascending ST segments. Further assessment of the EKGs of relatively sedentary victims of aborted sudden cardiac arrest reveals that notched J-waves or terminal slurring of the QRS >0.2 mV accompanied by horizontal or down-sloping ST segments are associated with the highest risk of adverse cardiac events. Whereas, J-point elevation with ascending ST segments in athletes is likely physiological. In our experience, J-point elevation followed by horizontal or down-sloping ST segments is not related to athletic training and should be investigated in athletes with syncope.[20]

Impact of Gender, Type of Sporting Discipline, Ethnicity, and Age

Gender and endurance athletes

The electrical patterns of athletic training are influenced by the gender, the type of sport, the ethnicity, and the age of the athlete.[21,22] In general, male athletes

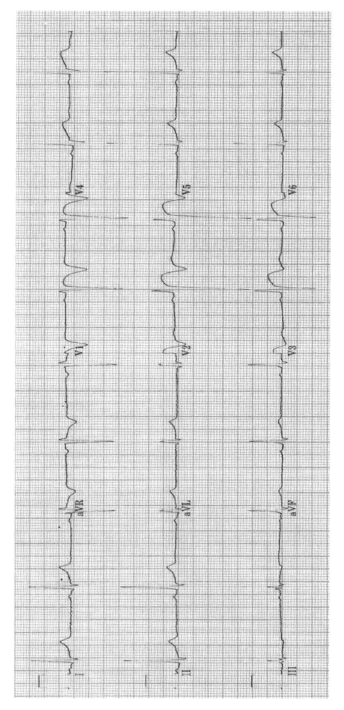

Figure 4.   EKG from an African/Afro-Caribbean athlete demonstrating convex ST segment elevation with T-wave inversion in V1–V3.

engaging in endurance sports reveal the most profound EKG patterns and show a considerably higher prevalence of bradyarrhythmias, voltage criteria for left or right ventricular hypertrophy, and early repolarization. In any given sporting discipline, female athletes demonstrate qualitatively similar electrical patterns, but to a lesser extent.[16,23–25] A recent study comparing 251 endurance athletes and 1,010 non-endurance athletes revealed that the prevalence of sinus bradycardia, early repolarization patterns, and voltage criteria for LVH was 68%, 72%, and 36%, respectively, in endurance athletes, compared with 51%, 37%, and 24% in non-endurance athletes. Additionally, 14.3% of endurance athletes showed a relatively high prevalence of TWI in the anterior precordial leads beyond V2 which is currently considered abnormal by most consensus panels for EKG interpretation in athletes.[23]

Athletes of African/Afro-Caribbean origin

Ethnicity has an important role in governing the electrical response to athletic training. African/Afro-Caribbean athletes have a higher prevalence of early repolarization compared with Caucasian athletes. A study comparing EKGs among 904 African/Afro-Caribbean male athletes, 1,819 Caucasian male athletes, and 119 sedentary African/Afro-Caribbean men showed that ST segment elevation was almost 3-fold more common in African/Afro-Caribbean athletes compared to the Caucasian athletes (63.2% vs. 26.5%). The prevalence of ST segment elevation in the African/Afro-Caribbean sedentary controls was similar to that in African/Afro-Caribbean athletes (65.5%) suggesting that early repolarization anomalies in African/Afro-Caribbean individuals are a normal ethnic variation. Detailed inspection of the morphology of the ST segments between African/Afro-Caribbean athletes and sedentary men revealed that the concave/saddle-shaped patterns simulating acute pericarditis were common in both groups, but that the convex ST segment elevation in leads V1–V4 simulating acute anterior myocardial infarction or the Brugada EKG pattern were 6-fold more common in athletes, indicating a physiological response to training.[15]

The same study showed that 23% of all African/Afro-Caribbean athletes exhibited a high prevalence of TWI compared with just 4% of Caucasian athletes. Almost 60% of the TWI was observed in leads V1–V4 and was usually preceded by convex ST segment elevation. Comprehensive assessment of the athletes with this particular EKG pattern with echocardiography, cardiac MRI, exercise stress test, and Holter monitoring failed to identify any cardiac pathology. TWI resolved with exercise in all patients when heart rates exceeded 80% of their maximum predicted for age suggesting that there is a vagal component to this repolarization abnormality. Resolution of the TWI was seen within 4 weeks in several athletes who agreed to detrain. Based on these observations, TWI in leads V1–V4 preceded by convex ST segment elevation is considered benign and does not warrant investigation in asymptomatic African/Afro-Caribbean athletes, unless there is a specific family history of cardiac disease or an abnormality on cardiac examination.[26,27]

The adolescent athlete

The adolescent athlete's heart has not been studied in detail, however, a plethora of reports on relatively large populations of such athletes demonstrate that adolescent athletes show a combination of EKG patterns reflecting athletic training, some of which are normal variants in the juvenile population. A report of 1,000 adolescent athletes aged 14–18 years old showed that these athletes develop changes similar to adult athletes.[4] The Sokolow–Lyon voltage criteria for LVH was detected in a significantly greater proportion of athletes compared to non-athletes of similar age (45% vs. 23%). While the increased prevalence of voltage criteria for LVH in athletes may be explained by an increased left ventricular (LV) size, a moderate proportion of the non-athletes (23%) also had voltage criteria for LVH, suggesting that the size and shape of the chest wall (reduced subcutaneous fat and thinner pectoral muscles) may also contribute to the greater QRS voltages.

All voltages in the QRS complex are increased in adolescent athletes. Deep Q-waves (>0.3 mV) are more frequent in adolescent athletes compared with adult athletes and do not warrant investigation in asymptomatic athletes without a family history of hypertrophic cardiomyopathy (HCM), unless the Q-wave duration is >40 ms or if the Q/R ratio is >0.25 (see section on Q-waves). In our experience, voltage criteria for left and right atrial enlargement are present in 14% and 16% of adolescent athletes, respectively,[4] and when present in isolation or with other electrical EKG patterns of an athlete's heart, only warrant investigation in symptomatic individuals or in those with an abnormal precordial examination.

TWI in leads V1–V3 (the so called "juvenile EKG pattern") is a normal variant in children and regresses with age (Figure 5). The prevalence of this particular EKG pattern ranges from 9% in children aged <14 years [28] to 4% in the adolescent Caucasian population aged 14–16 years.[4,11,28] The juvenile EKG pattern is not influenced by athletic training and the prevalence is similar in athletes and non-athletes. In an Italian study of 2,765 consecutive asymptomatic children, incomplete pubertal development was the only predictor of the persistent juvenile EKG pattern.[28] In our experience the persistence of TWI beyond V2 is present in 0.1–0.2% of children aged >16 years and warrants further investigation if present.[11] TWI in the inferior and lateral leads is uncommon regardless of age and warrants further investigation.[29]

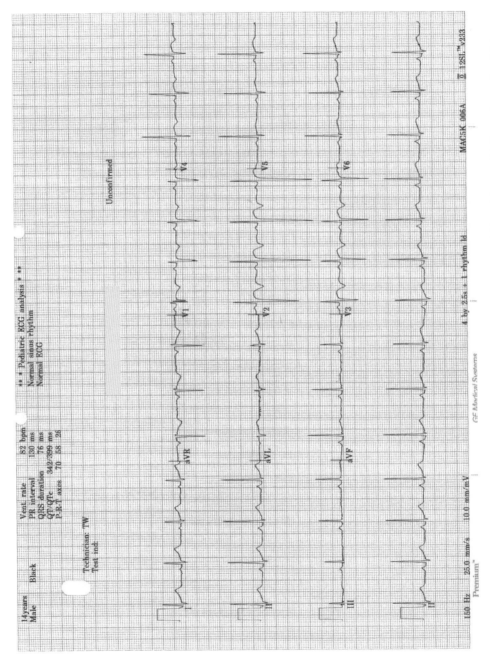

Figure 5.   EKG demonstrating a "Juvenile" pattern of T-wave inversion in V1–V3 in a 14-year-old Caucasian male athlete.

T-wave morphology is also affected by age. Notching of the T-waves in leads V1–V3 may be present in up to 25% of adolescent children aged <16 years and does not warrant any investigation if the QTc is not abnormally prolonged. African/Afro-Caribbean adolescent athletes frequently demonstrate ST segment elevation and TWI in leads V1–V4 similar to African/Afro-Caribbean adult athletes.[10,16]

Electrical Patterns Suggestive of Cardiac Pathology

ST segment depression and left bundle branch block (LBBB) are not consistent with athletic training and should always be considered abnormal irrespective of the athlete's demographics or lack of symptoms.

T-wave inversion

The prevalence and significance of TWI in athletes is not clear. T-wave inversion is generally observed in 3–4% of adults. Data suggesting that TWI may be a normal variant have been generally derived from small cohorts of athletes engaged in extreme endurance sports for prolonged periods.[2] With the exception of the aforementioned accounts in adolescent athletes and African/Afro-Caribbean athletes, TWI extending beyond V2 in the anterior leads, in contiguous inferior leads or affecting the lateral leads, should be considered abnormal and warrants further investigation. One exception is TWI up to V3, preceded by convex ST segment elevation in endurance athletes.[23]

Most athletes with TWI do not show structural abnormalities with echocardiography, but TWI may herald future cardiomyopathy. A large Italian study of 12,550 athletes found TWI in 123 athletes. Of these, 24 athletes had either cardiomyopathy or another cardiac abnormality diagnosed by echocardiography. Eighty-one had no echocardiographic features of cardiomyopathy at baseline initial investigation, but five developed hypertrophic cardiomyopathy ($n = 3$), dilated cardiomyopathy ($n = 1$), and arrhythmogenic right ventricular cardiomyopathy ($n = 1$) during a follow-up of 9 ± 7 years.[30]

The specific distribution of TWI seems important. The current literature suggests that TWI affecting the lateral leads is highly suggestive of cardiac pathology regardless of age or ethnicity. All five athletes who developed cardiomyopathy as mentioned above showed baseline lateral TWI. We have identified five athletes with HCM in our experience with >5,000 athletes studied with EKG and echo. All HCM athletes had lateral TWI.[27] We also found lateral TWI in 87% of 103 patients with HCM.[27] In a more recent study of 6,372 athletes including a relatively large proportion of African/Afro-Caribbean, 155 athletes

(24%) showed TWI. Of these athletes 69 (44%) were ultimately diagnosed with cardiac disease, predominantly HCM (*n* = 55) following a comprehensive investigation using echocardiography, exercise stress testing, 24-h Holter monitoring, and cardiac MR imaging. Importantly, 88% of the athletes diagnosed with a cardiomyopathy showed deep lateral TWI.[24]

Pathological Q-waves

Pathological Q-waves are a recognized manifestation of cardiomyopathy and previous myocardial infarction. The prevalence of pathological Q-waves is dependent on the definition. Definitions based purely on the depth of the Q-wave (>0.3 mV) lack specificity especially in adolescent athletes who frequently show large QRS complexes involving deep Q-waves (as discussed above). Although the definition of a pathological Q-wave (>0.3 mV deep or >40 ms duration) has a 35% sensitivity and 95% specificity for detecting genotype positive individuals with presumed HCM, this study was composed of numerous related probands with the same genetic mutation, which is not representative of the genetic heterogeneity of HCM.[26,31] We consider a Q-wave duration of ≥40 ms or the depth of the Q-wave more than or equal to 25% of the height of the proceeding R-wave (Q/R ratio ≥0.25) to be more specific. Our unpublished data demonstrate that among 200 patients with HCM, 55 (28%) had pathological Q-waves, defined as either a Q-wave duration ≥40 ms or a Q/R ratio ≥0.25. In contrast, none of the HCM patients showed Q-waves >0.4 mV in isolation.

Long QT interval

A prolonged QT interval raises concerns about congenital long QT syndromes (LQTS) which are genetic ion channel diseases that can cause polymorphic ventricular tachycardia (VT) and sudden cardiac death (Figure 6). The normal upper limit of the QT interval is 440 ms in males and 460 ms in females. The QT interval is usually corrected for heart rate using the Bazett's formula (QTc = QT/√RR interval).

Measurement of the QT interval in athletes can be difficult in the presence of sinus arrhythmia, prominent U-waves, or indistinct termination of the T-wave. When sinus arrhythmia is present, an average RR and QT interval should be used when correcting the QT interval for heart rate. The most accurate method to identify the end of the QT interval is to identify the intercept of the tangent of the downslope of the T-wave, (Figure 7) which is often best performed in leads II or V5.

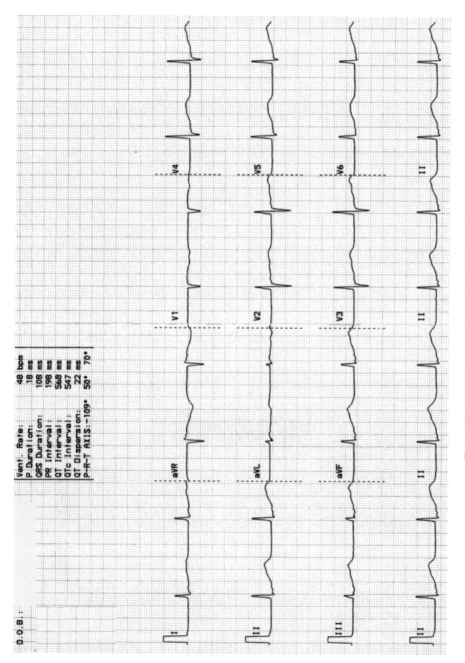

Figure 6.   EKG demonstrating a long QT interval.

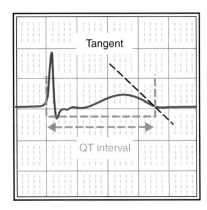

Figure 7.   Measuring the QT interval using the "Tangent" method. The end of the QT is defined as the intercept between the iso-electric baseline and the line drawn along the downslope of the T-wave.

Athletes generally exhibit a longer QT interval than controls.[32] Up to 3% of athletes could be considered to have a mildly prolonged QT interval based on the upper limits of the normal population.[33] The American Heart Association recommends an upper limit of the corrected QTc >470 ms in males and >480 ms in females.[34] These values represent the 99th percentile above the mean for the general population, but have a positive predictive accuracy for LQTS of <10% in isolation.[35]

Our own experience suggests that a corrected QT interval ≥500 ms is highly suggestive of long QT syndrome in athletes. A study of 2,000 athletes found that only three athletes (0.15%) had a QTc >500 ms. All three athletes had either paradoxical QTc prolongation with exercise, a family member with a long QT interval, or tested positive for a disease causing mutation.[32] Based on the above we suggest that in asymptomatic athletes with a QT interval 470–490 ms, a diagnosis of LQTS should only be considered if accompanied by one of the following: notched or bifid T-waves, paradoxical QT prolongation with exercise, a family history of sudden adult death syndrome, a family history of LQTS in a 1st degree relative, evidence of *torsades de pointes*, or unheralded syncope.

Short QT interval

The short QT interval is an extremely rare and poorly characterized condition. A short QT is defined as <370 ms to <320 ms according to different consensus panels.[1,36–38] In our experience the prevalence of a short QT interval <320 ms is 0.1%.[39] The association between a short QT interval and athletic training is weak and over a 5-year follow-up period we have not observed any adverse cardiac events in our athletes with a QT <320 ms. Therefore, the significance of a short QT is unclear.

Brugada EKG Pattern

Brugada syndrome (BrS) is a hereditary cardiac sodium channel disorder associated with fatal ventricular arrhythmias during resting conditions when the heart rate is slow. Theoretically, deaths from BrS should not occur during intense exercise, however, the risk of sudden death may be increased in athletes because exercise promotes a resting bradycardia due to increased vagal tone. Furthermore, VF may be precipitated by hyperpyrexia in BrS, and endurance sports such as the marathon, Ironman, and other triathlons can result in a core temperature >39°C. The diagnostic type 1 Brugada pattern comprises of a high J-point (≥0.2 mV), a coved ST segment, and TWI in ≥2 right precordial leads (V1–V3) (Figure 8). The non-diagnostic type 2 pattern is described as "saddle-back" ST elevation (>0.1 mV) with J-point elevation (≥0.2 mV) and either a biphasic or positive T-wave, which may convert to the classic type 1 pattern when leads V1 and V2 are placed in the second intercostal spaces, or after a challenge with a sodium ion channel blocker agent such as ajmaline or flecanide. We only recommend a provocation test in athletes with the type 2 EKG pattern if there is a history of unheralded syncope, a relevant family history, or the conversion of a type 2 pattern to a type 1 pattern when the EKG is repeated with leads V1 and V2 in higher intercostal spaces.

The type 1 pattern may resemble repolarization changes observed in African/ Afro-Caribbean athletes. The key difference is that the ST segment after the J-point descends abruptly in Brugada syndrome, whereas the ST segment in the African/Afro-Caribbean athlete is convex and elevated following the J-point. Additionally, measurement of the ST segment elevation at the J-point (STJ) and also 80 ms after the J-point (ST80) results in a STJ/ST80 ratio >1 in BrS and <1 in the African/Afro-Caribbean athlete with repolarization changes in V1–V3 (Figure 9). Brugada can often mimic incomplete RBBB, however, a differentiating feature is J-point elevation confined to V1–V2 without reciprocal S-waves in I and V6.

Wolff–Parkinson–White EKG Pattern

The Wolff–Parkinson–White (WPW) EKG pattern is due to the presence of an accessory pathway known as the Bundle of Kent. This pathway by-passes the AV

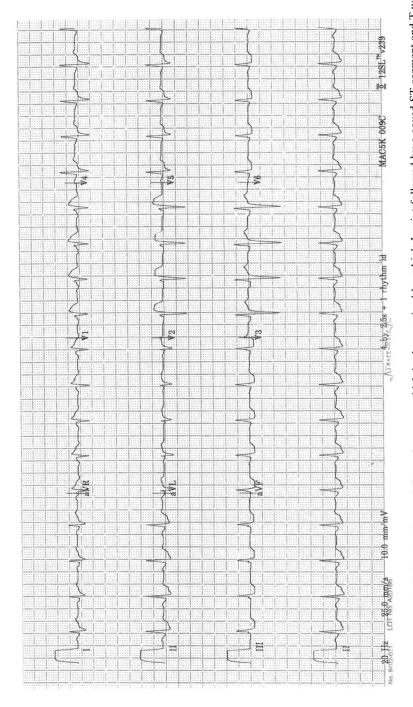

Figure 8.   EKG from an individual with type 1 Brugada pattern which is characterized by a coved ST segment and T-wave inversion in lead V1.

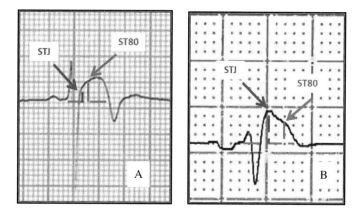

Figure 9.   Differentiation between the type 1 Brugada pattern and repolarization changes observed in African/Afro-Caribbean athletes. (A) Early repolarization in an African/Afro-Caribbean athlete with a STJ/ST80 ratio <1 and convex ST segment elevation after the J-point. (B) Type 1 Brugada pattern with a STJ/ST80 ratio >1 and the ST segment descending abruptly after the J-point. ST segment elevation at the J-point = STJ; ST segment elevation 80 ms after the J-point = ST80.

node resulting in a short PR interval (<120 ms), a slurred upstroke of the QRS (delta-wave), and a prolonged QRS duration (>120 ms) (Figure 10). The prevalence of the WPW EKG pattern in athletes is similar to that of the normal population (0.3%). Patients with WPW syndrome are prone to atrioventricular re-entrant tachycardia. In some instances the development of atrial fibrillation (AF) can result in VF due to rapid 1:1 conduction through an accessory pathway with an extremely short refractory period. The risk of sudden death from WPW syndrome in asymptomatic patients is 0.1% per year.

The management of symptomatic athletes with WPW is radiofrequency ablation of the accessory pathway. In such cases, an athlete may return to competition 6 weeks after treatment. Risk stratification is required for all other asymptomatic athletes with WPW. Non-invasive methods include an exercise stress test and 24-h EKG monitoring (to assess for intermittent pre-excitation, associated with a lower risk of developing VF and the presence of polymorphic pre-excited complexes suggestive of multiple pathways, associated with a higher risk of a potentially lethal arrhythmia). The disappearance of the delta-wave at a high heart rate during an exercise test suggests that the refractory period of the accessory pathway is not short enough to allow rapid AV conduction that can result in fatal ventricular arrhythmias. An electrophysiological (EP) study to demonstrate the refractory period of the accessory pathway and the ease of inducibility of AF is the best method for risk stratification. A refractory period ≤250 ms is considered to represent a high risk pathway. There is some controversy regarding the management of an asymptomatic athlete. An EP study is mandatory in all athletes with

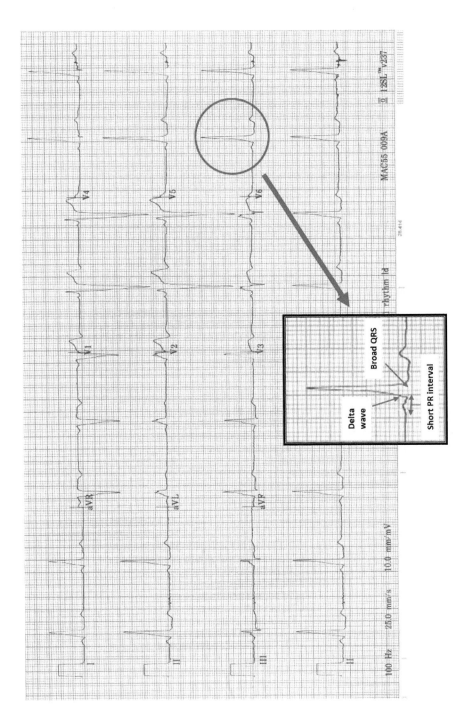

Figure 10.   EKG demonstrating Wolff–Parkinson–White syndrome demonstrating a short PR interval, delta-wave, and prolonged QRS duration.

pre-excitation that persists during an exercise test by the European guidelines.[40] In contrast, the American guidelines only recommend an EP study in athletes participating in moderate-high level competitive sports or if symptomatic.[34]

Current EKG Interpretation Recommendations in Athletes

2010 ESC guidelines

The European Society of Cardiology in 2010 published recommendations for interpretation of the athlete's EKG.[1] EKG patterns were divided into two categories: "Group 1" changes, which were representative of benign physiological alterations; "Group 2" changes, which were indicative of potential cardiac disease (Table 1). This document has proved a useful starting point in the evaluation of athletes, but is marred by a high false positive rate of 11–25% in some studies.[23,27,41–43] The data was derived from almost 33,000 unselected, largely Caucasian Italian athletes,[44] so the high prevalence of TWI in African/Afro-Caribbean athletes was not considered. Furthermore, upper limits of QT ranges were based on data in sedentary patients whereas we have shown that athletes have a longer QTc interval than sedentary individuals.[32] Certain non-specific anomalies not indicative of cardiac pathology such as axis deviation and voltage criteria for atrial enlargement or RVH were considered abnormal primarily because they were observed in <5% of athletes. Such changes constitute over 40% of the athletes' false positive results[33,45,46] and have a very poor diagnostic yield for cardiac disease in asymptomatic athletes.

Table 1.   ESC recommendations for EKG interpretation in young athletes.[1]

Group 1 criteria	Group 2 criteria
• Sinus bradycardia	• T-wave inversion
• 1st degree AV block	• ST segment depression
• Early repolarization	• Pathological Q-waves
• Incomplete RBBB	• Left atrial enlargement
• Isolated QRS voltage criteria for left ventricular hypertrophy	• Left axis deviation/left anterior hemiblock
	• Right axis deviation/left posterior hemiblock
	• Right ventricular hypertrophy
	• Ventricular pre-excitation
	• Complete LBBB/RBBB
	• Long or short QT interval
	• Brugada-like early repolarization

Note: AV = atrioventricular; LBBB = left bundle branch block; RBBB = right bundle branch block.

Table 2.   Seattle criteria for normal EKG findings in an athlete.[47]

Normal EKG findings in an athlete

- Isolated QRS voltage criteria for LVH (i.e. in the absence of non-voltage criteria for LVH such as left atrial enlargement, left axis deviation, ST segment depression, TWI, or pathological Q-waves)
- Sinus bradycardia (≥30 bpm)
- Sinus arrhythmia
- Ectopic atrial rhythm
- Junctional escape rhythm
- 1st degree AV block (PR interval >200 ms)
- 2nd degree AV block: Mobitz type 1 (Wenckebach)
- Incomplete RBBB
- Early repolarization (ST segment elevation, J-point elevation, J-waves, terminal QRS slurring)
- TWI V1–V4 in African/Afro-Caribbean athletes combined with convex ('domed') ST segment elevation
- TWI V1–V2 in Caucasian athletes

Note: AV = atrioventricular; LVH = left ventricular hypertrophy; RBBB = right bundle branch block; TWI = T-wave inversion.

Seattle guidelines

The "Seattle guidelines" were produced in 2012 by a convention of international experts in sports cardiology and sports medicine.[26,36,47] These criteria considered TWI in V1–V4 as a normal variant in African/Afro-Caribbean athletes if preceded by convex ST segment elevation. They also accepted TWI in V1 and V2 as a normal variant in athletes of all nationalities (Table 2). The Seattle criteria did not advise further investigation in athletes with right axis deviation or right atrial enlargement and only suggested further investigation in athletes with voltage criteria for RVH with co-existent right axis deviation. Finally, the Seattle criteria adopted the AHA recommendations for the upper limits of a QT interval as defined above (Tables 3(a) and (b)), Several recent studies have shown that the Seattle criteria reduce the number of positive EKGs and improve specificity without compromising sensitivity.[16,42,48,49]

"Refined criteria" guidelines

Our experience suggests that voltage criteria for RVH by the Sokolow–Lyon criteria (R-wave in V1 + largest S-wave in V5 or V6 >1.05 mV) is present in 11.8% of athletes and is frequently associated with right axis deviation.[46] Axis deviation

Table 3. (a) Seattle criteria for abnormal EKG findings in an athlete, unrelated to exercise and indicative of cardiomyopathy.[26] (b) Seattle criteria for abnormal EKG findings in an athlete, unrelated to exercise and indicative of primary electrical disease.[36]

(a) EKG findings indicative of cardiomyopathy

- **T-wave inversion:** >0.1 mV in depth in ≥2 leads V2–V6, II and AVF or I and AVL (not in III, V1, or AVR)
- **ST segment depression:** ≥0.05 mV in depth in ≥2 leads
- **Pathological Q-waves:** >0.3 mV in depth or >40 ms in duration in ≥2 leads (except III and AVR)
- **Complete LBBB:** QRS ≥120 ms, predominantly negative QRS in V1, and upright monophasic R-wave in I and V6
- **Intraventricular conduction delay:** QRS duration ≥140 ms
- **Left axis deviation:** −30° to −90°
- **Left atrial enlargement:** P-wave prolonged duration >120 ms in I or II with negative portion of P-wave ≥0.1 mV in depth and ≥40 ms in duration in V1
- **Right ventricular hypertrophy:** R in V1 + S in V5 >1.05 mV AND right axis deviation >120°
- **Premature ventricular ectopics:** ≥2PVCs per 10 s trace
- **Ventricular arrhythmia:** Couplets, triplets, NSVT

(b) EKG findings indicative of primary electrical disease

- **Ventricular pre-excitation:** PR interval <120 ms, delta-wave, wide QRS (>120 ms)
- **Long QT interval:** QTc ≥470 ms (male); QTc ≥480 ms (female); QTc ≥500 ms (marked QT prolongation)
- **Short QT interval:** QTc ≤320 ms
- **Brugada-like EKG:** High take off and down-sloping ST segment elevation followed by negative T-wave ≥2 leads in V1–V3
- **Profound sinus bradycardia:** <30 bpm or sinus pause ≥3 s
- **Atrial tachyarrhythmia:** Supraventricular tachycardia, AF, atrial flutter
- **Premature ventricular ectopics:** ≥2PVCs per 10 s trace
- **Ventricular arrhythmia:** Couplets, triplets, NSVT

Notes: LBBB = left bundle branch block; NSVT = non-sustained ventricular tachycardia; PVC = premature ventricular complex. AF = atrial fibrillation; NSVT = non-sustained ventricular tachycardia; PVC = premature ventricular complex.

and voltage criteria for atrial enlargement are the most common causes of ESC Group 2 changes and account for over 40% of false positive tests.[45] Left axis deviation and left atrial (LA) dilation are considered abnormal by the Seattle criteria, but we consider these borderline anomalies based on our examination of >12,000 young individuals (2,533 athletes) using EKG and echocardiography. Of these 139 athletes (5.5%) showed either isolated left or right axis deviation or voltage criteria for left or right atrial enlargement. Echocardiography in this group failed to detect sinister pathology and the prevalence of minor congenital abnormalities was similar in these individuals to those with normal EKGs.[45] We have since proposed the "Refined criteria" whereby we categorize left or right axis deviation, voltage criteria for left or right atrial enlargement, and RVH as borderline anomalies which only require further assessment in symptomatic athletes or if more than one of these five borderline anomalies are present in combination[27] (Figure 11). Although TWI in V1–V4 is a normal variant in African/Afro-Caribbean athletes, we categorized it as a borderline anomaly since our group has reported these anomalies as benign and there is limited data from others in this regard. As more groups report similar findings, it is anticipated that this specific repolarization pattern will become fully incorporated into the normal pattern category.[10,42,50]

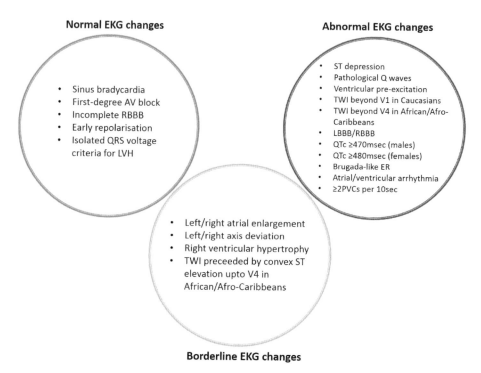

Figure 11.   The Refined criteria.[27] Athletes with physiological EKG changes in patterns do not warrant investigation in the absence of symptoms. Athletes with abnormal EKG patterns require further investigation irrespective of symptomatic status. Athletes with borderline EKG patterns only require further investigation if ≥2 borderline variants are identified on the same EKG. AV = atrioventricular; ER = early repolarization; ECG = electrocardiogram; LBBB = left bundle branch block; LVH = left ventricular hypertrophy; PVCs = premature ventricular complexes; RBBB = right bundle branch block; TWI = T-wave inversion.

The 2010 ESC, Seattle, and "Refined criteria" were compared retrospectively in 5,505 elite athletes, including 1,208 African/Afro-Caribbean athletes. The ESC recommendations suggested a cardiac abnormality in 40.4% of African/Afro-Caribbean athletes and 16.2% of Caucasian athletes. This high positive rate in African/Afro-Caribbean athletes was driven by a high prevalence of TWI in these individuals. The Seattle criteria reduced abnormal EKGs to 18.4% in African/Afro-Caribbean athletes and 7.1% in Caucasian athletes. The "Refined criteria" reduced abnormal EKGs further to 11.5% in African/Afro-Caribbean athletes and 5.3% in Caucasian athletes. All three criteria were tested in 103 athletes with HCM and identified 98.1% of athletes with HCM. Compared to ESC recommendations, the "Refined criteria" improved specificity from 40.3% to 84.2% in African/Afro-Caribbean athletes and from 73.8% to 94.1% in Caucasian athletes, without compromising the sensitivity of the EKG in detecting all pathology, which was similar with all three criteria (70% for African/Afro-Caribbean athletes, 60% for Caucasian athletes). The sensitivity for detecting serious pathology was also similar with all three criteria. Despite these improvements, the numbers of positive rates in African/Afro-Caribbean athletes remain high, calling for large prospective studies in this group with particular reference to the significance of TWI in leads other than V1–V4.

Overlap with Cardiac Disease

Hypertrophic cardiomyopathy (HCM)

The cardiac adaptations to exercise training include modest increases in chamber wall thickness and cavity size. The left ventricular wall thickness is increased by 15–20% and left ventricular cavity size may be increased by 10%.[51] Some male athletes, including 1.6–4% of Caucasians and 13–18% of African/Afro-Caribbean athletes, exhibit left ventricular wall thicknesses of 13–16 mm[5,15,52] which is within the range observed in individuals with mild HCM, the predominant cause of sudden cardiac death in persons <35 years old worldwide. Abnormalities on the 12-lead EKG may provide crucial information to differentiate HCM from physiologic hypertrophy. The detection of deep TWI in any lead other than V2 in Caucasian athletes and V1–V4 in African/Afro-Caribbean athletes, pathological Q-waves, ST segment depression, and LBBB favor pathological left ventricular hypertrophy (Figure 12). Conversely, the presence of Sokolow–Lyon voltage criteria for LVH, without associated features of LVH including ST segment depression, TWI, left axis deviation, or voltage criteria for LA enlargement, supports physiological LVH.

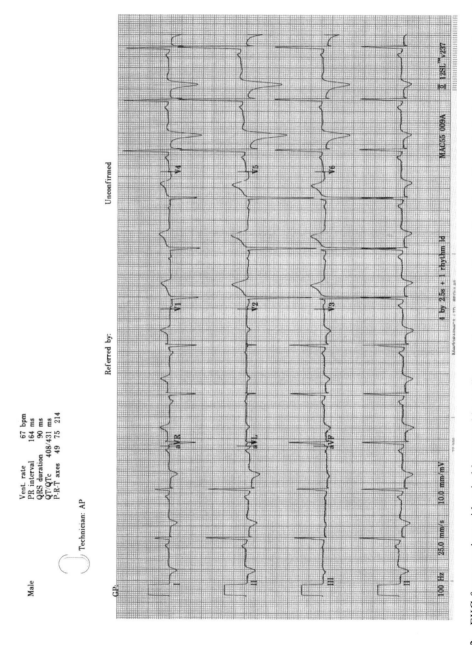

Figure 12.   EKG from a patient with apical hypertrophic cardiomyopathy showing voltage criteria for left ventricular hypertrophy, T-wave inversion in leads V4–V6, II, III, AVF, I and AVL, and ST segment depression in V4–V6, II, III, AVF.

Arrhythmogenic right ventricular cardiomyopathy (ARVC) and dilated cardiomyopathy

Right ventricle enlargement and ventricular extra-systoles of right ventricular origin may occur in some highly trained endurance athletes raising the possibility of ARVC,[53–55] the commonest cause of sudden cardiac death in Italian athletes, accounting for 25% of all young sudden deaths during sport in Italy.[56,57] ARVC should be considered when there is anterior TWI beyond lead V2 particularly when followed by isoelectric or depressed ST segments, epsilon waves, and >500 ventricular extra-systoles over a 24-h period with LBBB morphology suggesting right ventricular origin.[12,58] Additionally, in a recent study comparing athletes with TWI and ARVC patients, the presence of pathological Q-waves and small QRS complexes in the precordial leads (sum of the R-wave and the nadir of the S-wave <1.8 mV) were strong discriminators of ARVC, as was the presence of >1,000 ventricular extra-systoles (or >500 of non-RV outflow tract origin) (Figure 13).[59]

Endurance athletes may also develop an enlarged left ventricle with a low-normal ejection fraction.[60] In a large study of Tour de France cyclists, almost 50% exhibited a LV cavity size end diastole ≥60 mm and of these, 12% showed a LV ejection fraction (LVEF) <52%.[60] In contrast with most endurance athletes, individuals with dilated cardiomyopathy (DCM) often also display TWI, LBBB, or a non-specific intraventricular conduction delay. The diagnosis of DCM is more likely when there are also regional wall motion abnormalities, a failure of the LVEF to improve by 10% with exercise (unpublished data), and the inability to achieve a peak oxygen consumption >50 mL/kg/min or >120% predicted value on cardio-pulmonary exercise testing (Figure 14).

Ion channel diseases

A QT interval exceeding the upper limits for the general population is present in up to 6% of athletes, but a QT interval ≥500 ms is highly suggestive of long QT syndrome. A type 1 Brugada pattern is always considered abnormal. The significance of a short QT interval <320 ms is uncertain, but may be relevant in an athlete with paroxysmal atrial fibrillation, syncope, or a family history of sudden death in the presence of a structurally normal heart. Early repolarization is common in athletes, but J-point elevation ≥0.2 mV in an athlete with unheralded syncope or a family history of premature sudden cardiac death with a normal cardiac autopsy, and especially when associated with down-sloping/horizontal ST segments, should be viewed with a high degree of suspicion and evaluation should

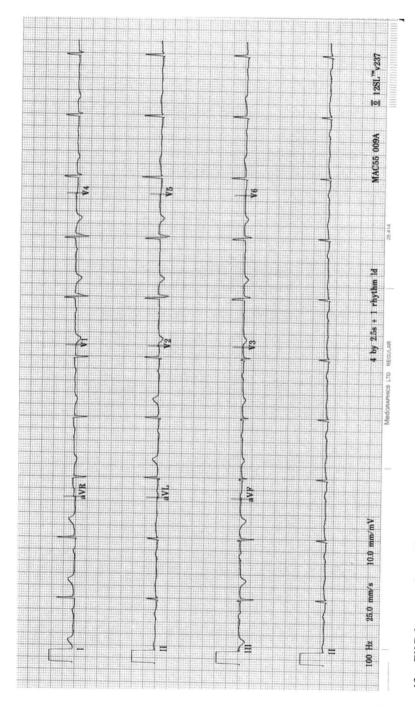

Figure 13.   EKG from a patient with arrhythmogenic right ventricular cardiomyopathy: TWI V1–V4 with an iso-electric ST segment and small QRS complexes in the precordial leads.

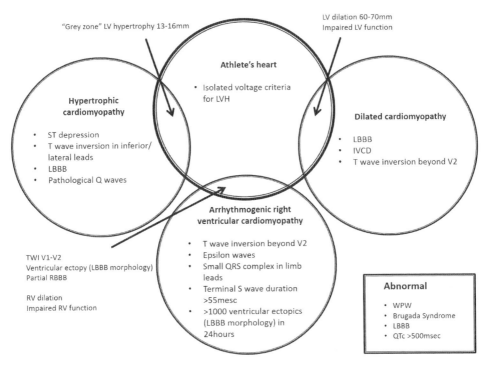

Figure 14.   The role of the EKG in facilitating a diagnosis where there is structural overlap between the athlete's heart and cardiomyopathy. IVCD = intraventricular conduction delay; LBBB = left bundle branch block; LVH = left ventricular hypertrophy; RBBB = right bundle branch block; RV = right ventricle; TWI = T-wave inversion; WPW = Wolff–Parkinson–White syndrome.

be sought from a specialist. Figure 15 provides a traffic light system whereby repolarization changes in green are considered benign whereas those in red are highly suggestive of either a cardiomyopathy or an ion channelopathy. There is a borderline amber group which may be considered pathological in the presence of palpitations, syncope, or a relevant family history.

Summary

Participation in intense physical training is associated with EKG changes likely produced by changes in autonomic tone and chamber size. General cardiologists are frequently required to evaluate athletes' cardiovascular health because many athletes are now screened prior to participation with an EKG, which are often considered abnormal. The ability to differentiate physiological EKG patterns from pathological changes will reduce false positive results and, more importantly, minimize the risk of false reassurance.

Normal variants	Possible abnormal variants	Abnormal variants
• J-point elevation • ST segment elevation • Tall T waves • T-wave inversion V2-V4 in African/ Afro-Caribbean athletes • T-wave inversion V2-V3 in children ≤14 years old • T-wave inversion V2-V3 preceeded by ST segment elevation in endurance athletes	• Early repolarization >0.2mV with down-sloping or horizontal ST segments • QT interval 480-490msec • Type 2 Brugada pattern	• ST segment depression • T-wave inversion inferior/laterally • T-wave inversion beyond V2 in adult Caucasian athletes • QT interval >500msec • Short QT interval <320msec • Type 1 Brugada pattern

Figure 15.   Interpretation of repolarization changes on an EKG of an athlete. "Normal" variants in the green box are commonly observed in athletes and do not require further investigation. "Possibly abnormal" variants are in the amber box and should be investigated if there was a clinical suspicion of a cardiomyopathy/electrical disorder from symptoms or family history. "Abnormal" variants in the red box always require further investigation regardless of symptoms and family history to exclude cardiac disease.

Personal Perspectives

Sanjay Sharma

A professor of inherited cardiac diseases and sports cardiology, Dr. Sanjay Sharma has studied athletes for almost 17 years. His research has helped characterize the adolescent athlete's heart and cardiac adaptation in athletes of African/Afro-Caribbean origin. Professor Sharma was responsible for the cardiac evaluation of Great Britian's Olympic team prior to the 2012 London Olympics. Additionally, he is the medical director of the London marathon and enjoys running recreationally.

Keerthi Prakash

A cardiology senior resident subspecailizing in non-invasive imaging, Dr. Keerthi Prakash has interests in inherited cardiac disease and sports cardiology. She was a research fellow in sports cardiology and inherited heart disease with Professor Sharma when she wrote this chapter.

References

1. Corrado D, Pelliccia A, Heidbuchel H, *et al*. Recommendations for interpretation of 12-lead electrocardiogram in the athlete. *Eur Heart J* 2010;31(2):243–259.
2. Huston TP, Puffer JC, Rodney WM. The athletic heart syndrome. *N Engl J Med* 1985;313(1):24–32.
3. Zehender M, Meinertz T, Keul J, Just H. ECG variants and cardiac arrhythmias in athletes: Clinical relevance and prognostic importance. *Am Heart J* 1990;119(6):1378–1391.
4. Sharma S, Whyte G, Elliott P, *et al*. Electrocardiographic changes in 1000 highly trained junior elite athletes. *Bret J Sports Med* 1999;33(5):319–324.
5. Basavarajaiah S, Boraita A, Whyte G, *et al*. Ethnic differences in left ventricular remodeling in highly-trained athletes relevance to differentiating physiologic left ventricular hypertrophy from hypertrophic cardiomyopathy. *J Am Coll Cardiol* 2008; 51(23):2256–2262.
6. Ryan MP, Cleland JG, French JA, *et al*. The standard electrocardiogram as a screening test for hypertrophic cardiomyopathy. *Am J Cardiol* 1995;76(10):689–694.
7. Melacini P, Cianfrocca C, Calore C, *et al*. Abstract 3390: Marginal Overlap between electrocardiographic abnormalities in patients with hypertrophic cardiomyopathy and trained athletes: Implications for preparticipation screening. *Circulation* 2007; 116(II):765.
8. Maron BJ, Wolfson JK, Ciró E, Spirito P. Relation of electrocardiographic abnormalities and patterns of left ventricular hypertrophy identified by 2-dimensional echocardiography in patients with hypertrophic cardiomyopathy. *Am J Cardiol* 1983;51(1): 189–194.
9. Savage DD, Seides SF, Clark CE, *et al*. Electrocardiographic findings in patients with obstructive and nonobstructive hypertrophic cardiomyopathy. *Circulation* 1978;58(3 Pt 1):402–408.
10. Di Paolo FM, Schmied C, Zerguini YA, *et al*. The athlete's heart in adolescent Africans: An electrocardiographic and echocardiographic study. *J Am Coll Cardiol* 2012;59(11):1029–1036.
11. Papadakis M, Basavarajaiah S, Rawlins J, *et al*. Prevalence and significance of T-wave inversions in predominantly Caucasian adolescent athletes. *Eur Heart J* 2009; 30(14):1728–1735.
12. Marcus FI, McKenna WJ, Sherrill D, *et al*. Diagnosis of arrhythmogenic right ventricular cardiomyopathy/dysplasia: proposed modification of the task force criteria. *Circulation* 2010;121(13):1533–1541.
13. Kim JH, Noseworthy PA, McCarty D, *et al*. Significance of electrocardiographic right bundle branch block in trained athletes. *Am J Cardiol* 2011;107(7):1083–1089.
14. Noseworthy PA, Weiner R, Kim J, *et al*. Early repolarization pattern in competitive athletes: Clinical correlates and the effects of exercise training. *Circ Arrhythm Electrophysiol* 2011;4(4):432–440.
15. Papadakis M, Carre F, Kervio G, *et al*. The prevalence, distribution, and clinical outcomes of electrocardiographic repolarization patterns in male athletes of African/Afro-Caribbean origin. *Eur Heart J* 2011;32(18):2304–2313.

16. Sheikh N, Papadakis M, Carre F, *et al.* Cardiac adaptation to exercise in adolescent athletes of African ethnicity: An emergent elite athletic population. *Brit J Sports Med* 2013;47(9):585–592.
17. Sheikh N, Sharma S. Impact of ethnicity on cardiac adaptation to exercise. *Nat Rev Cardiol* 2014;11(4):198–217.
18. Haïssaguerre M, Derval N, Sacher F, *et al.* Sudden cardiac arrest associated with early repolarization. *N Engl J Med* 2008;358(19):2016–2023.
19. Tikkanen JT, Anttonen O, Junttila MJ, *et al.* Long-term outcome associated with early repolarization on electrocardiography. *N Engl J Med* 2009;361(26):2529–2537.
20. Mellor GJ, Ghani S, Li A, Sharma S, Behr E. Early repolarisation in young adults: A dose-dependent relationship with physical activity. *Europace* 2014;16(suppl_3): iii2.
21. Sharma S. Physiological Society Symposium — the Athlete's Heart. *Exp Physiol* 2003;88(5):665–669.
22. Papadakis M, Wilson MG, Ghani S, Kervio G, Carre F, Sharma S. Impact of ethnicity upon cardiovascular adaptation in competitive athletes: Relevance to preparticipation screening. *Br J Sports Med* 2012;46(1):i22–i28.
23. Brosnan M, La Gerche A, Kalman J, *et al.* Comparison of frequency of significant electrocardiographic abnormalities in endurance versus nonendurance athletes. *Am J Cardiol* 2014;113(9):1567–1573.
24. Schnell F, Riding N, O'Hanlon R, *et al.* The recognition and significance of pathological T-wave inversions in athletes. *Circulation* 2014;131(2):165–173.
25. Wilson MG, Sharma S, Carré F, *et al.* Significance of deep T-wave inversions in asymptomatic athletes with normal cardiovascular examinations: Practical solutions for managing the diagnostic conundrum. *Brit J Sports Med* 2012;46(1):i51–i58.
26. Drezner JA, Ashley E, Baggish AL, *et al.* Abnormal electrocardiographic findings in athletes: Recognising changes suggestive of cardiomyopathy. *Brit J Sports Med* 2013;47(3):137–152.
27. Sheikh N, Papadakis M, Ghani S, *et al.* Comparison of electrocardiographic criteria for the detection of cardiac abnormalities in elite black and white athletes. *Circulation* 2014;129(16):1637–1649.
28. Migliore F, Zorzi A, Michieli P, *et al.* Prevalence of cardiomyopathy in Italian asymptomatic children with electrocardiographic T-wave inversion at preparticipation screening. *Circulation* 2012;125(3):529–538.
29. Calò L, Sperandii F, Martino A, *et al.* Echocardiographic findings in 2261 peripubertal athletes with or without inverted T waves at electrocardiogram. *Heart* 2015;101(3):193–200.
30. Pelliccia A, Di Paolo FM, Quattrini FM, *et al.* Outcomes in athletes with marked ECG repolarization abnormalities. *N Engl J Med* 2008;358(2):152–161.
31. Konno T, Shimizu M, Ino H, *et al.* Diagnostic value of abnormal Q waves for identification of preclinical carriers of hypertrophic cardiomyopathy based on a molecular genetic diagnosis. *Eur Heart J* 2004;25(3):246–251.
32. Basavarajaiah S, Wilson M, Whyte G, Shah A, Behr E, Sharma S. Prevalence and significance of an isolated long QT interval in elite athletes. *Eur Heart J* 2007; 28(23):2944–2949.

33. Chandra N, Bastiaenen R, Papadakis M, *et al*. Prevalence of electrocardiographic anomalies in young individuals: Relevance to a nationwide cardiac screening program. *J Am Coll Cardiol* 2014;63(19):2028–2034.

34. Zipes DP, Ackerman MJ, Estes NAM, Grant AO, Myerburg RJ, Van Hare G. Task Force 7: arrhythmias. *J Am Coll Cardiol* 2005;45(8):1354–1363.

35. Schwartz PJ, Ackerman MJ. The long QT syndrome: A transatlantic clinical approach to diagnosis and therapy. *Eur Heart J* 2013;34(40):3109–3116.

36. Drezner JA, Ackerman MJ, Cannon BC, *et al*. Abnormal electrocardiographic findings in athletes: Recognising changes suggestive of primary electrical disease. *Brit J Sports Med* 2013;47(3):153–167.

37. Priori SG, Wilde A a, Horie M, *et al*. HRS/EHRA/APHRS expert consensus statement on the diagnosis and management of patients with inherited primary arrhythmia syndromes: Document endorsed by HRS, EHRA, and APHRS in May 2013 and by ACCF, AHA, PACES, and AEPC in June 2013. *Heart Rhythm* 2013;10(12): 1932–1963.

38. Rautaharju PM, Surawicz B, Gettes LS, *et al*. AHA/ACCF/HRS recommendations for the standardization and interpretation of the electrocardiogram: Part IV: The ST segment, T and U waves, and the QT interval: A scientific statement from the American Heart Association Electrocardiography and Arrhythmias C. *J Am Coll Cardiol* 2009;53(11):982–991.

39. Dhutia H, Malhotra A, Parpia S, *et al*. The prevalence and significance of a short QT interval in low risk populations: Have we got it right? *Br J Sports Med* 2016;50(2):124–129.

40. Pelliccia A, Fagard R, Bjørnstad HH, *et al*. Recommendations for competitive sports participation in athletes with cardiovascular disease: A consensus document from the Study Group of Sports Cardiology of the Working Group of Cardiac Rehabilitation and Exercise Physiology and the Working Group of Myocerdial and Pericardial Diseases of the Eropean Society of Cardiology. *Eur Heart J* 2005;26(14): 1422–1445.

41. Weiner RB, Hutter AM, Wang F, *et al*. Performance of the 2010 European Society of Cardiology criteria for ECG interpretation in athletes. *Heart* 2011;97(19):1573–1577.

42. Riding NR, Sheikh N, Adamuz C, *et al*. Comparison of three current sets of electrocardiographic interpretation criteria for use in screening athletes. *Heart* 2015;101(5):384–390.

43. Baggish AL, Hutter AM, Wang F, *et al*. Cardiovascular screening in college athletes with and without electrocardiography: A cross-sectional study. *Ann Intern Med* 2010;152(5):269–275.

44. Pelliccia A, Maron BJ, Culasso F, *et al*. Clinical significance of abnormal electrocardiographic patterns in trained athletes. *Circulation* 2000;102(3):278–284.

45. Gati S, Sheikh N, Ghani S, *et al*. Should axis deviation or atrial enlargement be categorised as abnormal in young athletes? The athlete's electrocardiogram: Time for re-appraisal of markers of pathology. *Eur Heart J* 2013;34(47):3641–3648.

46. Zaidi A, Ghani S, Sheikh N, *et al*. Clinical significance of electrocardiographic right ventricular hypertrophy in athletes: Comparison with arrhythmogenic right

ventricular cardiomyopathy and pulmonary hypertension. *Eur Heart J* 2013;34(47): 3649–3656.

47. Drezner JA, Fischbach P, Froelicher V, *et al.* Normal electrocardiographic findings: Recognising physiological adaptations in athletes. *Brit J Sports Med* 2013; 47(3):125–136.

48. Brosnan M, La Gerche A, Kalman J, *et al.* The Seattle Criteria increase the specificity of preparticipation ECG screening among elite athletes. *Brit J Sports Med* 2014; 48(15):1144–1150.

49. Bessem B, de Bruijn MC, Nieuwland W. The ECG of high-level junior soccer players: Comparing the ESC vs. the Seattle criteria. *Br J Sports Med* 2015;49(15): 1000–1006.

50. Riding NR, Salah O, Sharma S, *et al.* ECG and morphologic adaptations in Arabic athletes: Are the European Society of Cardiology's recommendations for the interpretation of the 12-lead ECG appropriate for this ethnicity? *Brit J Sports Med* 2014; 48(15):1138–1143.

51. Maron BJ, Pelliccia A. The heart of trained athletes: Cardiac remodeling and the risks of sports, including sudden death. *Circulation* 2006;114(15):1633–1644.

52. Basavarajaiah S, Wilson M, Whyte G, Shah A, McKenna W, Sharma S. Prevalence of hypertrophic cardiomyopathy in highly trained athletes: Relevance to pre-participation screening. *J Am Coll Cardiol* 2008;51(10):1033–1039.

53. Zaidi A, Ghani S, Sharma R, *et al.* Physiological right ventricular adaptation in elite athletes of African and Afro-Caribbean origin. *Circulation* 2013;127(17): 1783–1792.

54. La Gerche A, Burns AT, Mooney DJ, *et al.* Exercise-induced right ventricular dysfunction and structural remodelling in endurance athletes. *Eur Heart J* 2012; 33(8):998–1006.

55. Heidbüchel H, Hoogsteen J, Fagard R, *et al.* High prevalence of right ventricular involvement in endurance athletes with ventricular arrhythmias. Role of an electrophysiologic study in risk stratification. *Eur Heart J* 2003;24(16):1473–1480.

56. Corrado D, Basso C, Rizzoli G, Schiavon M, Thiene G. Does sports activity enhance the risk of sudden death in adolescents and young adults? *J Am Coll Cardiol* 2003;42(11):1959–1963.

57. Corrado D, Basso C, Schiavon M, Thiene G. Screening for hypertrophic cardiomyopathy in young athletes. *N Engl J Med* 1998;339(6):364–369.

58. Steriotis AK, Bauce B, Daliento L, *et al.* Electrocardiographic pattern in arrhythmogenic right ventricular cardiomyopathy. *Am J Cardiol* 2009;103(9):1302–1308.

59. Zaidi A, Sheikh N, Jongman J, *et al.* Clinical differentiation between physiological remodeling and arrhythmogenic right ventricular cardiomyopathy in athletes with marked electrocardiographic repolarization anomalies. *J Am Coll Cardiol* 2015; 65(25):2702–2711.

60. Abergel E, Chatellier G, Hagege AA, *et al.* Serial left ventricular adaptations in world-class professional cyclists: Implications for disease screening and follow-up. *J Am Coll Cardiol* 2004;44(1):144–149.

Chapter 7

Echocardiography and the Athlete

Antonio B. Fernandez[*,†] **and Lovely Chhabra**[‡,§]

Director, Cardiac Intensive Care Unit
Hartford Hospital, Hartford, CT, USA
[†]*Assistant Professor of Medicine*
University of Connecticut, Farmington, CT, USA
[‡]*Chief Cardiology Fellow, Hartford Hospital*
Hartford, CT, USA
[§]*University of Connecticut, Farmington, CT, USA*

Echocardiography in the Evaluation of Athletes

Echocardiography provides extremely useful data in the management of cardiac problems in athletes because it can evaluate exercise-induced cardiac adaptations, identify myocardial and valvular pathologies, and simultaneously examine cardiac anatomy and function. Echocardiography is indicated when the clinical history, physical examination, or electrocardiogram (ECG) raise the possibility of structural heart disease including valvular disease, hypertrophic cardiomyopathy, or prior myocardial infarction. Traditional echocardiography provides useful information, but only if the exam and measurements of cardiac dimensions and performance are performed carefully. There are also newer techniques developed during the past two decades that aid in assessing cardiac structures and function in athletes. In this chapter, we discuss traditional and novel echocardiographic techniques that might be helpful in the clinical evaluation of cardiac problems in athletes.

Basic Principles of Echocardiography

Knowledge of the basic ultrasound principles is useful for interpreting echocardiographic images and Doppler data obtained from athletes. The basic ultrasound imaging modalities are: M-mode — a graph of depth vs. time, 2D — a sector scan in a tomographic image plane with real-time motion, and 3D — a selected cutaway real-time image in a 3D display format.

M-mode (motion based) ultrasonography in athletes

M-mode recordings allow identification of very rapid intracardiac motion due to its high sampling rate of approximately 1,800 times/s, compared to a 2D frame rate of 30 frames/s. M-mode provides an "ice-pick view" displaying the location and motion of the heart (Figure 1). M-mode dimensions are limited because M-mode measurements are influenced by the location of the available acoustic

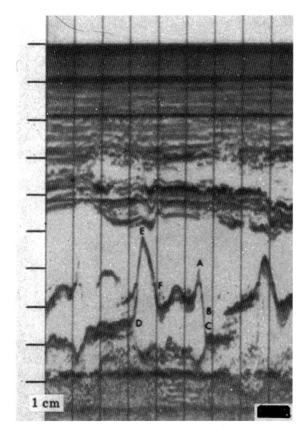

Figure 1.   Normal mitral valve M-mode.[1]

windows. Thus, the M-mode left ventricular (LV) diameter is rarely the true dimension because the dimension varies depending on the location of the acoustic window. In addition, the M-mode view is stationary although the heart is moving. 2D measurements overcome these shortcomings and provide a more correct anatomic shape and size of the cardiac structures. Consequently, the M-mode technique is considered to be obsolete by many. In our experience it remains particularly helpful in making a more accurate, cost-effective, and complete diagnosis in certain pathologies that can be seen in athletes. This imaging modality is particularly useful in detecting events that occur too fast for the naked eye to detect. Some cardiac structures, especially the valves and inter-ventricular septum, move quickly. In these circumstances, temporal resolution and sampling rate can be critical in detecting very rapid or subtle motion. The fastest moving cardiac structure is the mitral valve. Figure 1 describes an M-mode recording of a normal valve. A reduced A-wave amplitude, with a less steep slope of the mitral motion after the peak of the A-wave, is consistent with a more gradual closure of the mitral valve (Figure 2). This is particularly helpful in identifying patients with an elevated LV end-diastolic pressure (LVEDP).[1] In cases of elevated LVEDP, the atrium contracts against a stiff or already fully dilated ventricle. There is an earlier and rapid increase in the LV pressure during diastole, causing

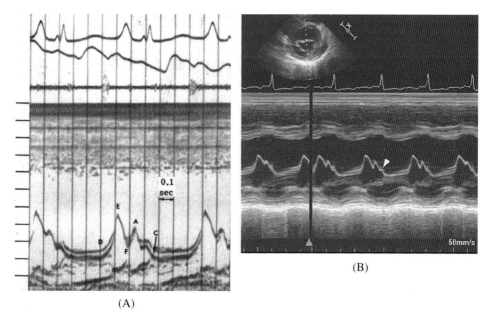

(A)

(B)

Figure 2. An old 2,000 samples/s mitral valve M-mode recording (A) and a recent 1,000 samples/s M-mode mitral valve recording (B) in patients with elevated LV end-diastolic pressure.[1,33]

the peak of the mitral valve A-wave to occur earlier. This causes a more pro-longed closure of the mitral valve before ventricular contraction with a frequent interruption or plateau caused by equalization of the pressures. This interruption is called a "B-bump" or "notch" or "shoulder" between the A and C points of the mitral valve (Figure 2). This is a very specific, yet non-quantitative, measure of elevated LVEDP (more than 20 mm Hg).[2] An M-mode B-bump is never present with normal filling pressures. A B-bump is often overlooked, but potentially helpful when differentiating normal adaptations to exercise training from pathology.

M-mode is also helpful in identifying systolic anterior motion (SAM) of the mitral valve, which is indicative of LV outflow tract obstruction.[3] SAM is fre-quent in hypertrophic cardiomyopathy (HCM), but rarely seen in athletes' heart (Figure 3). With SAM there is early apposition of the mitral valve to the

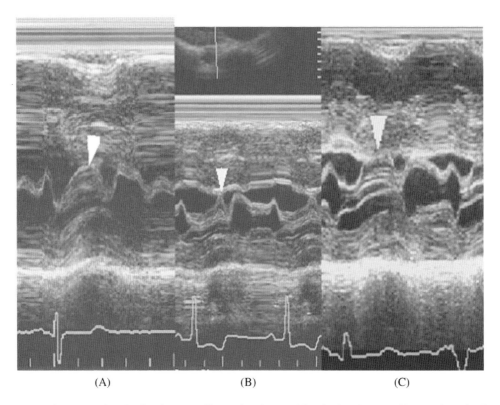

(A)   (B)   (C)

Figure 3.   M-mode mitral valve recordings of patients with mitral valve systolic anterior mitral valve motion. (A) The mitral valve touches the interventricular septum in mid-systole. (B) The mitral valve touches the septum only briefly in late systole. (C) The mitral valve strikes the septum in early systole and stays in contact with the septum almost throughout systole in this patient with hyper-trophic cardiomyopathy and severe LV outflow tract obstruction.[1]

interventricular septum, and the valve stays in contact with the septum during systole. The duration of contact between the mitral valve and the septum correlates with the severity of the obstruction,[4] but Doppler measurements are now used to assess more accurately the obstruction. Nevertheless, the M-mode recordings help understand the mechanism of the obstruction and to confirm the presence of dynamic LV outflow obstruction, especially if the 2D and Doppler data are equivocal.

M-mode recording of the aortic valve also provides useful clinical information in the echocardiographic evaluation of athletes. An abrupt closure of the valve in the latter half of systole represents a dynamic obstruction of flow, usually as a result of subaortic obstruction (Figure 4). Doppler flow velocity is usually

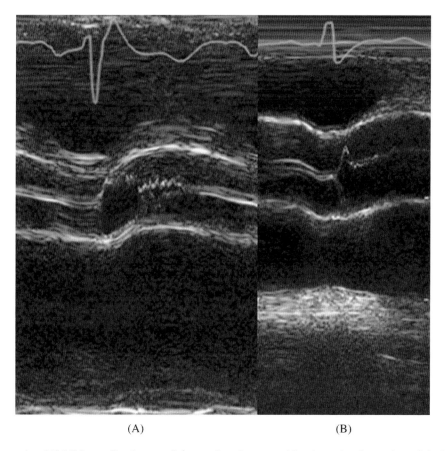

(A)   (B)

Figure 4.   (A) Mid-systolic closure of the aortic valve caused by dynamic obstruction of the LV outflow tract in a patient with hypertrophic, obstructive cardiomyopathy. (B) M-mode aortic valve recording in a patient with discreet membranous subaortic stenosis. The valve initially opens fully and then abruptly closes.[1]

diagnostic after demonstrating a late systolic peaking Doppler flow velocity. However, with severe HCM, the systolic peak flow velocity can be holosystolic and the dynamic nature of the obstruction might be more difficult to identify without seeing this M-mode phenomenon of the aortic valve. A subaortic membrane is a congenital anomaly that represents a fixed form of subaortic obstruction (subaortic stenosis) and, contrary to a dynamic obstruction, it causes an abrupt and early systolic closure of the valve after it initially opens fully. This is an important addition to the 2D exam, because the differentiation between valvular and subvalvular aortic stenosis is not always obvious. The membrane could be very thin and not recorded well by echocardiography or angiography. Furthermore, early- or mid-systolic closure of the aortic valve rules out significant valvular obstruction.

Another important use of the M-mode technique is to evaluate rapid interventricular septal motion such as seen with left bundle branch block and paradoxical septal motion. One of the most difficult diagnoses to make in echocardiography is the diagnosis of constrictive pericarditis. M-mode often demonstrates a "septal bounce" which helps confirm the 2D diagnosis.[5] M-mode measurement of tricuspid annular motion is useful as a measure of the right ventricular function. Tricuspid annular motion correlates with the right ventricular (RV) ejection fraction determined by Simpson's rule and has high specificity and negative predictive value for detecting abnormal RV systolic function.[6]

Doppler ultrasonography

Doppler ultrasound is based on the principle that ultrasound backscattered from moving red blood cells will appear higher or lower in frequency than the transmitted frequency depending on the speed and direction of blood flow. Accurate blood flow measurements depend on a parallel intercept angle between the ultrasound beam and the direction of blood flow. There are three basic Doppler modalities: pulse Doppler, color flow imaging, and continuous wave Doppler ultrasound. All three modalities are complementary and help in the assessment of flow velocities, the calculation of pressure gradients, and the assessment of valve regurgitation or stenosis severity. Doppler valvular assessment does not differ between athletes and non-athletes and will not be covered by this chapter.

Doppler is useful in the assessment of diastolic function. Diastolic function is preserved in most athletes but is impaired in HCM, hypertensive heart disease, and other cardiac diseases. Doppler interrogation of the mitral inflow provides useful information about diastolic function in athletes. Endurance athletes tend to have longer isovolumic-relaxation times[7] leading to rapid ventricular filling represented by the E-wave measured by Doppler echocardiography. Diastasis occurs after early diastolic filling. This tends to be quite long in athletes with slow heart rates, but it progressively shortens as the heart rate increases. Finally, atrial contraction occurs generating an additional pressure gradient. The A-wave measured by Doppler echocardiography represents the atrial contraction contribution to the LV filling. Historically, the E/A mitral inflow velocity ratio have been used to evaluate diastolic function. The E/A ratio of virtually all endurance athletes is >1.0, but can be as high as 4.8 in some athletes. The increased ratio is mainly due to a decrease in the A-wave velocity. This implies that at rest, the relative contribution of the atrial contraction is lower in trained athletes, since most of the LV filling occurs in the early diastole and during diastasis, particularly at slower HR.[7] These filling patterns can mimic the restrictive filling pattern seen in cardiomyopathies, but should not raise suspicion of pathology even in the presence of left atrial enlargement. In contrast, E/A ratio values <1.0 suggest a non-physiological condition in a trained athlete.

The E/A ratio, however, is not specific and is affected by heart rate, loading conditions, and pressure gradients. The normal Doppler tissue imaging (DTI), a normal calculated pulmonary artery systolic pressure, and the overall clinical picture should be used to avoid misclassifying diastolic indices in athletes as pathological.

LV filling is intrinsically related to systolic function. In fact, systolic twisting of the myocardium is necessary prior to untwisting and the initiation of diastolic suction. The untwisting of the LV during the isovolumic relaxation and early filling phases releases elastic energy stored by the preceding systolic twisting and contributes to the initial atrioventricular pressure gradient. The storage of energy during LV twisting appears to be fundamental in supporting diastolic filling during maximal exercise by creating a suction-aided, filling effect.[8]

2D and 3D echocardiography in the evaluation of cardiac adaptations — Chamber dimensions quantification and function

Left ventricular hypertrophy on an ECG is the most common trigger for an echocardiogram in asymptomatic athletes, and HCM is the most common differential. Therefore, it is paramount to quantify accurately the chamber dimensions and wall thicknesses. Inaccurate measurements can miss HCM with its increased risk of exercise-related SCD in athletes or lead to inappropriately restricting athletes from sport participation.

The American Society of Echocardiography (ASE) has recently published updated guidelines to standardize cardiac measurements.[9] The most commonly used parameters to quantify LV cavity size are linear internal dimensions and volumes. These measurements are reported for end-diastole and end-systole, which are then used to derive parameters of global LV function. Linear measurements should be carefully obtained perpendicular to the LV long axis and measured at, or immediately below, the level of the mitral valve leaflet tips in the parasternal long-axis view. Volumetric measurements can be obtained with 2D echocardiography, but they rely on the assumption of a fixed geometric LV shape, usually a prolate ellipsoid, which does not apply in a variety of cardiac conditions. Echo contrast agents can help define cardiac dimensions in individuals with sub-optimal acoustic windows, thereby helping to determine more accurate cardiac dimensions.[10] 3D echocardiography has additional advantages because it can provide volumetric measurements without geometrical assumptions, is unaffected by foreshortening, and is accurate and reproducible. Therefore, 3D is useful in athletes with difficult to determine cardiac dimensions if 3D is available and the lab is experienced with its use.[9] The recommended method for LV measurements by the ASE, however, is the 2D volumetric biplane method of disks summation technique.

Echocardiographic studies have demonstrated that the cardiac chamber adaptations to chronic endurance and strength exercise training mimic the cardiac response to volume and pressure overload, respectively.[11] Prospective exercise training studies demonstrate that endurance (aerobic) training and sports (for example, long-distance running) increase left ventricular internal dimensions with little change in LV wall thickness. Chronic endurance training predominantly produces a volume load on the left and right ventricles and the greatest changes in cavity size and wall thickness, resulting in eccentric hypertrophy.[12,13] In contrast, chronic static or strength sports (such as weight lifting, wrestling) produce only small increases in oxygen consumption (VO_2) and minimal changes in cavity size. Strength sports may be associated with mild to modest increases in wall thickness, some of which could be due to increased body mass in such athletes. These changes in wall thickness with little change in chamber dimensions mimic the changes produced by pressure load on the left and right ventricles, resulting in concentric hypertrophy.[14] Combination athletes typically display a phenotype with overlapping features of endurance and strength-trained athletes.[12] Among 1,300 Italian athletes, 45% had LV end-diastolic internal diameters (LVEDD) ≥55 mm, the upper limit of normal (ULN) used in most clinical echocardiographic laboratories, and 14% had an LVEDD ≥60 mm.[13] In contrast to the increases in chamber diameter among 738 male and 209 female Italian athletes, only 16 men had an LV wall thickness >12 mm, the ULN generally used for this parameter.[12] Racial differences exist in the propensity to develop hypertrophy in response to exercise, and as many as 12% of Afro-Caribbean athletes demonstrate wall thicknesses of more than 12 mm.[15] The upper limit of physiological hypertrophy in athletes of all ethnicities appears to be a wall thickness of 16 mm.[12] Asymmetric hypertrophy is rarely seen in athletes.

The right ventricle (RV) also increases in size with exercise training. 2D RV measurements are challenging because of the complex geometry of the RV and the lack of specific right-sided anatomic landmarks to be used as reference points. Multiple views including the short axis, left parasternal RV inflow, and subcostal views are required for a comprehensive assessment of RV size and function. An RV-focused view from the apical four chamber view, provides visualization of the entire RV free wall and is recommended as the best single view to evaluate the RV. 3D RV volumes may be clinically important and should be measured in experienced laboratories if available.

Douglas *et al.* described increased right ventricular size in 41 Ironman finishers 13 and 28 min after the race using 2D echocardiography.[16] Subsequent magnetic resonance studies have confirmed an increase in RV size and volume both acutely and chronically with exercise training and suggested that the RV changes might be relatively greater than the LV changes.[17] RV ejection fraction, fractional area change, and RV global strain and strain rates support this hypothesis. These cardiac adaptations should not be misinterpreted as arrhythmogenic right ventricular dysplasia.

Some athletes competing in endurance sports demonstrate markedly enlarged left atrial (LA) diameters, but LA function is typically preserved when measured by speckle tracking echocardiography. Patients with HCM also display increased LA volumes, but they have a significant impairment in LA myocardial deformation, strain, and strain rates.[18]

There is overlap between exercise-induced physiologic changes and pathology, therefore, it is important to consider the sport discipline, the type of training, the body surface area (BSA), and the athlete's gender and ethnicity in the interpretation of these data. All LV measurements in athletes should be indexed by BSA.

Novel echo imaging techniques — Strain, strain rate, torsion

The distinction between adaptive physiology and pathologic remodeling requires an understanding of the evolving myocyte changes during the development of disease. In most structural heart diseases, there is a transition from normal to abnormal myocyte function, which initially manifests as a reduction in the early diastolic mitral annular tissue velocity [e'] measured by DTI, strain, and strain rate, twist dysfunction, and global systolic strain. Strain and strain rate offer a greater sensitivity than DTI velocity or displacement for detecting subtle abnormalities in the longitudinal myocardial contraction very early in the disease course. In addition, strain imaging offers the advantage of differentiating an active myocardial contraction from passive motion such as that caused by tethering.

Strain imaging has provided great insight into the properties of myocardial function in athletes. The term "strain" refers to the myocardial deformation throughout the cardiac cycle and is calculated by the Lagrangian formula as the ratio of the change in myocardial length (L1–L2) and baseline length (L1). Strain is measured as a percentage (%) (strain = L1–L2/L1). The "strain rate" is another marker of deformation and is the ratio of the change in the velocity between the two points and the length between those two reference points (strain rate = V1–V2/L). The strain rate is measured as 1/s. The strain and strain rates can be derived by tissue Doppler imaging techniques, which are characterized by angle dependency and a low signal to noise ratio, and require great experience for data interpretation. A newer form of strain imaging is speckle-tracking echocardiography (STE), which is a relatively simple, reliable, reproducible, and angle-independent technique. Using STE, kernels or blocks of speckles are semi-automatically traced frame by frame, providing local displacement information, used to calculate all the spatial components of myocardial strain and strain rate without requiring a lot of experience.

The human heart has a complex arrangement of myocardial fibers and hence a complex contraction mechanism. LV subendocardial and subepicardial fibers are in oblique longitudinal orientation (subepicardial being clockwise while subendocardial are counter-clockwise), from the apex to the base, thus drawing a spiral around the ventricle.[19] The mid-wall LV fibers are circumferential. Thus, systole and diastole result in a complex deformation and movement of the LV wall fibers. In addition, the LV also has a wringing or twisting motion around its long axis during systole. Four types of myocardial strain patterns can thus be evaluated: circumferential, radial, longitudinal, and torsion/twisting/rotational. Longitudinal strain refers to shortening of myocardial walls in apical views, and by convention negative values represent contraction or shortening. Circumferential strain refers to shortening of LV cavity size in short-axis and negative values represent contraction or shortening. Radial strain refers to thickening of LV walls in short axis and positive values represent contraction or shortening. Torsion or rotational strain enables determination of the velocity and direction of LV wall rotation, also referred to as the twisting and untwisting motion the LV.

The study of LV mechanical deformation in athletes with these techniques has helped differentiate the physiological (adaptive or athletic) vs. pathological (maladaptive) LV hypertrophy such as seen in patients with essential hypertension and non-obstructive HCM. A reduction in the longitudinal strain is the earliest marker of LV dysfunction and is ubiquitous in patients with hypertensive heart disease and HCM, but absent in athletes' heart. This finding may be explained by the fact that the subendocardium is often first affected by most structural heart diseases (such as ischemic, diabetic, hypertensive, and valvular heart diseases) and longitudinal strain primarily represents the deformation of subendocardial fibers. Conversely, circumferential and radial strain may remain normal until the disease progresses.[20] STE can be applied to both ventricles and atria. However, signal quality may be suboptimal for atria and the right ventricle, because of their thin walls. Longitudinal and circumferential strain can be measured relatively easily, but the measurement of radial strain is more challenging and therefore less likely to be used clinically.[21]

Different studies have shown slightly variable data when comparing strain values in athletes and normal, non-athletic control populations. A comparison of strain patterns in 29 professional soccer players, 26 patients with HCM, and 17 sedentary controls revealed that radial and transverse strains were significantly higher in athletes whereas longitudinal strain was slightly lower, *albeit* normal. The professional athletes had higher values for transverse, radial, and circumferential strain when compared to HCM patients.[22] Caselli *et al.* also showed slightly lower but normal longitudinal strain scores in athletes compared to normal non-athletes.[23] In contrast, other studies demonstrated no significant difference in global LV longitudinal, radial, and circumferential strain patterns, among athletes (top level cyclists, rowers, and handball players) and healthy controls.[24,25] In fact, one study examining wrestlers found higher values of global longitudinal strain in athletes as compared to controls.[26] This variance might be due to the type of athlete population studied. These discordant results are not surprising and are likely due to the lack of standardization of different speckle-tracking algorithms among vendors. These conflicting data make it difficult to establish normal values in athletes and non-athletes when comparing data generated by different centers. However, these studies taken together suggest that below normal strain values should prompt further investigation in athletes (Figure 5).

Other studies have used strain-rate imaging to distinguish between individuals with hypertensive LVH and those with LVH from strength training. Systolic and diastolic strain and strain rate were reduced in hypertensive individuals, but not in athletes.[27] Patients with hypertensive LVH have reduced global longitudinal strain compared to athletes.[28] Strain rates also appear to be different in different athletic groups. LV apical circumferential strain in particular is lower in endurance athletes compared to the strength group athletes and normal controls.[29] In summary, the peak myocardial systolic velocities, strain, and strain rate are typically normal or supranormal in athletes with physiologic hypertrophy in contrast to HCM, in which longitudinal strain, both regional and global, are impaired.[30] LV global longitudinal strain (the earliest marker for LV dysfunction) in athletes is within the

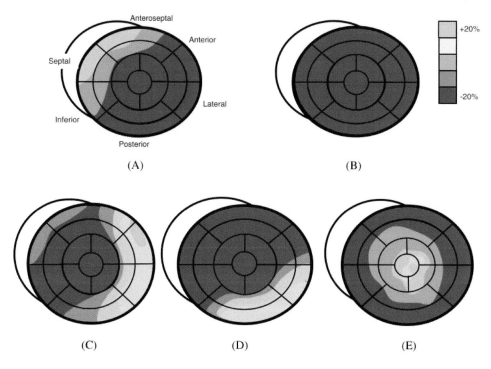

Figure 5.   Representative peak systolic strain maps in various forms of left ventricular hypertrophy. (A) A patient with hypertrophic cardiomyopathy and asymmetric septal hypertrophy, demonstrating a reduction in strain most prominent in the hypertrophied basal and mid-anteroseptal, septal, and inferior segments. (B) An athlete with physiological hypertrophy, demonstrating normal strain values in all segments. (C) A patient with cardiac amyloid, demonstrating a reduction in strain in the basal and mid-segments, with relative apical sparing. (D) A patient with Anderson–Fabry disease, demonstrating the characteristic reduction in strain in the basal and mid-posterolateral segments. (E) A patient with left ventricular non-compaction cardiomyopathy, demonstrating a reduction in strain in the mid and apical segments.[34]

normal range and comparable to that of normal controls. Thus, a significantly reduced LV strain in an athlete should prompt further evaluation.

Twisting and untwisting

LV twisting and untwisting are strain-derived and represent one of the most intriguing novel parameters in assessing athletes' heart physiology. This technique has been evaluated in cross-sectional studies of professional soccer players[31] and elite cyclists.[25] LV twist was lower in the cyclists, who demonstrated lower apical strain with no change in global LV diastolic and systolic function. The reduction in LV twist was driven by a reduction in apical rotation. This is presumed to be related to the LV apex being more sensitive to sympathetic activity than the LV base, likely related to a greater density of beta-adrenergic receptors in the apex.[32]

A study comparing endurance and strength athletes demonstrated a lower LV twisting and untwisting in endurance athletes compared to the strength group and control group.[30] The reduction in apical rotation and LV twisting observed in athletes could be related to training-induced changes in sympathovagal balance. This imbalance could provide cardiovascular functional reserve by increasing the radial strain and torsional response to exercise, a key element of diastolic filling and thus of cardiac performance.[20]

LV twisting and untwisting could help distinguish physiological adaptations from pathology, but its role in the differential diagnosis and identification of pathological hypertrophy deserves further investigation.

Conclusion

The diagnostic value of echocardiography as an imaging modality for a specific diagnosis depends both on the reliability of the echocardiographic data and on integration with other clinical information in a systematic manner. The framework for echocardiographic data acquisition and reporting is a structured diagnostic approach to the question posed by the requesting physician. Despite the use of a systematic approach, some athletes have cardiac dimensions that fall in a "gray-zone" between pathologic and normal measurements. M-mode and novel imaging techniques, such as DTI, strain, and strain rate, can help differentiate normal adaptations in athletes from pathological changes produced by disease.

Personal Perspectives

Antonio B. Fernandez

My interest in sports medicine stems from my involvement in sports during my childhood. I am a former mountain climber and triathlete. During my high school years I became the director of a hiking club in the city of Caracas, Venezuela. I was fascinated by the physiological adaptations to exercise training and altitude. This fascination led me, among a group of climbers, to train and complete expeditions in the Andes and the Himalayas. We conquered the summit of local peaks including the Pokalde, Humboldt Peak, the North and South Iliniza Peaks, the Cotopaxi and Tunguragua volcanos, amongst others.

I believe it was these sports that motivated me to learn more about cardiology and cardiac adaptations, but it was not until residency that my passion for sports cardiology was ignited. I continue to develop a career path in sports cardiology under the guidance of Dr. Paul Thompson at Hartford Hospital. At this point in my career, there is no other place I'd rather be!

Lovely Chhabra

Dr. Lovely Chhabra is the Chief Cardiology fellow at Hartford Hospital, University of Connecticut School of Medicine, CT (USA). Dr. Chhabra has received numerous awards for his clinical and academic work during his medical training. He has 140 publications in several international, peer-reviewed medical journals and has also authored and co-authored numerous abstracts and book chapters. His areas of research interest include electrocardiography, pericardial diseases, novel echocardiographic imaging techniques, and Takotsubo cardiomyopathy. Due to his special clinical interest on echocardiographic strain imaging, he has co-authored the section on the role of strain imaging in the evaluation of athletes, which has indeed emerged as a powerful diagnostic tool to differentiate adaptive/athletic cardiac hypertrophy from pathological hypertrophic states related to different systemic diseases.

References

1. Feigenbaum H. Role of M-mode technique in today's echocardiography. *J Am Soc Echocardiogr* 2010;23(3):240–257, 335–337.
2. Konecke LL, Feigenbaum H, Chang S, Corya BC, Fischer JC. Abnormal mitral valve motion in patients with elevated left ventricular diastolic pressures. *Circulation* 1973;47(5):989–996.
3. Henry WL, Clark CE, Griffith JM, Epstein SE. Mechanism of left ventricular outflow obstruction in patients with obstructive asymmetric septal hypertrophy (idiopathic hypertrophic subaortic stenosis). *Am J Cardiol* 1975;35(3):337–345.
4. Pollick C, Rakowski H, Wigle ED. Muscular subaortic stenosis: The quantitative relationship between systolic anterior motion and the pressure gradient. *Circulation* 1984;69(1):43–49.
5. Candell-Riera J, Garcia del Castillo H, Permanyer-Miralda G, Soler-Soler J. Echocardiographic features of the interventricular septum in chronic constrictive pericarditis. *Circulation* 1978;57(6):1154–1158.
6. Miller D, Farah MG, Liner A, Fox K, Schluchter M, Hoit BD. The relation between quantitative right ventricular ejection fraction and indices of tricuspid annular motion and myocardial performance. *J Am Soc Echocardiogr* 2004;17(5):443–447.
7. Caselli S, Di Paolo FM, Pisicchio C, Pandian NG, Pelliccia A. Patterns of left ventricular diastolic function in Olympic athletes. *J Am Soc Echocardiogr* 2015; 28(2):236–244.
8. Santoro A, Alvino F, Antonelli G, Cameli M, Bertini M, Molle R, Mondillo S. Left ventricular strain modifications after maximal exercise in athletes: A speckle tracking study. *Echocardiography* 2014;32(6):920–927.

9. Lang RM, Badano LP, Mor-Avi V, Afilalo J, Armstrong A, Ernande L, Flachskampf FA, Foster E, Goldstein SA, Kuznetsova T, Lancellotti P, Muraru D, Picard MH, Rietzschel ER, Rudski L, Spencer KT, Tsang W, Voigt JU. Recommendations for cardiac chamber quantification by echocardiography in adults: An update from the American Society of Echocardiography and the European Association of Cardiovascular Imaging. *J Am Soc Echocardiogr* 2015;28(1):1–39, e14.

10. Mulvagh SL, Rakowski H, Vannan MA, Abdelmoneim SS, Becher H, Bierig SM, Burns PN, Castello R, Coon PD, Hagen ME, Jollis JG, Kimball TR, Kitzman DW, Kronzon I, Labovitz AJ, Lang RM, Mathew J, Moir WS, Nagueh SF, Pearlman AS, Perez JE, Porter TR, Rosenbloom J, Strachan GM, Thanigaraj S, Wei K, Woo A, Yu EH, Zoghbi WA. American society of echocardiography consensus statement on the clinical applications of ultrasonic contrast agents in echocardiography. *J Am Soc Echocardiogr* 2008;21(11):1179–1201.

11. Eijsvogels TM, Fernandez AB, Thompson PD. Are there deleterious cardiac effects of acute and chronic endurance exercise? *Physiol Rev* 2016;96(1):99–125.

12. Pelliccia A, Maron BJ, Spataro A, Proschan MA, Spirito P. The upper limit of physiologic cardiac hypertrophy in highly trained elite athletes. *N Engl J Med* 1991;324(5):295–301.

13. Pelliccia A, Culasso F, Di Paolo FM, Maron BJ. Physiologic left ventricular cavity dilatation in elite athletes. *Ann Intern Med* 1999;130(1):23–31.

14. Morganroth J, Maron BJ, Henry WL, Epstein SE. Comparative left ventricular dimensions in trained athletes. *Ann Intern Med* 1975;82(4):521–524.

15. Papadakis M, Carre F, Kervio G, Rawlins J, Panoulas VF, Chandra N, Basavarajaiah S, Carby L, Fonseca T, Sharma S. The prevalence, distribution, and clinical outcomes of electrocardiographic repolarization patterns in male athletes of African/Afro-Caribbean origin. *Eur Heart J* 2011;32(18):2304–2313.

16. Douglas PS, O'Toole ML, Hiller WD, Reichek N. Different effects of prolonged exercise on the right and left ventricles. *J Am Coll Cardiol* 1990;15(1):64–69.

17. La Gerche A, Heidbuchel H, Burns AT, Mooney DJ, Taylor AJ, Pfluger HB, Inder WJ, Macisaac AI, Prior DL. Disproportionate exercise load and remodeling of the athlete's right ventricle. *Med Sci Sports Exer* 2011;43(6):974–981.

18. Gabrielli L, Enriquez A, Cordova S, Yanez F, Godoy I, Corbalan R. Assessment of left atrial function in hypertrophic cardiomyopathy and athlete's heart: A left atrial myocardial deformation study. *Echocardiography* 2012;29(8):943–949.

19. Buckberg GD. Architecture must document functional evidence to explain the living rhythm. *Eur J Cardiothorac Surg* 2005;27(2):202–209.

20. D'Ascenzi F, Caselli S, Solari M, Pelliccia A, Cameli M, Focardi M, Padeletti M, Corrado D, Bonifazi M, Mondillo S. Novel echocardiographic techniques for the evaluation of athletes' heart: A focus on speckle-tracking echocardiography. *Eur J Prev Cardiol* 2016;23(4):437–446.

21. Mor-Avi V, Lang RM, Badano LP, Belohlavek M, Cardim NM, Derumeaux G, Galderisi M, Marwick T, Nagueh SF, Sengupta PP, Sicari R, Smiseth OA, Smulevitz B, Takeuchi M, Thomas JD, Vannan M, Voigt JU, Zamorano JL. Current and evolving echocardiographic techniques for the quantitative

evaluation of cardiac mechanics: ASE/EAE consensus statement on methodology and indications endorsed by the Japanese Society of Echocardiography. *J Am Soc Echocardiogr* 2011;24(3):277–313.

22. Richand V, Lafitte S, Reant P, Serri K, Lafitte M, Brette S, Kerouani A, Chalabi H, Dos Santos P, Douard H, Roudaut R. An ultrasound speckle tracking (two-dimensional strain) analysis of myocardial deformation in professional soccer players compared with healthy subjects and hypertrophic cardiomyopathy. *Am J Cardiol* 2007;100(1):128–132.

23. Caselli S, Montesanti D, Autore C, Di Paolo FM, Pisicchio C, Squeo MR, Musumeci B, Spataro A, Pandian NG, Pelliccia A. Patterns of left ventricular longitudinal strain and strain rate in Olympic athletes. *J Am Soc Echocardiogr* 2015;28(2):245–253.

24. Cappelli F, Toncelli L, Cappelli B, De Luca A, Stefani L, Maffulli N, Galanti G. Adaptative or maladaptative hypertrophy, different spatial distribution of myocardial contraction. *Clin Physiol Funct Imaging* 2010;30(1):6–12.

25. Nottin S, Doucende G, Schuster-Beck I, Dauzat M, Obert P. Alteration in left ventricular normal and shear strains evaluated by 2D-strain echocardiography in the athlete's heart. *J Physiol* 2008;586(19):4721–4733.

26. Simsek Z, Hakan Tas M, Degirmenci H, Gokhan Yazici A, Ipek E, Duman H, Gundogdu F, Karakelleoglu S, Senocak H. Speckle tracking echocardiographic analysis of left ventricular systolic and diastolic functions of young elite athletes with eccentric and concentric type of cardiac remodeling. *Echocardiography* 2013;30(10):1202–1208.

27. Saghir M, Areces M, Makan M. Strain rate imaging differentiates hypertensive cardiac hypertrophy from physiologic cardiac hypertrophy (athlete's heart). *J Am Soc Echocardiogr* 2007;20(2):151–157.

28. Galderisi M, Lomoriello VS, Santoro A, Esposito R, Olibet M, Raia R, Di Minno MN, Guerra G, Mele D, Lombardi G. Differences of myocardial systolic deformation and correlates of diastolic function in competitive rowers and young hypertensives: A speckle-tracking echocardiography study. *J Am Soc Echocardiogr* 2010;23(11): 1190–1198.

29. Santoro A, Alvino F, Antonelli G, Caputo M, Padeletti M, Lisi M, Mondillo S. Endurance and strength athlete's heart: Analysis of myocardial deformation by speckle tracking echocardiography. *J Cardiovasc Ultras* 2014;22(4):196–204.

30. Vinereanu D, Florescu N, Sculthorpe N, Tweddel AC, Stephens MR, Fraser AG. Differentiation between pathologic and physiologic left ventricular hypertrophy by tissue Doppler assessment of long-axis function in patients with hypertrophic cardiomyopathy or systemic hypertension and in athletes. *Am J Cardiol* 2001;88(1):53–58.

31. Zocalo Y, Bia D, Armentano RL, Arias L, Lopez C, Etchart C, Guevara E. Assessment of training-dependent changes in the left ventricle torsion dynamics of professional soccer players using speckle-tracking echocardiography. *Conf Proc IEEE Eng Med Biol Soc* 2007;2007:2709–2712.

32. Mori H, Ishikawa S, Kojima S, Hayashi J, Watanabe Y, Hoffman JI, Okino H. Increased responsiveness of left ventricular apical myocardium to adrenergic stimuli. *Cardiovasc Res* 1993;27(2):192–198.

33. Feigenbaum H. *Echocardiography*, 1st (Edn.), Philadelphia: Lea and Eebiger, 1972.

34. Robert LM, Goldstein SA. *ASE's Comprehensive Echocardiography. Cardiomyopathies*. New York: Elsevier, 2015.

Chapter 8

Exercise at High Altitude

Eugene E. Wolfel

Professor of Medicine, Section of Advanced Heart Failure
and Transplant Cardiology
Medical Director, Cardiac Rehabilitation and Exercise/
Stress Testing Laboratory
Division of Cardiology
University of Colorado School of Medicine
Anschutz Medical Campus
Aurora, CO, USA

Exposure to the hypobaric hypoxia of high altitude creates a number of physiological stresses that affect exercise and athletic performance. The reduction in barometric pressure causes a decrease in the partial pressure of oxygen in the alveoli, arteries, capillaries, and peripheral veins that causes a dramatic reduction in the oxygen cascade when compared to sea level. There are compensatory responses in the cardiovascular, autonomic nervous, respiratory, skeletal muscle, and hematologic systems that will modulate this response, especially over time of exposure to a given altitude, that will lead to improvements in exercise performance, but exercise capacity at high altitude will never equal that at sea level, despite ideal acclimatization and training techniques. However, climbers have been able to reach the summit of Mount Everest at 8,850 m (29,028 ft) without oxygen, where the VO_2 max is reduced by 80%, compared to sea level. This is an extreme example of adequate adaptation to exercise at extreme high altitude, but many athletic events are conducted each year at more modest altitudes. In fact, 140 million people live and recreate at altitudes >2,500 m. Last year 11 million people came to Colorado's ski resorts where altitude varies from 3,050 to 3,980 m in elevation. Interest in athletic performance at high altitude was first heightened with the Olympic games in Mexico City in 1968, where the altitude was 2,290 m. In South America, professional football games occur in La Paz, Bolivia (3,600 m); Bogota, Columbia (2,640 m); Cusco, Peru (3,400 m); and Quito, Ecuador (2,800 m). Competition at these altitudes is particularly challenging for teams who travel from sea level cities in Argentina and Brazil. Several of the stages of the Tour de France also occur at high altitude. In Colorado, there are several running events including the Bolder Boulder, Mount Evans Run, Pikes Peak Marathon, and the Leadville 100 that involve exercise at altitudes up to 4,300 m (14,100 ft). Both elite and recreational athletes are able to compete and demonstrate a high level of performance at these altitudes, although their performance never approaches that at sea level. In this chapter, the effect of high altitude exposure on physiological measurements of both maximal and submaximal exercise performance will be examined, along with a review of some of the factors affecting both marathon and distance running performance. Although the data from extreme altitude (>5,000 m) will be referenced, the focus of this treatise will be on exercise performance at more moderate altitudes (500–4,500 m). The cardiovascular responses to both acute and more sustained hypoxia will be reviewed and related to exercise performance. The role of the autonomic nervous system will also be discussed as this has a major impact on cardiovascular functioning at high altitude. In addition, the ventilatory, metabolic, and hematologic adaptations to high altitude will be presented. Methods of exercise training at high altitude will be examined as applied to both sea level and high altitude exercise performance. High altitude illness can be a major factor in limiting exercise performance, and approaches to improving symptoms from especially acute high altitude exposure will be presented. Finally, the effect of high altitude on exercise capacity in patients with cardiovascular disease will be reviewed. Current recommendations concerning the risk stratification of patients with cardiovascular disease who plan to travel and exercise at moderate high altitude will also be presented. During the following discussion, altitude will be referenced as meters above sea level and barometric pressure will not be presented. To convert meters to feet, one needs to multiply meters (m) by 3.28. The mountains and areas of higher terrestrial elevation are beautiful to behold and adaptations in our human physiology allow us to exercise and participate in physical activities in a lower oxygen environment.

Exercise Performance at High Altitude

Maximal oxygen consumption ($\dot{V}O_2$ max) represents the most accurate and predictive measurement of aerobic exercise performance. Utilizing the Fick equation (cardiac output = VO_2/arterial – venous oxygen content difference), it is obvious that three major physiologic variables influence maximal exercise capacity. Acute and sustained exposure to altitudes >1,500 m will affect blood flow (cardiac output and skeletal muscle blood flow) and arterial oxygen content, both of which will determine oxygen delivery. In addition, mixed venous oxygen content, as a determinant of peripheral oxygen extraction, can also play a role in the determination of exercise capacity at high altitude. Each of these variables will be discussed separately, but the overall effect of high altitude is a reduction in VO_2 max.

The most dramatic decreases in exercise capacity occur, as expected, at the highest attainable terrestrial altitudes where barometric pressure is greatly reduced. At altitudes >8,000 m there is a substantial reduction in the partial pressure of oxygen with downstream effects throughout the entire oxygen cascade. During a simulated, hypobaric chamber experiment that mimicked the ascent of Mount Everest (Operation Everest II), there was progressive decrease in VO_2 max, despite a gradual altitude ascent.[1] As shown in Table 1, the VO_2 max decreased from 49.1 ± 2.9 mL/kg/min at sea level to 15.3 ± 1.3 mL/kg/min at a simulated altitude of 8,848 m in the five subjects who were tested at all altitude elevations. This represented a 69% decrease in VO_2 max. There were significant decreases in arterial oxygen saturation (SaO_2) and heart rate but no significant change in exercise minute ventilation (V_E) with progressive altitude. The average age of these male subjects was 28 ± 2 years and their sea level VO_2 max varied from 41.6 to 63 mL/kg/min. The two subjects with the higher VO_2 max at sea level (most athletic) had evidence of a drop in SaO_2 at maximal exercise at sea level. These two subjects were unable to complete the simulated ascent. Their data are not included in Table 1. The remaining subjects with the highest VO_2 max at sea level had the highest VO_2 max values at each altitude, but they also had the greatest reductions in VO_2 max. The reductions in VO_2 max were associated with a decrease in

Table 1. Operation Everest II: maximal exercise measurements.

Altitude	Barometric pressure mmHg	VO_2 max mL/kg/min	V_E L/min	Heart rate bpm	SaO_2 %
Sea level	760	49.1 ± 3.0	176.8 ± 7.0	175 ± 2	95 ± 2
4,270 m	464	35.6 ± 2.0	206.9 ± 5.0	165 ± 4	67 ± 2
6,100 m	347	27.9 ± 1.5	196.8 ± 9.0	141 ± 2	52 ± 3
7,620 m	289	21.4 ± 1.0	191.8 ± 8.1	136 ± 5	42 ± 3
8,849 m	240	15.3 ± 1.3	185.3 ± 13.0	127 ± 6	35 ± 3

Means ± SE; $n = 5$; V_E = minute ventilation (BTPS); SaO_2 = arterial O_2 saturation. All measurements at maximal exercise on a cycle ergometer at simulated altitude in hypobaric chamber. Data derived from subjects who were studied at all altitudes in Ref. 1.

maximal heart rate and cardiac output; however, the relationship between cardiac output and oxygen consumption appeared to be similar to that at sea level.[2] Although the results of this experiment are most relevant to mountain climbers, these relationships between cardiac function, ventilation, and exercise performance (VO_2 max) at extreme altitude provide a framework to understand the maladaptations and compensatory mechanisms that influence exercise capacity at more moderate high altitude.

There appears to be a curvilinear relationship between increasing altitude elevation and a reduction in VO_2 max. This has been shown in an analysis of 67 research studies, utilizing both laboratory or field research at high altitude.[3] At altitudes >1,500 m, there appears to an approximate 1% reduction in VO_2 max for each additional 100 m of altitude. There is definite variation in this predicted reduction in VO_2 max and this "rule of thumb" can only serve as an estimate. There are no reported differences between men and women, when matched by sea level aerobic capacity, in the effects of high altitude on limitations of maximal exercise performance. There does appear to be a major influence of sea level aerobic fitness on the decrement in VO_2 max at high altitude. Elite athletes appear to be more susceptible to the deleterious effects of high altitude on exercise performance. At 4,000 m, an untrained individual was reported to have a 13% reduction in VO_2 max, compared to a 22% reduction in a trained individual.[4] Reductions in VO_2 max have been observed to occur in elite athletes as low as 580 m.[4] An analysis of the studies involving male, non-acclimatized, elite athletes at high altitude has determined that there is a different rate of decline in VO_2 max with progressive altitude.[5] In subjects with a mean VO_2 max >60 mL/kg/min, there was a 7.7% reduction in VO_2 max per 1,000 m of increasing altitude. However, the reduction in VO_2 max appeared to begin at a lower altitude of 800 m. The reasons for the greater susceptibility in athletes to reductions in VO_2 max may be explained by the greater degree of arterial oxygen desaturation during exercise[4,6] compared to unfit individuals. Data from the Operation Everest II Project[7] demonstrated ventilation–perfusion mismatch and significant capillary diffusion limitations that could explain this phenomenon. In the most athletic subject in that trial, the VO_2 max decreased from 63.3 mL/kg/min at sea level to 42.6 mL/kg/min at 3,790 m, a 33% reduction. His SaO_2 at maximal exercise was 85% at sea level and 29% at 3,790 m. This reduction in VO_2 max was consistent with the range predicted by Wehrlin and colleagues (29%) at 3,790 m.[5] Based on these physiological data, one might expect that there is a particular phenotype that would predict tolerance and ability to perform physical activity at extreme altitude. However, an analysis of six elite mountain climbers, who successfully summited at least one of the four highest peaks in the world, did not demonstrate any physiological advantages to be able to achieve such remarkable performances.[8] Although these elite climbers had VO_2

max values similar to an amateur marathon runner, they did not approach values seen in elite long-distance runners. There was a suggestion that their SaO_2 may not have dropped as much as expected during exercise during both normoxia and normobaric hypoxia, but the results of a non-invasive cardiac evaluation, pulmonary function tests, ventilatory control, and analysis of skeletal muscle fiber type and morphometry did not elucidate any physiological advantage. Thus, it is difficult to predict from sea level physiological investigations alone, how exercise performance will be affected by high altitude. Genetic factors may be another explanation for the variation in the VO_2 max at high altitude. In an analysis of 11 studies examining the potential role of genetic factors on human hypoxic exercise performance, 4 of 13 genetic polymorphisms were found to have an association with decreased exercise performance at altitude.[9] The exercise phenotypes evaluated were mountaineering performance, running performance, and VO_2 max. The genetic polymorphisms included the adenosine monophosphate deaminase (AMPD1) C34T, the beta$_2$-adrenergic receptor (ADRB2) Gly16Arg, the androgen CAG repeat polymorphisms, and the angiotensin I-converting enzyme (ACE) insertion/deletion polymorphism. The strongest association was with the ACE I/D polymorphism. In another study involving Belgian lowlanders with the determination of VO_2 max at sea level and acute normobaric hypoxia, there was an association between a low and high reduction in VO_2 max and six single nucleotide polymorphisms (SNP).[10] These six SNPs were vascular endothelial growth factor A (VEGFA), peroxisome proliferator-activated receptor alpha (PPARA), endothelial PAS domain-containing protein 1 (EPASI), angiotensin converting enzyme polymorphism (ACE), and two different Beta$_2$-adrenergic receptor G-protein (ADRB2) genotypes. These genes are involved in the hypoxia-induced factor (HIF), oxygen signaling pathway (EPASI, PPARA), angiogenesis and vascular permeability (VEGFA), epinephrine responses (ADRB2), and aspects of endurance performance (ACE I allele) with a higher VO_2 max at altitude. A genetic disposition score (GPS) was devised with a protective effect of $0.11 LO_2$/min per each additional allele. The GPS was shown to discriminate between low vs. high delta VO_2 max subgroups (normoxia–hypoxia) with a receiver operator curve AUC of 0.78. The GPS explained 23% of the overall variance in hypoxia-induced reductions in VO_2 max and also discriminated between the high vs. low delta VO_2 max subgroups. These data suggest that there may be genetic influences that interact with other physiological factors in determining the degree of exercise impairment with high altitude exposure. It is unclear at this time whether these genetic factors are altered to improve exercise performance at high altitude.

Although acclimatization to altitude allows for greater tolerance, there are limited data that VO_2 max improves over time at high altitude. With acute exposure to high altitude, there is a significant decrease in the arterial oxygen content

(CaO$_2$) that cannot be compensated by an increase in heart rate and cardiac output. Thus, conductive oxygen delivery (cardiac output × CaO$_2$) is reduced. Despite the improvements in CaO$_2$ resulting from initial ventilatory and later hematologic acclimatization, in the absence of exercise training, VO$_2$ max has not been demonstrated to improve in the majority of studies at moderate high altitude. At extreme high altitude, VO$_2$ max does not improve over time (Table 1). Thus, VO$_2$ max at high altitude is always reduced compared to sea level. Factors that may prevent an improvement in VO$_2$ max at high altitude include the severity of hypoxic exposure (extreme vs. moderate altitude), level of activity at altitude, mechanism of fatigue (central vs. cardiovascular), and development of muscle wasting.[11] At modest altitudes, augmentation of CaO$_2$ by either erythropoietin (EPO) or blood transfusions, can result in a greater VO$_2$ max with relatively acute to short-term exposure to moderate but not extreme high altitude.[12-14] This dichotomy relates to the probable different mechanisms of reduced exercise capacity related to the severity of hypoxia. At moderate altitudes oxygen delivery mechanisms seem to predominate, but at extreme altitude there appears to be a direct effect of severe hypoxia on the central nervous system with "central fatigue" related to the inability to excite motor neurons in an adequate manner.

The maintained reduction in VO$_2$ max over time at high altitude has a major impact on submaximal exercise performance as exercise performed at an absolute workload (VO$_2$, power output) will always occur at a higher relative percent of VO$_2$ max at high altitude (Figure 1). From a physiological and potentially clinical

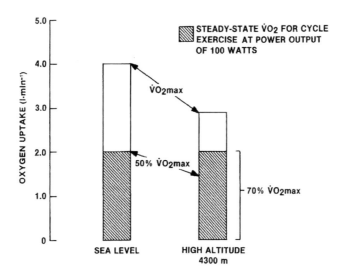

Figure 1.   Absolute vs. relative workloads at high altitude. VO$_2$ of 2.0 L/min is 50% VO$_2$ max at sea level but 70% VO$_2$ max at high altitude. Data derived from combined data from Refs. 18, 36, and 52.

perspective, relative workload is primarily responsible for the degree of sympathetic stimulation, metabolic responses, and cardiovascular activation during exercise. However, exercise capacity is also reduced at the same relative workload at high altitude within the first few days of arrival at high altitude.[15,16] The results of most studies at moderate altitude demonstrate improvement in submaximal exercise performance over several weeks' residence at the same altitude, manifested as prolonged endurance time at a given workload.[15,17] At more modest elevations (2,340 m) this could be due to an increase in VO_2 max and thus a reduced relative exercise intensity,[15] but this is not the explanation for improved submaximal exercise performance at higher altitudes (4,300 m). With high altitude acclimatization there is an increase in minute ventilation during submaximal exercise and an increase in hemoglobin concentration that is initially due to hemoconcentration and later to actual increased RBC mass. These adaptations lead to an increase in CaO_2 during a given submaximal workload. VO_2 does not change from sea level values and there is a corresponding decrease in cardiac output, resulting in less cardiac work during exercise. In a study of seven men who were studied over a 21-day period at 4,300 m, there were no changes in VO_2 at a given submaximal workload; however, the workload was 65% of VO_2 max at both acute and sustained altitude exposure, compared to only 50% VO_2 max at sea level.[18] Over 21 days at 4,300 m, there was a decrease in oxygen delivery despite an improvement in CaO_2 related to both ventilatory acclimatization and an increase in RBC volume. Both cardiac output and leg blood flow were decreased during exercise at high altitude compared to sea level values. Submaximal exercise duration was not evaluated in this study, but with a significant increase in relative exercise intensity at high altitude, submaximal exercise performance would be reduced compared to sea level. In two other studies at 4,300 m there was a 59% improvement in performance at the same absolute workload in one study[17] and no improvement in the other study.[16] These findings occurred in the absence of exercise training and only reflect the influence of hypobaric hypoxia. In all these studies, subjects were required to maintain the same level of physical activity as at sea level to avoid the confounding influence of deconditioning and muscle wasting.

One additional factor that could influence endurance exercise capacity at high altitude is an alteration in muscle mechanical efficiency. This is manifested by the relationship between VO_2 and workload. It is a cardinal rule of exercise physiology that this ratio remains constant under most physiological perturbations. If VO_2 at a given power output was decreased at high altitude, this could adversely affect submaximal exercise performance. A thorough review of studies involving both total body and leg VO_2 measurements did not support a change in the muscle mechanical efficiency or VO_2 economy at altitudes up to 4,300 m.[19] However, at substantially higher altitudes (5,260 m) there were decreases in VO_2 at a given submaximal workload, both with acute exposure and after 9 weeks of acclimatization. This finding with more profound hypoxia may be caused by an alteration in substrate utilization in skeletal muscle, but does not appear to be related to anatomical or physiological adaptations over time at greater altitudes since the lower VO_2 was evident on arrival. Thus, for the average person who exercises at moderate high altitude, alterations in exercise economy do not explain a reduction in submaximal exercise capacity.

The physiological changes that occur during exercise at high altitude have a major impact on exercise performance in athletic events that are greater than 800 m and involve aerobic metabolism. The longer the duration of an event, the more likely that altitude will prolong the time to complete the event.[3] High altitude is a particular challenge for long-distance running. In a study of 27 elite men and women athletes who performed a 3,000 m time trial at sea level and 48 h after arrival at an altitude of 2,500, there were significant increases in time to complete the distance at altitude.[20] There was a 48.4 ± 14.6 s increase in men and a 48.6 ± 8.9 s increase in women. This represented a 9.6% reduction in time trial performance in men and 8.6% reduction in women. At a simulated altitude using 16.3% oxygen at sea level there were expected reductions in VO_2 max compared to normoxic conditions. Athletes with a decrease in SaO_2 at maximal exercise at sea level had greater reductions in both VO_2 max and 3,000 m time at high altitude compared to those athletes who did not develop arterial oxygen desaturation during maximal exercise at sea level. Thus, the physiology of exercise at sea level in endurance athletes may predict the degree of impairment in exercise performance at moderate high altitude. Performance in longer endurance events, such as the marathon (42.2 km) is even more reduced than at shorter distances. In a review of 16 popular marathons performed at different altitudes above sea level there was a direct correlation between the finishing times and the altitude where the event occurred.[21] When the runners who finished from the 21st to 100th position were evaluated, there was a 10.8 ± 0.6% increase in race time in men and 12.3 ± 0.7% increase in women for every 1,000 m above sea level. The adverse effect of altitude was seen at elevations as low as 700 m. In elite and good runners who ran marathons at sea level, 4,300 and 5,200 m, there were expected increases in race time in both groups at high altitude.[22] The estimated VO_2 max at sea level was 71.5 ± 5.2 mL/kg/min in the elite runners and 59.3 ± 3.1 mL/kg/min in the good runners. The race speed was decreased by 29% at 4,300 m and 33% at 5,200 m in elite runners. In the good runners with a lower VO_2 max there was a 43% decrease in running speed at 4,300 m, compared to sea level. They did not participate in the marathon at 5,200 m. In these runners, marathon performance was primarily affected by the reduction in VO_2 max estimated at higher altitude. However, the elite runners were able to perform at a higher percent of VO_2 max than less skilled athletes. It was postulated that the work of breathing may have been greater in the less skilled runners, but differences related to training, duration of acclimatization, and innate physiological ability could not be evaluated. These studies indicate a significant impediment in endurance exercise performance at altitude with a direct correlation to the degree of elevation and thus severity of hypoxia.

Events of shorter duration that involve higher rates of speed, anaerobic metabolism, throwing, or lifting are associated with enhanced performance at high altitude.[23,24] Wind resistance is decreased and this results in the ability of the athlete to exceed sea level performance. However, as pointed out by Lundby[11] there may be expected problems with aerodynamics at high altitude that could affect the presumed trajectory of a flying ball. Overall, for short-term events, the favorable effects of activity at high altitude outweigh the disadvantages.

Cardiovascular Responses to Acute and Sustained High Altitude Exposure

The role of the cardiovascular system is to provide appropriate oxygen and substrate delivery to exercising muscle beds for maintenance of VO_2 and exercise performance. At more moderate high altitudes (500–4,500 m), the limiting factor in exercise performance is the inability of oxygen supply or delivery to offset the deficits in CaO_2 related to a hypoxic environment. At extreme altitudes (>5,000 m) there is a central nervous system effect that also limits performance. The main driver of the cardiovascular responses at high altitude, both with acute and more sustained exposure, is the autonomic nervous system with sympathetic stimulation playing the major role. The responses of the cardiovascular system to both acute and more sustained high altitude exposure are listed in Table 2.[25] During acute exposure to high altitude (hours to a few days), the cardiovascular system is mostly responsible for compensation for decrease in PaO_2 and CaO_2. However, with more sustained exposure (days to weeks), the cardiovascular system responds to adaptations in other organ systems during the process of acclimatization with resulting increases in CaO_2.

Acute hypoxia

In acute hypoxia with a sudden drop in PaO_2 and CaO_2, there is an attempt by the cardiovascular system to compensate for this sudden drop in convective O_2 delivery by increasing cardiac output and muscle blood flow. The degree of augmentation of cardiac output is directly related to the degree of hypoxia with no significant increase at altitudes <700 m and as great as 75% higher than sea level values at altitudes >5,000 m. This occurs primarily by an increase in heart rate with little

Table 2.   Cardiovascular responses to acute and sustained hypoxia during submaximal exercise at 4,300 m, compared to sea level.

	Acute hypoxia	Sustained hypoxia
Heart rate (bpm)	Increased	Increased
Stroke volume (mL)	No Change	Decreased
Cardiac output (L/min)	Increased	Decreased
MAP (mmHg)	No Change	Increased
SVR (wu)	No Change	Increased
CaO_2 (vol%)	Decreased	Improved*
O_2 delivery (L O_2/min)	Decreased	Decreased
$CmvO_2$ (vol%)	Decreased	Decreased
Leg blood flow (L/min)	Increased	Decreased
Leg O_2 delivery (L O_2/min)	Decreased	Decreased
VO_2 (L/min)	Unchanged	Unchanged
Leg VO_2 (mL/min)	Unchanged	Unchanged

Notes: All parameters are compared to sea level values. Data derived from combined studies on Pikes Peak at 4,300 m. Submaximal exercise: 51% VO_2 max at sea level; 67–68% VO_2 max at 4,300 m. *Increase in CaO_2 compared to acute hypoxia but still lower than sea level. Data derived from Refs. 18 and 36.

change in stroke volume. The increase in heart rate is primarily related to enhanced sympathetic nervous system activity, although there is also a lesser effect from parasympathetic withdrawal. Intrinsic heart rate does not change. A decrease in PaO_2 stimulates the carotid bodies and results in an increase in sympathetic nervous system activity that leads to the increase in heart rate. The heart rate increases significantly, both at rest and during submaximal exercise. Resting heart rate is higher, while stroke volume is either slightly diminished (first few hours of exposure) or unchanged. Thus, the increase in resting cardiac output is primarily related to increases in heart rate. Exercise at a constant workload at high altitude occurs at a higher relative workload (% VO_2 max) and heart rate is accordingly increased. However, heart rate is also increased, compared to sea level, at the same relative workload.[26] At maximal exercise with acute hypoxic exposure, heart rate is similar to sea level. Stroke volume does not change despite augmented myocardial contractility and decreases in end-systolic volume due to simultaneous decreases in end-diastolic volume. This occurs within the first few hours of altitude exposure. In subjects with no cardiac disease, there is no decrease in myocardial contractility and thus stroke volume, due to coronary vasodilation with increased myocardial blood flow[27,28] and perhaps a shift in myocardial metabolism from the more O_2 requiring free fatty acids to glucose.[29] Despite the increase in cardiac output with acute hypoxic exposure, maximal exercise capacity (VO$_2$ max) is still decreased due to the inability of cardiac output to normalize convective oxygen delivery. With no ability for tissues to acutely increase oxygen extraction, the significant decreases in PaO$_2$ and CaO$_2$ results in reduced exercise capacity.

There are also systemic vascular effects that influence the cardiovascular responses to acute altitude exposure. Despite heightened sympathetic stimulation, vasoconstriction only occurs in the pulmonary vascular bed during the first few hours of acute hypoxic exposure. In the systemic vascular beds, especially where metabolic demand is great, vasodilation occurs. In the coronary circulation, this response is neurally-mediated,[30] but this does not appear to be the mechanism in the peripheral circulation. Studies with beta-blockade in the forearm did not abolish the vasodilator response to acute hypoxia.[31] This physiologic response in the peripheral circulation is termed "functional sympatholysis" and it is related to local factors that result in a decrease in systemic vascular resistance and blood pressure while cardiac output and muscle blood flow increase. There is a direct relationship between the decrease in CaO$_2$ and an increase in muscle blood flow. CaO$_2$ and not PaO$_2$ appears to be the signal responsible for this local, metabolic vasodilation. Factors involved in this response include endothelial derived hyperpolarization factor (EDHF) and nitric oxide (NO). The red blood cell appears to be the main oxygen sensor, responding to decreases in CaO$_2$.[32] However, other factors such as neuropeptide Y and the alpha$_2$-adrenergic receptor may also play a role. Systemic blood pressure is influenced by the balance between the local vasodilation caused by "functional sympatholysis" and sympathetically driven vasoconstriction. This balance is important both at rest and during exercise. This balance is affected by the timing of ascent to high altitude, the degree of elevation and thus the severity of hypoxia, and the rapidity of early acclimatization responses. This local vasodilatory response is most prominent during the first few hours of acute hypoxic exposure and diminishes somewhat with more prolonged exposure, when factors such as increase minute ventilation and hemoconcentration with an increase in hematocrit result in some increase in both PaO$_2$ and CaO$_2$. It remains unclear which factors have a major influence on the control of blood pressure during the early exposure to high altitude.

In applying this knowledge of the cardiovascular changes that occur with early exposure to high altitude (acute hypoxia), a person can expect a reduction in maximal exercise capacity (VO$_2$ max) due to the inability of increased cardiac output and muscle blood flow to compensate for the significant reduction in PaO$_2$ and CaO$_2$ caused by a low inspiratory oxygen availability. Thus, all submaximal workloads will occur at a higher relative workload (% VO$_2$ max) compared to sea level. Heart rate will be increased at rest and during submaximal exercise, but heart rate at maximal exercise will be similar to sea level. This augmented heart rate response during exercise occurs at both absolute and relative work intensities and is mostly related to sympathetic stimulation,[32] although some increase in heart rate still occurs in the setting of beta-blockade.[31] Stroke volume plays a minor role in the increase in cardiac output response to acute hypoxia, but factors that would decrease stroke volume, such as dehydration, could further limit exercise capacity upon arrival. In addition, anemia with a resulting decrease in CaO_2 would also affect exercise performance at high altitude.

Sustained hypoxia

With more sustained exposure to high altitude (days to weeks), the cardiovascular system adapts to the gradual improvements in CaO_2 that result from ventilatory acclimatization, hemoconcentration, and an increase in RBC mass. Compared to acute hypoxia where the cardiovascular system responds to hypoxia itself, in sustained hypoxia the cardiovascular system reacts to changes in various organ systems that improve but do not correct the reduction in CaO_2 that results from breathing a low inspired oxygen tension (PiO_2). There is a cardiovascular sparing effect with reductions in cardiac output and muscle blood flow related to increases in CaO_2 and improved oxygen extraction. At altitudes between 2,500 and 4,500 m there is a decrease in cardiac output to VO_2 relationship, when compared to sea level, in the majority of studies.[18,33–36] This finding appears to be related to less hypoxic vasodilation and alterations in sympathetic activity with sustained exposure to high altitude. The reported magnitude of this reduction varies widely from no change to a reduction of 23% during submaximal exercise, but is uniformly present at maximal exercise. However, at extreme altitudes the cardiac output to VO_2 relationship is similar to sea level.[2,37] The reasons for the alteration in this relationship are not clear but are probably related to the severity of hypoxia with its resulting effects on peripheral vascular function. The cause of the reduction in cardiac output is primarily related to a decrease in stroke volume. This reduction in stroke volume is seen at rest and during exercise. Combined data from studies in normal men on Pikes Peak, Colorado at 4,300 m clearly demonstrate a reduction in stroke volume during the same absolute workload between initial ascent and 21 days' residence at this altitude (Figure 2). The character of the response in stroke volume is similar to the decrease in cardiac output. CaO_2 increases due to acclimatization and this adaption supports oxygen delivery to offset the reduction in cardiac output and muscle blood flow. The reduction in stroke volume is related to reductions in cardiac pre-load. Cardiac contractile function is preserved, both at more modest elevations of 3,100–4,300 m and even in the setting of extreme hypoxia, equivalent to the summit of Mount Everest.[38,39] The mechanisms responsible for preserved or enhanced myocardial contractile function at high altitude

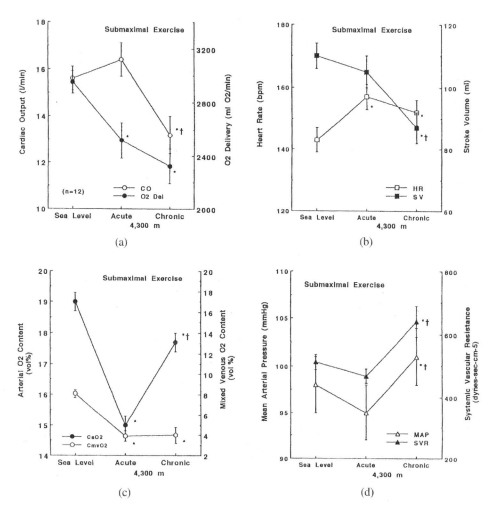

Figure 2. Submaximal exercise hemodynamic responses in 12 male subjects at 4,300 m. Submaximal exercise was at same absolute workload (100 watts) but this was 50% VO_2 max at sea level and 65% VO_2 max at high altitude. (a) Cardiac output and O_2 delivery; (b) heart rate and stroke volume; (c) arterial O_2 content and mixed venous O_2 content; (d) mean arterial pressure and systemic vascular resistance. * $p < 0.05$ vs. sea level. † $p < 0.05$ vs. acute hypoxia. Date are ± SE. Data derived from Refs. 18 and 36.

have not been clearly defined. Possibilities include enhanced sympathetic stimulation, a switch in myocardial metabolism with increased yield of ATP per molecule of oxygen, increases in myocardial blood flow, and transcriptional changes in nuclear and mitochondrial genes. The reduction in stroke volume is related to reductions in left ventricular end-diastolic volume (LVEDV), which is determined by cardiac filling. Although late LV diastolic filling is enhanced, it does not offset the reduction in early diastolic filling at altitude. There is diminished early diastolic filling and this is caused primarily by decreases in plasma volume. Plasma volume is reduced by 20–30% over the first few hours to days of high altitude exposure,[40] and prevention of this reduction in plasma volume reduced the decrease in stroke volume.[41] However, impaired LV filling is not completely explained by reduction in plasma volume since intravenous volume supplementation does not completely restore stroke volume.[34] Other possibilities that could explain a decrease in LVEDV include the increase in heart rate, similar to the effect of ventricular pacing, and impaired right ventricular function. Reductions in stroke volume during exercise are similar at both submaximal and maximal exercise, but reductions in heart rate also lead to a reduced cardiac output at maximal exercise.

Heart rate remains elevated compared to sea level, but it does decrease over time at high altitude. The magnitude of heart rate elevation appears to be related to the degree of altitude elevation. The mechanism responsible for the reduction in heart rate during submaximal exercise appears related to CaO_2 as administration of supplemental oxygen during submaximal exercise further reduces heart rate.[2] At maximal exercise, heart rate is clearly reduced and is related to the duration and severity of sustained hypoxia, especially at more extreme altitudes (Table 1). This reduction in heart rate at maximal exercise has been proposed to be related to several factors including a direct depressant effect of hypoxia on the sinus node, a depressant effect on central cortical irradiation (central command of cardiovascular responses), and under the control of exercising skeletal muscle in the setting of reduced work capacity. Alterations in autonomic nervous system control have also been considered but are unproven. Supplemental oxygen increases maximal heart rate, cardiac output, and VO_2 at 4,300 m, but the cardiac output is still less than at sea level.[42] The blunting of the heart rate response to exercise during sustained hypoxia occurs despite enhanced sympathetic activity.[32,43] This could be due to down regulation of myocardial beta-adrenergic receptors that occurs with sustained hypoxia exposure.[44,45] Enhanced parasympathetic activity may also play a role as the administration of atropine restored sea level values for maximal heart rate.[46] However, the responsiveness of heart rate to parasympathetic blockade is more prominent in subjects with the greatest reduction in sympathetic responsiveness, indicating a dual role of diminished sympathetic and enhanced parasympathetic activity.[47] Both atropine and glycopyrrolate have been used to augment parasympathetic activity and thus maximal heart rate at high altitude. However, there was no accompanying increase in VO_2 max. Thus, reduction in work capacity appears to be the primary cause of the reduction in maximal heart rate. Stroke volume remains the major determinant in the reduction in cardiac output during sustained hypoxia.

There are significant changes that occur in the systemic and coronary vascular beds that influence exercise capacity during sustained hypoxia. Since oxygen

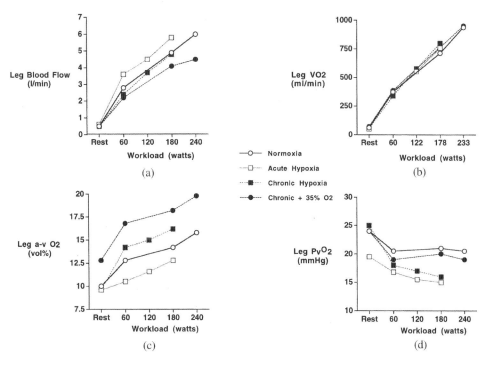

Figure 3.   Leg hemodynamics and oxygenation parameters in 7 men studied at 4,300 m. (a) leg blood flow by thermodilution; (b) leg VO_2 calculated from the Fick equation; (c) leg arteriovenous oxygen content difference; (d) femoral vein O_2 content. Data derived from Ref. 52.

delivery is the product of blood flow (cardiac output or leg blood flow) and CaO_2, changes in one factor will have a major impact on the other. At high altitude, oxygen delivery at rest and during exercise is reduced compared to sea level and this reduction does not change over time with sustained exposure to hypoxia. CaO_2 increases due to hyperventilation with a shift in the oxygen dissociation curve to the left that raises arterial O_2 saturation, and elevation in hemoglobin concentration by both hemoconcentration and eventfully an increase in RBC mass. As CaO_2 increases, there is a reduction in blood flow. This is seen in both cardiac output (Figure 2) and leg blood flow (Figure 3). There is also an increase in oxygen extraction related to both increased CaO_2 and a decrease in mixed venous and femoral venous O_2 content (Figure 2). If supplemental oxygen is given to further increase CaO_2, then there is a further decrease in blood flow (Figure 3). Hypocapnia may also play an important role in the regulation of blood flow during sustained hypoxia as there was no decrease in resting arm blood flow when hypoxia was induced in the setting of normocapnia.[48] It is unclear whether this is important during exercise. Similar physiology appears to occur in the coronary circulation despite the high degree of O_2 extraction at rest. With decreases in CaO_2 during acute hypoxia, coronary blood flow increases. In the setting of sustained hypoxia,

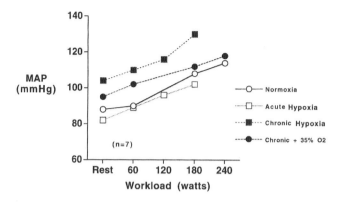

Figure 4.   Invasively determined mean arterial pressure (MAP) in 7 men studied at 4,300 m. Data obtained at rest and during exercise at sea level (normoxia) and acute and sustained hypoxia (18 days at 4,300 m). Acute normoxia was established after acclimatization with 35% oxygen. There was only partial restoration of sea level MAP. Figure derived from Ref. 52.

the myocardium is able to further increase the amount of O_2 extraction with a reduction in coronary blood flow. In a study of normal men at Leadville, Colorado (3,100 m), there was a 30% reduction in coronary blood flow, compensated by an increase in O_2 extraction over time at this altitude. All these adaptations result in a circulatory sparing effect.

Sympathetic stimulation increases over time at high altitude and results in increases in systemic blood pressure and systemic vascular resistance. This also occurs in the peripheral circulation and sympathetic vasoconstriction is no longer offset by "functional sympatholysis" or local metabolic vasodilation. This increase in systemic blood pressure has been shown to occur a rest, during 24-h ambulatory monitoring, and during exercise (Figure 4). The rise in systemic blood pressure is directly related to various indicators of enhanced sympathetic activity.[49,50] However, alpha- and beta-adrenergic blockade only modified but did not prevent the rise in systemic blood pressure with sustained hypoxia.[49,51] In addition, the administration of supplemental oxygen did not return blood pressure to sea level values (Figure 4).[52] The current mechanisms responsible for the increase in systemic blood pressure with sustained hypoxia have not been determined. Increases in both systemic and leg vascular resistance accompany the increase in system blood pressure with exposure to sustained hypoxia. Despite the increase in systemic vascular resistance and a decrease in blood flow and oxygen delivery, VO_2 is unchanged at a given workload. Even in the setting of beta-adrenergic blockade, similar physiologic changes occur (Figure 5). Femoral venous O_2 saturation during exercise approaches values measured at simulated altitudes >8,000 m.[36] This increased oxygen extraction offsets the decrease in oxygen delivery as a result of both sustained hypoxia and beta-adrenergic blockade.

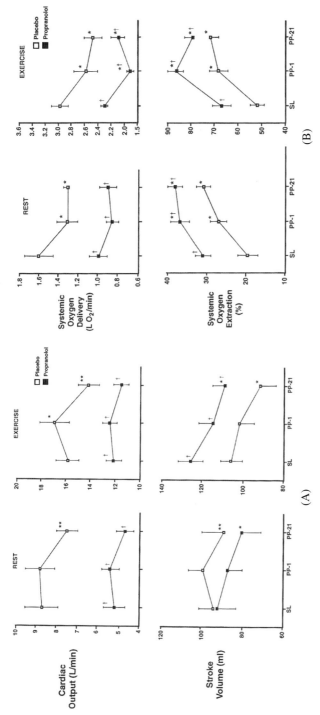

Figure 5. (A) Mean cardiac output and stroke volume responses at rest and during submaximal exercise at sea level, acute hypoxia (PP-1) and sustained hypoxia (PP-21) in 6 propranolol vs. 5 placebo treated subjects at 4,300 m. *Left upper and lower:* rest; *Right upper and lower:* submaximal exercise at 100 watts. $* p < 0.05$ vs. sea level. $** p < 0.05$ vs. sea level and PP-1. $+ p < 0.05$ vs. placebo. Taken from Ref. 36. (B) Mean systemic O_2 delivery (cardiac output $\times CaO_2$) and mean systemic O_2 extraction (arteriovenous O_2 content difference/$CaO_2 \times 100$) at rest and during submaximal exercise at sea level, PP-1 and PP-21 in six propranolol and five placebo treated subjects at 4,300 m. *Left upper and lower:* rest; *Right upper and lower:* exercise. $*p < 0.05$ vs. sea level. $+ p < 0.05$ vs. placebo. Taken from Ref. 36.

In applying the knowledge of these cardiovascular adaptations to exercise with sustained exposure to moderate altitude, a person can expect no significant increase in exercise capacity at the same altitude after short-term acclimatization. VO_2 max is unchanged and the VO_2 at a given submaximal workload is also unchanged. Heart rate may decrease somewhat but is still elevated compared to sea level. With acclimatization and an increase in CaO_2, cardiac output is decreased, while oxygen extraction increases. This results in a more "hypoxic tolerant" cardiovascular system. With a lower heart rate and improved blood volume, exercise may be better tolerated at altitude. In addition, there may be an advantage in improved exercise performance on the initial return to sea level.

Autonomic nervous system at high altitude

There are significant alterations in the autonomic nervous system with both acute and sustained exposure to hypoxia at high altitude. The peripheral chemoreceptors respond to the decrease in PaO_2 and there is enhanced sympathetic activation. This mechanism initiates ventilatory acclimatization. The arterial baroreceptors are also affected with decreased sensitivity to changes in pressure, causing a reduction in the gain of the heart rate response.[53] These peripheral receptors interact with several areas of the central nervous system including the nucleus *tractus solitarius* (NTS), the rostral ventromedulla, the C1 sympathoexcitatory region, the respiratory pre-Botzinger complex, the pons, and the hypothalamus. The exact mechanisms of these interactions have not been elucidated but the results of these interactions lead to enhanced sympathetic activity at high altitude. There are elevations in urinary and plasma catecholamines that begin with acute exposure and increase over time at high altitude.[32,54] Direct neural recordings from sympathetic nerves in skeletal muscle have also been shown to be elevated with acute[55] and sustained exposure to moderate altitudes.[43] Heart rate variability studies have demonstrated that there is a relative decrease in parasympathetic, compared to sympathetic, nerve activity on arrival at high altitude.[56,57] Over time at moderate altitude, this sympathetic predominance is enhanced. This enhanced sympathetic stimulation is also present during exercise with higher levels of arterial catecholamines. During acute exposure to hypoxia there are increased levels of epinephrine compared to norepinephrine. However, with continued exposure to the same altitude, epinephrine levels decrease while there is a significant increase in norepinephrine.[32] Both catecholamines have been postulated to have a major role in the cardiovascular adaptations that occur with sustained hypoxia at moderate altitudes (Figure 5). This hypothesis has led to the evaluation of the effects of both beta and alpha-adrenergic blockade on physiologic adaptations to high altitude. Beta-adrenergic blockade administered prior to ascent to altitude reduced the expected increase in heart rate, both at rest and during exercise, but there was no decrease in VO$_2$ max or ventilatory acclimatization.[36,58] Although there was a direct relationship between urinary norepinephrine levels and elevated mean arterial pressure (MAP) at 4,300 m, this relationship was not altered by beta-adrenergic blockade.[49] However, the correlation between urinary epinephrine and MAP was abolished. Studies with alpha-adrenergic blockade under conditions of sustained hypoxia have also produced conflicting results. While there was some reduction in diastolic and mean systemic pressure during exercise with the alpha-blocker prazosin in women after 48 h of hypoxia in a hypobaric chamber,[51] similar blockade after 12 days at 4,300 m only produced a mild reduction in systemic blood pressure observed with ambulatory monitoring.[59] Thus, although there is enhanced sympathetic activity that influences many of the cardiovascular responses to exercise at high altitude, selective adrenergic blockade has not significantly altered these adaptations. No studies have been performed utilizing combined adrenergic blockade. It should be noted that there have been no demonstrated reductions or enhancements in either submaximal or maximal exercise performance with adrenergic blockade at moderate high altitude. There are compensatory mechanisms that counteract the effects of these drugs on both alpha and beta-receptors. It is unclear whether downregulation of these adrenergic receptors may also be an important factor on the physiologic effects of adrenergic blockade at high altitude.

Parasympathetic nervous system activity is reduced with initial exposure to high altitude; however, it is unclear if parasympathetic activity is also responsible for some of the cardiovascular effects seen with sustained high altitude exposure. Atropine has been shown to restore heart rate at maximal exercise to sea level values,[46] but it appears that the response to atropine may depend on the extent of reduction in adrenergic responsiveness.[47] In studies where glycopyrrolate, a postganglionic anticholinergic drug, was shown to augment both resting and exercise heart rate, there was no increase in cardiac output during exercise and no improvement in VO$_2$ max at high altitude.[60] This effect is only seen at maximal exercise at high altitude as atropine increased heart rate during submaximal exercise at 4,300 m to the same extent as at sea level.[61] The interaction between the sympathetic and parasympathetic nervous system at high altitude is quite complex and both systems appear to play a role, especially in the heart rate responses, during exercise at high altitude (Figure 6).[93]

Respiratory, hematologic, and metabolic adaptations

Ventilatory acclimatization is the earliest and probably most important adaptation that occurs with exposure the hypoxia at high altitude. An increase in both resting

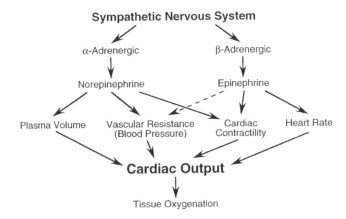

Figure 6.   Schematic of the effect of both norepinephrine and epinephrine on key cardiovascular factors that influence cardiac output and tissue oxygenation at high altitude.[93]

and exercise ventilation occurs within a few hours after arrival and continues for days to weeks with sustained exposure to a given altitude or with a gradual increase in elevation. The extent of enhanced ventilation depends on the hypoxic ventilatory response (HVR), initiated by peripheral chemoreceptors. This response can vary and is related to ventilatory responses to both hypoxia and CO_2. There is a greater susceptibility to a reduction in the HVR in elite athletes.[4,6] These athletes develop arterial O_2 desaturation at high levels of exercise and they may have a more difficult time adjusting to exercise at high altitude, especially with initial exposure to hypoxia. Ventilation during exercise is greater at high altitude than at sea level, but mostly during submaximal exercises. Ventilation at maximal exercise is usually not greatly affected at high altitude due to the reduction in VO_2 max. However, the ratio of ventilation to VO_2 is higher.[62] At progressive altitudes, there are minimal differences in ventilation at maximal exercise, despite progressive hypoxia. The most dramatic representation of this phenomenon is presented in Table 1. These data from the Operation Everest II study demonstrate minimal differences in minute ventilation, despite the decrease in VO_2 max with incremental increases in simulated altitude.[1] These data also demonstrate the ability of these normal subjects to exercise at maximal effort despite a mean arterial O_2 saturation (SaO_2) of 35 ± 3% at simulated 8,840 m. Work at a given power output during submaximal exercise occurs at a higher relative workload (% VO_2 max) as VO_2 max is reduced at high altitude. However, ventilation is also increased at the same relative workload. Minute ventilation during exercise increases in proportion to the degree of elevation or severity of hypoxia. Ventilatory acclimatization results in a leftward shift in the O_2 dissociation curve and increases the SaO_2 in the setting of a low inspired O_2 concentration. Thus, CaO_2 is increased with ventilatory acclimatization. With sustained exposure to moderate altitude, ventilation increases and contributes to the improvement in CaO_2 along with changes in blood volume and RBC mass.

Hemoglobin concentration is an important factor in CaO_2. An increase in CaO_2 will lead to an increase in oxygen delivery. On initial ascent to high altitude, this is accomplished by hemoconcentration with a decrease in plasma volume. With sustained hypoxia, there is a gradual increase in RBC mass. This increase is related to elevations in erythropoietin (EPO) that persist for the 1st 10 days at altitude. However, RBC mass has been shown to continue to rise for several months of sustained exposure to hypoxia at high altitude. There is considerable individual variation in this response and the factors responsible for this variation have not been clearly defined. Iron deficiency would be an impediment to developing an increase in RBC mass and, thereby, an increase in CaO_2. For most individuals who travel to high altitude, changes in RBC mass will not be a major factor in their exercise performance. Athletes need to consider several factors if they seek to improve their exercise performance by an increase in RBC mass from living or training at high altitude.[63] The altitude needs to be above 2,100 m and the duration of hypoxic exposure should be at least 13–14 h per day. There is substantial debate on the role of an increased RBC mass on exercise performance at high altitude. Studies utilizing both blood transfusions and EPO injections have shown either no improvement or only modest increases in exercise performance at moderate altitudes.[13,14] This is different than the known ergogenic effects of an increase in RBC mass at sea level.[64] At altitudes >4,500 m, there appears to be no significant improvement in exercise performance with an increased RBC mass. This suggests that oxygen delivery is not the limiting factor at these higher altitudes.

There is a shift in metabolism during exercise at high altitude. With both acute and sustained exposure to high altitude at 4,300 m there is an increased dependence of blood glucose at rest and during submaximal exercise.[65] This is a more O_2 efficient energy source than fatty acids or lipid with more ATP derived per unit O_2 consumed. Skeletal muscle was shown to be the predominant site of glucose disposal during exercise at high altitude. Some of this switch or crossover in metabolism may be related to the higher relative workload (% VO_2 max) at high altitude than at sea level. It is unclear whether changes in diet to enhance utilization of glucose at high altitude will result in enhanced exercise performance.

Exercise training approaches at high altitude

There are several aspects of high altitude acclimatization that may improve exercise performance in competitive endurance athletes. The most important of these adaptations is an increase in RBC mass that will lead to an increase in CaO_2 and thus improve oxygen delivery. In addition, ventilatory acclimatization that begins early after acute exposure to high altitude may be important in the athlete who travels from sea level to compete at high altitude. It is important to consider the goal of the athlete who wishes to use high altitude exposure in their training regimen. Is the goal to improve performance at high altitude or at sea level? Where should training occur, at high altitude or sea level? Finally, should the athlete have intermittent or more prolonged exposure to hypoxia in order to improve endurance performance?

For most endurance athletes who compete at high altitude, most of their training occurs at sea level. They will be exercising at the same absolute workload, but this will occur at a lower relative intensity at sea level, compared to high altitude. This higher relative exercise intensity is caused by the reduction in VO_2 max observed at high altitude. Thus, it may be advantageous to exercise at a greater intensity at sea level, but this is often impractical as they are already working at near maximal capacity. Timing of arrival and pre-acclimatization strategies become important approaches to improve performance at moderate to high altitude.[66] The ideal time for arrival prior to an endurance event at altitude is 14 days, as most short-term acclimatization effect will have occurred in this period of time. Within the 1st 14 days at 2,340 m there was a reported 4% per week increase in VO_2 max and a 6% per week increase in time to exhaustion.[15] A longer period or residence (14–21 days) did not result in any further improvement. This period of time should also prevent any loss of effects of sea level training. Usually during this time, the athlete will have reduced their training in preparation for an event. It is important to note that 14 days of residence at moderate altitude is not enough time to obtain a significant increase in RBC mass. In the study by Levine and colleagues, it required 4 weeks of residence at an altitude of 2,500 m to obtained a 7–8% increase in RBC mass.[67] Thus, the improvement in exercise performance during early altitude acclimatization occurs by a mechanism other than enhanced erythropoiesis. Some improvement in exercise performance can also be expected from a shorter residence at an altitude equivalent to where the event will occur. There will be a decrement and not an improvement in endurance performance if the athlete resides for 5 days at an altitude significantly greater than where the event will occur. However, short-term exposure to a lower high altitude elevation will lead to some pre-acclimatization with improved exercise performance. Subjects staying 6 days at 2,200 m had a 44% improvement in a time trial at 4,300 m, compared to acute hypoxic exposure.[68] This short-term lower altitude exposure led to ventilatory acclimatization and decreased symptoms of acute mountain sickness. Intermittent hypoxic exposure (IHE) using a small, enclosed, hypoxic environment, that can be set up in the athletes home at sea level, has been suggested to be an alternative approach to obtain altitude pre-acclimatization. This method allows exposure to normobaric hypoxia. However, exposure to IHE for 7 days did not improve cycle exercise performance.[69] Intermittent exposure to hypoxia in a hypobaric chamber did result in improved exercise performance at 4,300 m.[70] There is some evidence that intermittent hypoxic training at sea level may improve exercise performance at high altitude. This improvement has been seen in both cyclists and runners.[71,72] Finally, improvement in exercise performance upon arrival at high altitude is increased by administration of recombinant human erythropoietin (rhEPO). This administration has been shown to blunt the decrease in VO_2 max with acute exposure to hypoxia, but only at altitudes <3,500 m.[13] This form of "doping" is banned by all international sport governing bodies and is not a viable strategy for athletes seeking to improve their performance during high-altitude events. Another approach to minimizing the adverse effects of acute hypoxia exposure on endurance performance is to arrive as close to the event as possible. This is termed the "fly in, fly out" strategy and is widely used by professional teams in South America. It is unclear if this strategy is superior to whatever benefit that would be derived from short-term exposure by a day or overnight stay with resulting early ventilatory acclimatization. Most athletes will chose a given approach to enhance their exercise performance at high altitude based on multiple factors that are most advantageous to their situation. There are no comparative studies to determine which of the above approaches will lead to the greatest improvement in endurance performance.

The role of either training or residing at high altitude in improving endurance exercise performance at sea level has been the focus of multiple studies over the last 19 years. There are several approaches that have been used to investigate this important question. Athletes can both reside and train at high altitude. This has been the classical approach for many years and is termed "Live High-Train High" (LH–TH). This type of training should only be undertaken by an athlete who has been training at a high level for several years and cannot expect any significant increase in performance from continued training at sea level. The recommended altitude is between 1,800 and 2,500 m. At altitudes lower than 1,800 m, there are minimal stimuli for the important physiological adaptations that can result in improved exercise performance. The athlete needs to stay at high altitude for 3–4 weeks to obtain an improvement in exercise performance at sea level.[73] During this period of residence there is nearly complete ventilatory acclimatization and some increase in RBC mass. Longer duration of residence at high altitude is probably counterproductive with evidence of deterioration in exercise capacity. The main criticism of this type of training is that exercise training will occur at a lower absolute exercise intensity. Since VO_2 max is reduced at high altitude, any level of submaximal exercise will occur at a greater relative intensity than at sea level.

Therefore, the training stimulus will be less and this will reduce the expected improvement in exercise performance. However, there have been several approaches to address this issue. Athletes can exercise at a greater relative exercise intensity than at sea level.[74] This can be more feasible at altitude than at sea level as it can occur with less potential musculoskeletal trauma. Longer recovery times can be used and training can be instituted at a lower intensity, higher volume with interval training to maintain racing velocities. With acclimatization, the intensity of training can be increased.[75] It is important that athletes take iron supplements during this type of training since iron deficiency is common and will prevent the expected benefits of adaptations to sustained hypoxia. A recent meta-analysis of studies evaluating the LH–TH method has provided modest support for this type of training.[76] In uncontrolled studies there was a $1.9 \pm 2.3\%$ improvement in sea level performance; however, this improvement was reduced to $1.6 \pm 2.7\%$ in controlled studies. Although these changes appear small, they may be significant in a highly competitive athlete. Return to sea level and timing of an athletic event are also important issues with LH–TH.[77] Athletes can develop neocytolysis, which is a selective hemolysis of younger RBCs when erythropoietin levels fall below normal with deacclimatization. This process leads to a reduction in RBC mass and oxygen delivery with an expected decrease in exercise performance. In addition, the timing of the decay in ventilatory acclimatization and the potential effect of the increase in ventilatory work after altitude training on impairment of blood flow to exercising muscle at high workloads are unknown. All these factors make timing of the athletic event uncertain after descent from high altitude.

The other main approach to improving sea level performance utilizes the "Live High-Train Low" (LH–TL) technique. With this method athletes are able to attain the physiological benefits from acclimatization to high altitude but are able to train at a higher workload at lower altitude. The athlete can train at higher speeds with greater oxygen flux between the muscle capillary and mitochondria, compared to training at high altitude. In a study of athletes who lived at 2,500 m for 4 weeks but trained at a lower altitude of 1,250 m, there was a 7% increase in VO$_2$ max, a 1.5% improvement in a 3,000 m time trial, and a 3% improvement in a 5,000 m time trial.[67,78,79] These improvements were accompanied by a 7–8% increase in RBC mass. Subjects who trained and resided at 2,500 m had a similar increase in RBC mass but a slightly lower 6% improvement in VO$_2$ max and no improvement in the 3,000 and 5,000 m time trials. Despite these favorable results, there are other studies that do not demonstrate an improvement in sea level performance with the LH–TL method.[80] There are few double blinded, placebo-controlled studies available to make a firm conclusion about this type of training. Logistically, this type of training is challenging for an athlete to complete. The daily hypoxic exposure or dose needs to be ≥22 h at 1,800–2,500 m for a period of 3–4 weeks.[81] These conditions are difficult to attain using any type of nitrogen apartment or hypoxic tent at sea level.

High altitude illnesses and exercise

Many people who travel to higher altitude can develop various forms of illnesses directly related to the exposure to the hypoxic environment of high altitude. There are three main high altitude illnesses: acute mountain sickness (AMS), high altitude cerebral edema (HACE), and high altitude pulmonary edema (HAPE).[82] Acute mountain sickness is the most common and usually less severe form of high altitude illness. The main symptom is headache, but there are other associated symptoms including anorexia, nausea, malaise, dizziness, sleep disturbance, or a combination of these symptoms. AMS usually occurs at altitudes of >2,500 m (8,200 ft) with an incidence of 10–25% in unacclimatized individuals. However, cases have been reported between 2,000 and 2,500 m (6,560–8,200 ft). The greater the altitude, the more likely that AMS and other altitude illnesses can occur. There are several risk factors for the development of AMS and this assessment is important in determining a preventive strategy, especially in the competitive athlete who will be exercising at high altitude, whether for training or competition. These risk factors include a prior history of AMS or other altitude illnesses, rapid ascent to high altitude with lack of previous acclimatization, female sex, age <46 years, and a history of migraine headache. It is clear that exercise exacerbates the symptoms and a high level of aerobic fitness is not protective against AMS or other altitude illnesses. The symptoms usually begin within 6–12 h after arrival at altitude and last for 1–2 days. Unfortunately, many athletes or physically active people develop symptoms during their first arrival at high altitude and it is unclear how to estimate the risk of AMS or other altitude illnesses from information obtained at sea level. There is an association between abnormal ventilatory responses to hypoxic conditions at rest or during exercise at sea level and the development of severe AMS symptoms. Since exercise exacerbates AMS symptoms, a hypoxic cardiopulmonary exercise test has been proposed to identify subjects at increased risk and greater need for special preventive therapy.[83] However, these tests are not practical for the average person traveling to altitude and there is a great deal of overlap in the results between AMS and non-AMS subjects, making prediction of AMS difficult. There are several practical approaches that will reduce both the incidence and severity of AMS that apply to all persons planning on exercising at high altitude. If the planned activity is to occur at >3,000 m (9,840 ft), then a gradual ascent rate of 300–500 m (984–1,640 ft) per day is advised with a day of rest every 3–4 days. Gradual exposure to higher altitudes, either naturally by arriving at high altitude several days before an event or artificially using a hypobaric tent, will increase the ventilatory response to exercise and improve arterial oxygen saturation at rest. This usually occurs within a few days and should reduce the incidence of significant AMS symptoms. However, it is less clear whether exercise ventilation is improved and whether exercise performance is enhanced. Hydration is extremely important. High altitude exposure leads to a decrease in plasma volume, and hypovolemia from inadequate oral hydration can aggravate symptoms of AMS and adversely affect aerobic performance. Other factors including good nutrition with a higher carbohydrate intake and proper sleep hygiene are also important. There are several pharmacologic options to decrease the development of AMS. Acetylsalicylic acid and ibuprofen started several hours before ascent to altitude have been somewhat effective.[84] The more effective drug is acetazolamide, usually in low doses of 125 mg twice a day, started one day prior to arrival at altitude. This therapy has reduced the incidence of AMS in susceptible subjects by 44%. In subjects intolerant to acetazolamide due to side effects, or in subjects where acetazolamide is not effective, dexamethasone can be used. These drugs can be used in non-competitive athletes or in physically active people who travel to high altitude. However, both drugs have been banned by the World Anti-Doping Agency (WADA) and competitive athletes will be disqualified if they test positive for these substances. Other options include the supplement ginkgo biloba, but this may be contaminated with banned substances and again may lead to disqualification. For treatment of mild to moderate AMS symptoms, ibuprofen (600 mg) or acetylsalicylic acid (320 mg) can be taken, three times a day. For more severe symptoms with alteration of functional capacity, an antiemetic drug may be needed for nausea, and also supplemental oxygen for more severe malaise or concerns about the development of more severe altitude illnesses.

HACE and HAPE usually occur at altitudes >3,000 m (9,840 ft) and rarely occur at altitudes <2,500 m (8,200 ft). The principal signs of HACE include truncal ataxia, decreased consciousness, and mild fever. The development of recurrent vomiting and headache unresponsive to ibuprofen in a patient with severe AMS symptoms should alert one to the possible development of HACE. HAPE usually presents with worsening dyspnea, both at rest and during exercise, often with the initial development of a dry cough. There is loss of stamina and, often, obvious cyanosis. The cough will often progress to the development of pink, frothy sputum. Both these more serious forms of altitude illness usually develop after at least 2 days at high altitude and in the presence of more severe hypoxia at altitudes >10,000 ft. Obviously, both these conditions would prevent adequate physical performance by the athlete and exercise clearly exacerbates symptoms. Patients at risk of HACE have similar risk factors to those with AMS. In patients with HAPE, there is an association with an exaggerated pulmonary artery response to hypoxia and more frequent association with the major histocompatibility alleles HLA-DR6 and HLA-DQ4.[85] Of course this analysis was performed in subjects with a prior history of HAPE and routine genetic screening for risk of HAPE is not recommended. There are several drugs that have been shown to prevent the onset of HAPE in susceptible individuals. These include nifedipine, inhaled salmeterol, and tadalafil.[82,86] Tadalafil is a monitored substance by the WADA, but it has not been banned. Nifedipine is likely to unfavorably affect exercise performance, in part due to increased heart rate and lactate levels. There is limited information about the effectiveness of an inhaled beta-agonist in the prevention and treatment of HAPE. It does not appear to favorably or unfavorably affect exercise performance. As with any drug, the competitive athlete and coaching staff need to review the updated list of banned drugs by the WADA to avoid potential ineligibility. Thus, there are no good pharmacologic options for HAPE prevention in competitive athletes. Gradual acclimatization, adequate hydration, and appropriate nutrition remain the best options.

The most appropriate treatment for severe symptoms of both AMS and HAPE is rapid descent from high altitude, supplemental oxygen (2–4 L/min), and pulmonary vasodilators (nifedipine) for HAPE. For the competitive athlete, the balance of increased risk of a recurrent serious high altitude illness, especially when all preventive measures were undertaken, vs. the potential benefit from competing at high altitude needs to be seriously evaluated by the athlete and coaching staff.

The cardiovascular patient at high altitude

Exercise, especially with acute exposure to high altitude, results in a low arterial O_2 saturation, an increase in heart rate, enhanced sympathetic activity, a higher relative workload during submaximal exercise when compared to sea level, reduction in plasma volume, and elevation of systemic blood pressure. This sounds like the "perfect storm" for a coronary event in a cardiac patient who exercises at high altitude. In the patient with coronary artery disease there are several factors that could lead to instability of the coronary circulation and an acute coronary syndrome. These include the effect of hypoxia on plaque stability, the role of sympathetic stimulation, a direct hypoxic effect, and endothelial dysfunction. These factors influence both myocardial oxygen supply and demand. At sea level, myocardial ischemia occurs at a given heart rate and blood pressure product rate-pressure product (RPP) that occurs at a given submaximal workload. At high altitude, the VO_2 max is decreased and the same absolute workload occurs at a higher % of VO_2 max. Relative workload is responsible for the degree of sympathetic stimulation with elevations in heart rate and blood pressure rate-pressure product (RPP). Therefore, myocardial ischemia will occur at the same RPP but at a lower workload than at sea level. Thus, ischemia is caused by an increase in myocardial oxygen demand that exceeds the ability of coronary blood flow to supply the required oxygen for myocardial function.

Myocardial blood flow is also adversely affected by acute exposure to hypoxia. In normal individuals, coronary blood flow increases with hypoxia at high altitude.[28,87] However, in patients with atherosclerosis, there can be paradoxical coronary vasoconstriction with certain stimuli, such as exercise.[88] This paradoxical coronary vasoconstriction also occurs with acute hypoxia and is probably related to the increased sympathetic stimulation that occurs at high altitude.[89] Thus, there is also a decrease in myocardial oxygen supply and coronary obstruction becomes dynamic. Myocardial ischemia can occur at a lower heart rate and blood pressure than at sea level, independent of the workload during exercise. It can also occur at rest. This pattern of ischemia was seen in a study of elderly men at moderate altitude.[90] With acute hypoxic exposure, myocardial ischemia occurred at a lower heart rate and blood pressure than at sea level. However, with acclimatization ischemia occurred at the same heart rate and blood pressure as at sea level. Thus, acclimatization appears to diminish and possibly abolish paradoxical coronary vasoconstriction.

Heart rate may be one of the primary factors that could lead to myocardial ischemia at high altitude. There is an accelerated heart rate, especially with initial altitude exposure. Holter monitor recordings in downhill skiers in Colorado indicated that the mean heart rate was >80% of predicted maximum.[91] Blood pressure is also elevated during exercise at high altitude and this effect actually intensifies with an increased duration of altitude exposure.

Despite these potentially adverse physiological responses, cardiac patients can safely travel and exercise at high altitude. If a patient does not have ischemia at sea level, it is unlikely that unexpected ischemia will occur at high altitude, at least up to 2,500 m.[92] Patients who are stable, with good functional capacity at sea level, do not need any testing before traveling to high altitude. However, the patient who is elderly, has stable angina, limited exercise capacity at sea level, and decreased left ventricular systolic function at sea level, should undergo an exercise test before traveling to high altitude.

Cardiac patients with limited exercise capacity at sea level will also have difficulty with physical activity at high altitude. VO_2 max decreases by 1% for every 100 m of elevation above 1,500 m.[3] This magnitude of reduction was also seen in elderly patients[90] and patients with coronary disease.[92] At an altitude of 3,500–4,500 m, there is a 20–30% reduction in VO_2 max. If a patient with coronary disease has a peak VO_2 of less than 20 mL/kg/min, he or she will have very limited exercise capacity at high altitude. Information about a patient's exercise capacity

Table 3.   Guidelines for cardiac patients traveling to high altitude.

- Importance of stability and optimal fitness at sea level
- Consider exercise test in higher risk patients
- Importance of gradual acclimatization — 5 days
- On arrival — limit high intensity physical activity
- Maintain adequate hydration
- Check blood pressure, if possible
- Continue sea level medications (aspirin and statin)
- Need for nocturnal oxygen if sleep apnea at sea level
- Class III Heart Failure — avoid high altitude

can also be obtained by an exercise test at sea level. If the patient can improve his or her exercise capacity at sea level before they travel to high altitude, e.g. in a cardiac rehabilitation program, they will have greater functional capacity once they arrive.

Blood pressure should also be controlled at sea level before a patient travels to high altitude. It is likely that blood pressure will become further elevated, especially if the patient plans to stay for more than one week at high altitude. Some general guidelines for patients with coronary disease who travel to high altitude are included in Table 3.

Personal Perspective

Eugene E. Wolfel

I first became interested in exercise physiology while I was working in the Pulmonary Division at Ohio State while my wife was one of the chief residents in Pediatrics at Columbus Childrens' Hospital. I carried this interest with me when I started my cardiology fellowship at the University of Colorado. During the research years of my fellowship I worked with Hank Brammell, the medical director of our cardiac rehab program, on the effects of beta-adrenergic blockade on exercise training in normal subjects. I also worked with Lawrence Horwitz on a dog model investigating the role of the beta-adrenergic system in exercise performance. With this background, I was approached by Jack Reeves, one of the premier investigators in high altitude research, to join the group of investigators studying the physiology of exercise on Pikes Peaks (4,300 m) in Colorado. This collaboration led to nine years of productive research in this area of exercise physiology. My role in this research included performing skeletal muscle biopsies before and after exercise, evaluation of blood pressure and heart rate variability responses, and obtaining and interpreting the cardiovascular hemodynamics responses during exercise under a variety of physiologic and pharmacologic conditions. During this time, I had the privilege of working with several outstanding investigators including Robert Grover, George Brooks, Robert Mazzeo, Lorna Moore, Stacie Zamudio, Bert Groves, Allen Cymerman, Paul Rock, and Charles Fulco. Our research team was outstanding and our work would not have been successful without the expertise and experience provided by Rosann and Gene McCullough. I am also forever indebted to my deceased colleagues who contributed to my knowledge and success in these scientific endeavors. These former colleagues include John Sutton, Herbert Hultgren, Gail Butterfield, Amy Roberts, and especially Jack Reeves. I will never forget them and what they have contributed to my life and the field of high altitude physiology. I now carry this legacy forward in my role as the medical director of the cardiac rehabilitation program and exercise testing laboratory at the University of Colorado Hospital where our altitude is 5,280 ft (1,610 m). I am also using my knowledge of the physiology of exercise at high altitude in my additional role as a member of the Advanced Heart Failure and Cardiac Transplantation team at our institution. For me, the journey continues in both my clinical and scientific endeavors, to better understand the remarkable ability of humans to adapt and prosper under the physiologicial stresses imposed by visiting or living at high altitudes.

References

1. Cymerman A, Reeves JT, Sutton JR, Rock PB, Groves BM, Malconian MK, Young PM, Wagner PD, Houston CS. Operation Everest II: Maximal oxygen uptake at extreme altitude. *J Appl Physiol* 1989;66:2446–2453.
2. Reeves JT, Groves BM, Sutton JR, Wagner PD, Cymerman A, Malconian MK, Rock PB, Young PM, Houston CS. Operation Everest II: Preservation of cardiac function at extreme altitude. *J Appl Physiol* 1987;63:531–539.
3. Fulco CS, Rock PB, Cymerman A. Maximal and submaximal exercise performance at altitude. *Aviat Space Environ Med* 1998;69:793–801.
4. Gore CJ, Hahn AG, Scroop GC, *et al.* Increased arterial oxygen desaturation in trained cyclists during maximal exercise at 580 m altitude. *J Appl Physiol* 1996;80:2204–2210.
5. Wehrlin JP, Hallen J. Linear decrease in VO$_2$ max and performance with increasing altitude in endurance athletes. *Eur J Appl Physiol* 2006;96:404–412.
6. Mollard P, Woorons X, Letournel M, *et al.* Role of maximal heart rate and arterial O$_2$ saturation on the decrement in VO$_2$ max in moderate acute hypoxia in trained and untrained men. *Int J Sports Med* 2007;28:186–192.

7. Wagner PD, Sutton JR, Reeves JT, Cymerman A, Groves BM, Malconian MK. Operation Everest II: Pulmonary gas exchange during a simulated ascent of Mt Everest. *J Appl Physiol* 1987;63:2348–2359.

8. Oelz O, Howard H, DiPrampero PE, Hoppeler H, Claassen H, Jenni R, Buhlmann A, Ferretti G, Bruckner JC, Veicsteinas A, Gussoni M, Cerretelli P. Physiological profile of world-class high-altitude climbers. *J Appl Physiol* 1986;60:1734–1742.

9. Hennis PJ, O'Doherty AF, Levett DZH, Grocott MPW, Montgomery HM. Genetic factors associated with exercise performance in atmospheric hypoxia. *Sports Med* 2015;45:745–761.

10. Masschelein E, Puype J, Broos S, Thienen RV, Deldicque L, Lambrechts D, Hespel P, Thomis M. A genetic predisposition score associates with reduced aerobic capacity in response to acute normobaric hypoxia in lowlanders. *High Alt Med Biol* 2015;16:34–42.

11. Lundby C. *Exercise in High Altitude: Human Adaptation to Hypoxia.* Swenson, ER, Bartsch P (eds.), Springer: New York, Heidelberg, Dordrecht, London, 2014:301–323.

12. Lundby C, Damsgaard R. Exercise performance in hypoxia after novel erythyrpoiesis stimulating protein treatment. *Scand J Med Sci Sports* 2006;16:35–40.

13. Robach P, Calbet JAL, Thomsen JJ, Boushel R, Mollard P, Rasmussen P, Lundby C. The ergometric effect of recombinant human erythropoietin on VO$_2$ max depends on the severity of arterial hypoxemia. *PLoS One* 2008;3:e2996.

14. Young AJ, Slawka MN, Muza SR, Boushel R, Lyons T, Rock PB, *et al.* Effects of erythrocyte infusion on VO$_2$ max at high altitude. *J Appl Physiol* 1996;81:252–259.

15. Shuler B, Thomsen JJ, Gassmann M, Lundby C. Timing the arrival at 2340 m altitude for aerobic performance. *Scand J Med Sci Sports* 2007;17:588–594.

16. Beidleman BA, Muza SR, Rock PB, *et al.* Exercise responses after altitude acclimatization are retained during reintroduction to altitude. *Med Sci Sports Exer* 1997;29:1588–1595.

17. Horstman D, Weiskopf R, Jackson RE. Work capacity during a 3-wk sojourn at 4,300 m: Effects of relative polycythemia. *J Appl Physiol* 1980;49:311–318.

18. Wolfel EE, Groves BM, Brooks GA, Butterfield GE, Mazzeo RS, Moore LA, Sutton JR, Bender PR, Dahms TE, McCullough RE, McCullough RG, Huang SY, Sun SF, Grover RF, Hultgren HN, Reeves JT. Oxygen transport during stead-state submaximal exercise in chronic hypoxia. *J Appl Physiol* 1991;70:1129–1136.

19. Lundby C, Calbet JAL, Sander M, van Hall G, Mazzeo RS, Stray-Gundersen J, Stager JM, Chapman RF, Saltin B, Levine BD. Exercise economy does not change after acclimatization to moderate to very high altitude. *Scand J Med Sci Sports* 2007;17:281–291.

20. Chapman RF, Stager JM, Tanner DA, Stray-Gundersen J, Levine BD. Impairment of 3000-m run time at altitude is influenced by arterial oxyhemoglobin saturation. *Med Sci Sports Exerc* 2011;43:1649–1656.

21. Lara B, Salinero JJ, Del Coso J. Altitude is positively correlated to race time during the marathon. *High Alt Med Biol* 2014;15:64–69.

22. Roi GS, Giacometti M, Von Duvillard SP. Marathons in altitude. *Med Sci Sports Exer* 1999;31:723–728.

23. Dickinson ER, Piddington MJ, Brain T. Project olympics. *Schweiz Z Sport Med* 1966;14:305–308.

24. Peronnet F, Thibault G, Cousineau DL. A theoretical analysis of the effect of altitude on running performance. *J Appl Physiol* 1991;70:399–404.

25. Baggish Al, Wolfel EE, Levine BD. In *Exercise in High Altitude: Human Adaptation to Hypoxia*. Swenson ER, Bartsch P (eds.), Springer: New York, Heidelberg, Dordrecht, London, 2014:103–139.

26. Stenberg J, Ekblom B, Messin R. Hemodynamic response to work at simulated altitude, 4,000 m. *J Appl Physiol* 1966;21:1589–1594.

27. Kaufmann PA, Schirlo V Pavlicek V, *et al.* Increased myocardial blood flow during acute exposure to simulated altitudes. *J Nucl Cardiol* 2001;8:158–164.

28. Wyss CA, Koepfli P, Fretz G, Seenbauer M, Schirlo C, Kaufmann PA. Influence of altitude exposure on coronary flow reserve. *Circulation* 2003;108:1202–1207.

29. Chen CH, Liu YF, Lee SD, *et al.* Altitude hypoxia increases glucose uptake in human heart. *High Alt Med Biol* 2009;10:83–86.

30. Hackett JG, Abboud FM, Mark AL, Schmid PG, Heistad DD. Coronary vascular responses to stimulation of chemoreceptors and baroreceptors: Evidence for reflex activation of vagal cholinergic innervation. *Circ Res* 1972;31:8–17.

31. Richardson DW, Kontos HA, Raper AJ, Patterson JL Jr. Modification by beta-adrenergic blockade of the circulatory responses to acute hypoxia in man. *J Clin Invest* 1967;46:77–85.

32. Mazzeo RS, Bender PR, Brooks GA, Butterfield GE, Groves BM, Sutton JR, Wolfel EE, Reeves JT. Arterial catecholamine responses during exercise with acute and chronic high-altitude exposure. *Am J Physiol* 1991;261:E419–E424.

33. Klausen K. Man's acclimatization to altitude during the first week at 3,800 m. *Schweiz Z Sportmed* 1966;14:246–253.

34. Alexander JK, Hartley LH, Modelski M, Grover RF. Reduction of stroke volume during exercise in man following ascent to 3,100 m altitude. *J Appl Physiol* 1967;23:849–858.

35. Vogel JA, Hartley LH, Cruz JC, Hogan RP. Cardiac output during exercise in sea-level residents at sea level and high altitude. *J Appl Physiol* 1974;36:169–172.

36. Wolfel EE, Selland MA, Cymerman A, Brooks GA, Butterfield GE, Mazzeo RS, Grover RF, Reeves JT. O_2 extraction maintains O_2 uptake during submaximal exercise with beta-adrenergic blockade at 4,300 m. *J Appl Physiol* 1998;85:1092–1102.

37. Sutton JR, Reeves JT, Wagner PD, *et al.* Operation Everest II: Oxygen transport during exercise at extreme simulated altitude. *J Appl Physiol* 1988;64:1309–1321.

38. Fowles RE, Hultgren HN. Left ventricular function at high altitude examined by systolic time intervals and M-mode echocardiography. *Am J Cardiol* 1983;52:862–866.

39. Suarez J, Alexander JK, Houston CS. Enhanced left ventricular systolic performance at high altitude during Operation Everest II. *Am J Cardiol* 1987;60:137–142.

40. Prasad A, Popovic ZB, Arbab-Zadeh A, *et al*. Effects of age on plasma aldosterone levels and hemoconcentration at altitude. *Am J Cardiol* 2007;99:1629–1936.

41. Grover RF, Reeves JT, Maher JT, *et al*. Maintained stroke volume but impaired arterial oxygenation in man at high altitude with supplemental CO_2. *Circ Res* 1976;38: 391–396.

42. Pugh LG, Gill MB, Lahiri S, Milledge JS, Ward MP, West JB. Muscular exercise at great altitudes. *J Appl Physiol* 1964;19:431–440.

43. Hansen J, Sander M. Sympathetic neural overactivity in healthy humans after prolonged exposure to hypobaric hypoxia. *J Physiol* 2003;546(Pt 3):921–929.

44. Voelkel NF, Hegstrand L, Reeves JT, McMurty IF, Molinoff PB. Effect of hypoxia on density of beta-adrenergic receptors. *J Appl Physiol* 1981;50:363–366.

45. Richalet JP, Larmignat P, Rathat C, Keromes A, Baud P, Lhoste F. Decreased cardiac response to isoproterenol infusion in acute and chronic hypoxia. *J Appl Physiol* 1988;65:1957–1961.

46. Hartley LH, Vogel JA, Cruz JC. Reduction of maximal exercise heart rate at altitude and it reversal with atropine. *J Appl Physiol* 1974;36:362–365.

47. Savard GK, Areskog NH, Saltin B. Cardiovascular response to exercise in humans following acclimatization to extreme altitude. *Acta Physiol Scand* 1995;154:499–509.

48. Cruz JC, Grover RF, Reeves JT, Maher JT, Cymerman A, Denniston JC. Sustained venoconstriction in man supplemented with CO_2 at high altitude. *J Appl Physiol* 1876;40:96–100.

49. Wolfel EE, Selland MA, Mazzeo RS, Reeves JT. Systemic hypertension at 4,300 m is related to sympathoadrenal activity. *J Appl Physiol* 1994;76:1643–1650.

50. Reeves JT, Mazzeo RS, Wolfel EE, Young AJ. Increased arterial pressure after acclimatization to 4,300 m. Possible role of norepinephrine. *Int J Sports Med* 1992;13 (1):S18–S21.

51. Mazzeo RS, Carroll JD, Butterfield GE, Braun B, Rock PB, Wolfel EE, Zamudio S, Moore LG. Catecholamine responses to alpha-adrenergic blockade during exercise in woman acutely exposed to altitude. *J Appl Physiol* 2001;90:121–126.

52. Bender PR, Groves BM, McCullough RE, *et al*. Oxygen transport to exercising leg in chronic hypoxia. *J Appl Physiol* 1988;65:2592–2597.

53. Sagawa S, Torii R, Nagaya K, Wada F, Endo Y, Shiraki K. Carotid baroreflex control of heart rate during acute exposure to simulated altitudes of 3,800 m and 4,300 m. *Am J Physiol* 1997;273(4 Pt 2):R1219–R1223.

54. Cunningham WL, Becker EJ, Kreuzer F. Catecholamines in plasma and urine at high altitude. *J Appl Physiol* 1965;20:607–610.

55. Saito M, Mano T, Iwase S, Koga K, Abe H, Yamazaki Y. Responses in muscle sympathetic activity to acute hypoxia in humans. *J Appl Physio* 1988;65:1548–1552.

56. Hughson RL, Yamamoto Y, McCullough RE, Sutton JR, Reeves JT. Sympathetic and parasympathetic indicators of heart rate control at altitude as studied by spectral analysis. *J Appl Physiol* 1994;77:2537–2542.

57. Perini R, Milesi S, Biancardi L, Veicsteinas A. Effects of high altitude acclimatization on heart rate variability in resting humans. *Eur J Appl Physiol Occup Physiol* 1994;73:521–528.

58. Moore LG, Cymerman A, Huang SY, McCullough RE, McCullough RG, Rock PB, Young A, Young P, Weil JV, Reeves JT. Propranolol blocks metabolic rate but not ventilatory acclimatization to 4,300 m. *Respir Physiol* 1987;70:195–204.

59. Mazzeo RS, Dubay A, Kirsch J, Braun B, Butterfield GE, Rock PB, Wolfel EE, Zamudio S, Moore LG. Influence of alpha-adrenergic blockade on the catecholamine response to exercise at 4,300 m. *Metabolism* 2003;52:1471–1477.

60. Boushel R, Calbet JA, Radegran G, Sondergaard H, Wagner PD, Saltin B. Parasympathetic neural activity accounts for the lowering of exercise heart rate at high altitude. *Circulation* 2001;104:1785–1791.

61. Grover RF, Weil JV, Reeves JT. Cardiovascular adaptation to exercise at high altitude. *Exer Sport Sci Rev* 1986;14:269–302.

62. Lundby C, Calbet JAL, van Hall G, Saltin B, Sander M. Pulmonary gas exchange at maximal exercise in Danish lowlanders during 8 wk of acclimatization to 4,100 m and in high-altitude Aymara natives. *Am J Physiol* 2004;287:R1202–R1208.

63. Schmidt W, Prommer N. Effects of various training modalities on blood volume. *Scand J Med Sci Sports* 2008;18(1):57–69.

64. Buick FJ, Gledhill N, Froese AB, Spriet L, Meyers EC. Effect of induced erythrocythemia on aerobic work capacity. *J Appl Physiol* 1980;48:626–642.

65. Brooks GA, Butterfield GE, Wolfe RR, Groves BM, Mazzeo RS, Sutton JR, Wolfel EE, Reeves JT. Increased dependence on blood glucose after acclimatization to 4,300 m. *J Appl Physiol* 1991;70:919–927.

66. Chapman RF, Laymon AS, Levine BD. Timing of arrival and pre-acclimatization strategies for the endurance athlete competing at moderate to high altitude. *High Alt Med Biol* 2013;14:319–324.

67. Levine BD, Stray-Gundersen J. "Living high-training low": Effect of moderate altitude acclimatization with low altitude training on performance. *J Appl Physiol* 1997;83:102–112.

68. Fulco CS, Muza SR, Beidleman B, Jones J, Stabb J, Rock PB, Cymerman A. Exercise performance of sea-level residents at 4300 m after 6 days at 2200 m. *Aviat Space Environ Med* 2009;80:955–961.

69. Beidleman BA, Muza SR, Fulco CS, Jones JE, Lammi E, Staab JE, Cymerman A. Intermittent hypoxic exposure does not improve endurance performance at altitude. *Med Sci Sports Exerc* 2009;41:1317–1325.

70. Beidleman BA, Muza SR, Fulco CS, Cymerman A, Sawka MN, Lewis SF, Skrinar GS. Seven intermittent exposures to altitude improves exercise performance at 4300 m. *Med Sci Sports Exerc* 2008;40:141–148.

71. Roels B, Bentley DJ, Coste O, Mercier J, Millet GP. Effects of intermittenthypoxic training on cycling performance in well trained athletes. *Eur J Appl Physiol* 2007;101:359–368.

72. Dufoour SP, Ponsot E, Zoll J, Doutreleau S, Lonsdorfer-Wolf E, Geny B, Lampert E, Fluck M, Hoppeler H, Billat V, Mettauer B, Richard R, Lonsdorfer J. Exercise training

in normobaric hypoxia in endurance runners. I. Improvement in Aerobic performance capacity. *J Appl Physiol* 2006;100:1238–1248.

73. Rusko HK, Tikkanen HO, Peltonen JE. Altitude and endurance training. *J Sports Sci* 2004;22:928–944.

74. Friedmann-Bette B. Classical altitude training. *Scand J Med Sci Sports* 2008;18 (1):11–20.

75. Saunders PU, Pyne DB, ad Gore CJ. Endurance training at altitude. *High Alt Med Biol* 2009;10:135–148.

76. Bonetti DL, Hopkins WG. Sea-level exercise performance following adaptation to hypoxia: A meta-analysis. *Sports Med* 2009;39:107–127.

77. Chapman RF, Laymond Stickford AS, Lundby C, Levine BD. Timing of return from altitude training for optimal sea level performance. *J Appl Physiol* 2014;116: 837–843.

78. Chapman RF, Stray-Gundersen J, Levine BD. Individual variation in response to altitude training. *J Appl Physiol* 1998;85:1448–1456.

79. Levine BD. Intermittent hypoxic training: Fact and fancy. *High Alt Med Biol* 2002;3: 177–193.

80. Geiser J, Vogt M, Billeter R, Zuleger C, Belforti F, Hoppeler H. Training high-living low: Changes of aerobic performance and muscle structure with training at simulated altitude. *Int J Sports Med* 2001;22:579–585.

81. Wilber RL, Stray-Gundersen J, Levine BD. Effect of hypoxic "dose" on physiological responses and sea level performance. *Med Sci Sports Exerc* 2007;39:1590–1599.

82. Bartsch P, Swenson ER. Acute high altitude illnesses. *New Engl J Med* 2013;368:2294–2302.

83. Richalet JP, Canoui-Poitrine F. Pro: Hypoxic cardiopulmonary exercise testing identifies subjects at risk of severe high altitude illnesses. *High Alt Med Biol* 2014;15: 315–317.

84. Luks AM, McIntosh SE, Grissom CK. Wilderness medical society consensus guidelines for the prevention and treatment of acute altitude illnesses. *Wilderness Environ Med* 2010;21:146–155.

85. Hanaoka M, Kubo K, Yamazaki Y, Miyahara T, Matsuzawa Y, Kobayashi T, Sekiguchi M, Ota Y, Watanabe H. Association of high altitude pulmonary edema with the major histocompatibility complex. *Circulation* 1998;97:1124–1128.

86. Koehle MS, Cheg I, Sporer B. Canadian academy of sport and exercise medicine position statement: Athletes at high altitude. *Clin J Sport Med* 2014;24:120–127.

87. Beaudin AE, Brugniaux JV, Vohringer M, Flewitt J, Green JD, Friedrich MG, Poulin MJ. Cerebral and myocardial blood flow responses to hypercapnia and hypoxia in humans. *Am J Physiol Heart Circ Physiol* 2011;301:H1678–H1686.

88. Gordon JB, Ganz P, Nabel EG, Fish RD, Zebede J, Mudge GH, Alexander RW, Selwyn AP. Atherosclerosis influences the vasomotor response of epicardial coronary arteries to exercise. *J Clin Invest* 1989;83:1946–1952.

89. Arbab-Zadeh A, Levine BD, Trost JC, Lange RA, Keeley EC, Hillis LD, Cogarroa JE. The effect of acute hypoxemia on coronary arterial dimensions in patients with coronary artery disease. *Cardiology* 2009;113:149–154.

90. Levine BD, Zuckerman JH, deFilippi CR. Effect of high-altitude exposure in the elderly: The Tenth Mountain Division study. *Circulation* 1997;96:1224–1232.
91. Grover RF, Tucker CE, McGroarty SR, Travis RR. The coronary stress of skiing at high altitude. *Arch Intern Med* 1990;150:1205–1208.
92. Erdmann J, Sun KT, Masar P, Niederhauser H. Effects of exposure to altitude on men with coronary artery disease and impaired left ventricular function. *Am J Cardiol* 1998;81:266–270.
93. Wolfel, EE. Sympathy, Adrenal and Cardiovascular adaptation to hypoxia. In the 8th International Hypoxia Symposium Proceedings. Houston CS (eds.), Queen City Printer, Inc. Berlington, VT, 1993:62–80.

Chapter 9

Cardiovascular Problems
with Swimming and Diving

Alfred A. Bove

Emeritus Professor of Medicine
Temple University School of Medicine
Philadelphia, PA, USA

The Aquatic Environment

Swimming and diving underwater are activities that go back to ancient times. Ancient Greek images on an Assyrian Freize show divers swimming underwater with weapons suggesting that they were in some form of underwater combat.[1] Fishermen used spears underwater for many centuries to catch fish for sustenance, and in Japan the Ama divers (commercial female breathhold divers) have worked at harvesting marine life for many centuries.[2,3] In the late 19th century, equipment was developed to allow divers to remain underwater for prolonged periods to perform work tasks with breathing air supplied continuously from the surface. In the post-World War II era, self-contained underwater breathing equipment (SCUBA) became available to the public and the sport of recreational diving grew with estimates of over two million recreational divers in the US.[4] Breathhold diving also continues to be a sport followed by many divers. Single breath dives of over 500 ft have been reported. Breathhold diving for depth records has developed into a competitive sport.[2] In addition to these diving exposures, the triathlon (swim–bike–run) has become a popular sport with several hundred thousand individuals competing annually. The swimming phase of the triathlon produces unique physiological responses that can result in pulmonary edema.[5,6] Death in triathlons is almost entirely confined to the swimming phase of the event.[7] Exposure to the aquatic environment produces changes that result from immersion, breathholding, increased ambient pressure, heat loss, altered oxygen and carbon dioxide partial pressure, and changes in the kinetics of inert gases in blood and tissues.

The Physical Environment

The most evident change in the environment underwater is the increased ambient pressure. In sea water, ambient pressure increases by one atmosphere for each 33 ft (10 m) of depth. Since the pressure at the surface is one atmosphere, at 33 ft depth, the total ambient pressure is two atmospheres absolute (ATA). In water, pressure and depth are linearly related, thus pressure at any depth can be calculated from the relationship of 33 ft depth in sea water (FSW) = one atmosphere pressure. Table 1 shows the relationship between depth and pressure. Exposure to increased ambient pressure produces effects from two important physical principles: Boyle's law and Henry's law.

Boyle's law

In 1668, Robert Boyle demonstrated that the volume of a fixed mass of inert gas was inversely proportional to the ambient pressure.[8] In the body, this effect results in reduction of gas volume with increased ambient pressure. Paranasal sinuses, middle ear, and lungs are the most affected spaces when diving underwater.

Table 1.   Guage pressure at various depths in seawater.

Depth	Pressure	atm ata	P abs	PO_2
feet	psi	atm	ata	ata
0		0.0	1.0	0.21
33	14.7	1.0	2.0	0.42
66	29.4	2.0	3.0	0.63
99	44.1	3.0	4.0	0.84
132	58.7	4.0	5.0	1.05
165	73.4	5.0	6.0	1.26
198	88.1	6.0	7.0	1.47

Middle ear barotrauma due to inadequate equilibration of pressure during descent is the most common form of injury related to pressure,[9] while lung injury during ascent when breathing compressed air is the most dangerous injury related to pressure effects from Boyle's law (see next section). Breathhold divers undergo significant reductions in lung volume when immersed.

Henry's law

William Henry in 1803[10] described the increased dissolution of gases in liquids with increased gas partial pressure. As ambient pressure increases, inert gas (nitrogen) concentration in tissues and other body fluids is increased. On ascent, the increased nitrogen dissolved in the body can become supersaturated as pressure is reduced and will change to a gas phase, resulting in free gas in tissues and blood. This process results in a pathologic process labeled decompression sickness (see next section).

Immersion

Volume shifts and pulmonary edema

When an individual is immersed in water to the neck, the surrounding pressure opposes gravitational effects on the venous system and 600–700 mL of blood are shifted into the central circulation.[3,11] This additional blood expands lung vascular volume, and results in increased volume of the cardiac chambers. Atrial dilatation induces release of natriuretic hormones that increase urine production (swimmer's diuresis). In individuals with compromised cardiac function the fluid shift can result in acute pulmonary edema. Expansion of lung vascular volume, associated with immersion and increased exercise, a combination often experienced by triathletes and divers, can result in increased pulmonary venous pressure, which combined with the increased lung vascular volume, can result in increased pulmonary capillary pressure and pulmonary edema.[12–14] This effect has been identified as swimming induced pulmonary edema (SIPE[15]) or immersion pulmonary edema (IPE[13]), and is associated with onset of severe dyspnea, cough, blood tinged sputum, and evidence of lung congestion on physical examination and chest X-ray. In addition to these immersion effects, exercise itself can induce lung congestion and pulmonary edema.[16,17] West and co-workers[18] described exercise-induced pulmonary hemorrhage (EIPH) in race horses. Subsequent studies have described similar changes in humans at high levels of exercise.[16,17] Expansion of the atria during water immersion can also stimulate atrial arrhythmias.

Diving reflex

Air breathing marine mammals (whales, seals) are known to dive to profound depths while breathholding. During their diving exposure, they demonstrate profound bradycardia, with arterial vasoconstriction that limits blood flow to skeletal muscle, and preserves perfusion and oxygenation of the brain and heart.[19–21] The diving reflex is a vagally-mediated reflex that responds to cold and water sensations on the face.[22] Because skeletal muscle blood flow is limited during diving, significant lactate production occurs, and metabolic acidosis develops that requires post-dive hyperventilation to restore metabolic balance. The diving reflex is poorly developed in most humans, however, some individuals demonstrate significant bradycardia when their face is immersed in water. Attempts have been made to use the diving reflex to convert atrial tachycardia to sinus rhythm.[23]

Breathhold diving

While marine mammals have adapted to their existence underwater with structural, metabolic, and regulatory changes, for the most part, there is little adaptation to immersion and breathholding in humans. Marine mammals have cartilaginous ribs that allow the thorax to collapse as lung volume is reduced by increasing pressure, and as noted above, marine mammals have a well-developed diving reflex that shunts blood away from skeletal muscle during diving to preserve blood flow to brain and heart. Reduced muscle blood flow also reduces oxygen consumption and allows prolonged time underwater. Metabolic acidosis resulting from anaerobic metabolism appears to be better tolerated in marine mammals compared to humans.

Gas exchange

Immediately upon breathholding, blood and tissue oxygen stores begin to fall, and blood and tissue carbon dioxide content begins to rise.[2,24] During diving, muscle blood flow is not reduced as it is in diving marine mammals, and oxygen is rapidly consumed from available stores in blood and tissues. Increasing ambient pressure initially increases the partial pressure of oxygen and lowers the urge to breathe even though total oxygen stores are not increased. Upon ascent, oxygen partial pressure will fall suddenly as ambient pressure falls, and can reach levels that cannot sustain cerebral function resulting in loss of consciousness.[24] This phenomenon is called Shallow Water Blackout, because it does not require diving to occur. It is a common cause of drowning in breathhold divers. While rising carbon dioxide levels contribute to the urge to breath, the increased oxygen partial pressure suppresses the urge and breathholding can be prolonged enough to result in shallow water blackout upon ascent. Shallow water blackout can also occur in underwater swimmers especially if the swimmer hyperventilates to increase the tolerated time underwater. Hyperventilation reduces pre-dive carbon dioxide. Carbon dioxide increases during the swim, but may not reach the level which forces the swimmer to breathe before decreasing oxygen content producing unconsciousness and drowning.

Lung volume changes

During a breathhold dive, lung volume is reduced with depth according to Boyle's law. Thus, at a depth equivalent to five atmospheres (132 FSW), total lung volume will be reduced to 20% of its surface volume, and approaches residual volume. Because the thorax is rigid and cannot shrink to compensate for reducing lung volume as in marine mammals, the reduced gas volume is compensated by blood shifts into the pulmonary circulation.[25] As lung volume continues to shrink below residual volume with increasing depth, progressive engorgement of the pulmonary vasculature eventually causes capillary rupture, pulmonary edema, and alveolar hemorrhage. Findings of reduced arterial oxygen saturation, cough, and hemoptysis in breathhold divers seeking to set depth records supports this diagnosis.[26,27] While lung volume reduction with depth is predictable, and suggests that maximal breathhold depths should be in the range of 6–8 ATA (165–230 FSW), depth records have exceeded this range in a number of world record dives. Depths over 500 FSW have been achieved without serious lung injury. The record holders usually have low residual volume/total lung capacity (TLC) ratios, and forcefully expand their lung volume above usual TLC using "lung packing" techniques. These techniques allow significant volume reduction under pressure, and when accompanied by blood shifts into the pulmonary vasculature, will allow the 90–95% volume reduction without significant lung injury.

Injuries Due to Diving with Compressed Gas

The sport and occupation of diving usually involves underwater exposure with use of a life support system to supply breathing gas underwater and allow prolonged exposure underwater for work or recreation.[28] Breathing gas can be supplied from the surface through a hose attached to an air compressor (surface supplied diving), or can be carried with the diver in high pressure containers where gas can be compressed to 100 ATA and provided to the diver at ambient pressure through a pressure reduction regulator (self-contained diving). In both cases, the diver breathes oxygen-containing compressed gas at ambient pressure, and is subjected to both

Boyle's law effects due to changing volumes of gas, and to Henry's law effects due to increased dissolution of inert gas in blood and tissues.[29]

Direct and Indirect Effects of Pressure

Barotrauma

Changes in gas volume with increasing pressure result in changes in volume of the middle ear, paranasal sinuses, stomach, and other occult pockets of gas sometimes found around tooth roots, and occasionally within intervertebral discs.[30–33] Each of these spaces creates a specific syndrome when gas volume is reduced under pressure, unless equilibration of the space can be achieved during descent. Equalization of the middle ear can be accomplished by performing a Valsalva maneuver to force air into the Eustachian tubes and into the middle ear.[9] Similarly, equalization of paranasal sinuses can be accomplished by increasing the pressure in the nasopharynx with a Valsalva maneuver. On ascent, expanding gas in the maxillary sinus can injure the Trigeminal nerve.[30] Failure to equilibrate these spaces results in vascular engorgement, and hemorrhage into the space, and in the case of the middle ear, tympanic rupture. Rupture of the round window can also occur from barotrauma during descent with loss of perilymph and accompanying vertigo, hearing loss, and tinnitus. Tooth pain (barodontalgia) occurs on descent when a gas pocket around a tooth is compressed, or on ascent when gas in a trapped space expands. Failure to equilibrate the air in the face mask on descent can cause injury to the periorbital and orbital tissues.[31,32] Expansion of gas within an intervertebral disc results in a radiculopathy, often in the cervical or lumbar distribution. Expansion of gas in the stomach on ascent can result in overdistention and gastric rupture with an accompanying pneumoperitoneum.[34]

Pulmonary barotrauma

When breathing compressed gas underwater, gases in the lung must expand upon ascent according to Boyle's law. Thus, lung gas volume will double after breathing compressed air at 33 FSW, and the expanding volume must be ventilated appropriately or the expanding gas will distend and disrupt lung tissue.[34–38] Expanding gas in a damaged lung will dissect to the pleural surface and result in a pneumothorax, or will dissect into the mediastinum and to the soft tissues of the neck causing pneumomediastinum and subcutaneous emphysema.[36] Tension pneumothorax is an emergency as the expanding gas in the pleural space will compress venous return and result in shock.

The most serious of the lung barotrauma complications is arterial gas embolism.[36] When gas expands and injures the lung, capillaries are ruptured, gas enters the pulmonary capillary circulation, travels to the left atrium and to the arterial circulation. Chronic lung disorders can increase susceptibility.[37] Typical roentgenographic findings have been described.[38] Arterial gas embolism commonly affects the cerebral circulation causing stroke, and unconsciousness.[39] The unconscious diver often aspirates water and drowns. Coronary arterial gas embolism can result in transient coronary ischemia, but rarely causes a myocardial infarction. Large gas volumes injected into the arterial circulation can fill the left ventricle and proximal aorta with air, obstructing cardiac output, and resulting in shock and death.[40] Treatment requires urgent recompression in a hyperbaric chamber to reduce intravascular gas volume and provide increased oxygen partial pressure to oxygenate ischemic tissues.

Pulmonary barotrauma is prevented by careful training, focused on normal breathing during ascent from a dive. Some divers with focal lung disease can develop lung barotrauma due to local airway obstruction and overexpansion of a lung segment.[37] Candidates for diving with a history of lung disease (e.g. bronchiectasis, tuberculosis) should be evaluated for evidence of local airway obstruction using pulmonary function testing or computed tomographic imaging.

Decompression sickness

Henry's law dictates the increasing concentration of inert gas in tissues and blood that accompanies exposure to increased pressure. The molar concentration of nitrogen, for example, increases significantly when breathing air at increased pressure. Other inert gases follow the same principles, thus when helium is used in the breathing gas, tissue helium concentration increases. While oxygen and carbon dioxide content also increase with increased ambient pressure, oxygen is quickly consumed by metabolism, and the high solubility of carbon dioxide reduces the likelihood of supersaturation of this gas in tissues. Inert gas, however, rapidly becomes supersaturated when ambient pressure falls, and follows the kinetics of supersaturated solutions, where at a point in the degree of supersaturation, the solute will change phase.[41,42] In the case of dissolved solids, a solid, often crystalline form of the solute is formed, while in the case of a dissolved gas, the solute phase change results in free gas formation. Diffusion limitations dictate that gas enters and leaves tissues in an exponential fashion. Figure 1 shows a set of tissue nitrogen uptake and washout curves first described by Boycott *et al.*[41] who pointed out that the body could be considered to be made up of several tissue compartments, characterized by the rate at which gases entered and left the tissues with

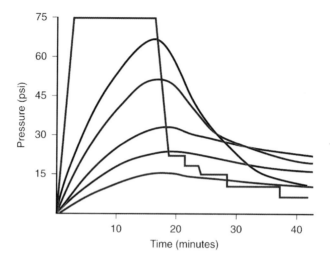

Figure 1. Tissue nitrogen concentration vs. time for five tissue compartments during exposure to 75 PSI environmental pressure for 18 min and stepwise return to atmospheric pressure. Pressure exposure profile is shown in red. The nitrogen concentration of five hypothetical tissue compartments expressed as partial pressure are shown by the black lines. Each compartment has a different rate of nitrogen uptake and washout. After Boycott et al.[42]

change in ambient pressure. They proposed a decompression protocol that established stops at different depths during ascent from diving to allow supersaturated tissues to eliminate nitrogen before it converted into the gas phase. These principles have been incorporated into computer algorithms that compute safe decompression schedules for different depth-time exposures.[42] These have been incorporated into small wrist-mounted computers that can be carried on a dive to provide a real-time calculation of decompression schedules and present them in a visible display to the diver.

The disorder that results from free gas formation in organs and tissues is called Decompression Sickness (DCS).[43,44] Symptoms and signs of DCS vary depending on where gas formation occurs and which tissue and organ function are affected by the expanding gas. Golding et al.[43] proposed a description of DCS that involved two levels of severity. Type I was less severe, did not affect neurologic function, and was often concentrated in large joints (musculoskeletal DCS[45]), type II or more severe DCS was associated with impaired neurologic function, particularly focused on the spinal cord, and severe respiratory distress. Musculoskeletal DCS is usually categorized as a type I disorder, a cutaneous form (*Cutis Marmorata*, Figure 2) is also grouped with type I DCS, while evidence of spinal cord or cerebral injury is considered type II DCS, as is respiratory DCS resulting from significant gas embolism to the pulmonary circulation and vascular obstruction. Inner

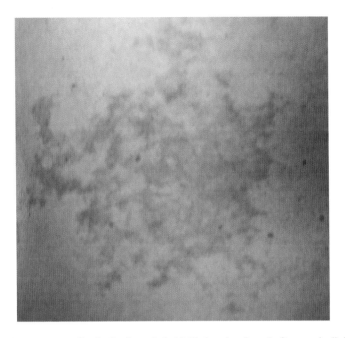

Figure 2.   *Cutis marmorata* (Latin for "mottled skin") that developed after an air diving exposure.

ear DCS associated with abrupt neurologic hearing loss is also considered to be type II DCS.[46,47] Table 2 provides a summary of signs and symptoms of DCS. Symptoms of DCS appear after surfacing from a dive that commonly exceeds safe boundaries for DCS risk. Symptoms can occur up to 24 h following the diving exposure, but most symptoms appear within the 1st 6 h after diving.[48] Exposure to altitude following diving can aggravate bubble formation and DCS symptoms due to further reduction in ambient pressure.[49,50] Osteonecrosis is a long-term consequence of diving thought to be related to obstruction by bubbles of bone vasculature.[51,52]

Factors affecting DCS risk

Various studies have been conducted to elucidate factors that can increase DCS risk. Depth-time profile is the most important factor affecting risk of DCS as it establishes the degree of supersaturation of tissue inert gas. Several studies have demonstrated that older divers seem to be more prone to DCS compared to younger divers.[53,54] Exercise immediately following diving also appears to increase risk of DCS.[55] Exposure to warm water also can increase risk of DCS.[56] An important controversy involves the role of a patent foramen ovale (PFO) in DCS risk. Several

Table 2.   Signs and symptoms of decompression syndrome.

Joint pain	%
Leg	30
Arm	70
Dizziness	5.3
Paralysis	2.3
Shortness of breath	1.6
Extreme fatigue	1.3
Unconsciousness	0.5

meta-analyses and clinical studies[57–60] suggest that a PFO increases risk for DCS. Because there is clear evidence that initial bubble formation is observed in the venous system,[61,62] there is concern that a right to left shunt at the atrial level would allow venous gas emboli (VGE) to arterialize and result in arterial embolization. The degree of VGE is related to the tissue gas load and the degree of supersaturation that occurs during ascent. To date, there have been no prospective studies demonstrating the value of PFO closure on DCS risk, however, the study of Honek *et al.*[63] suggests that a large PFO in the presence of large amounts of VGE would increase DCS risk. Large amounts of VGE are likely to cross the PFO resulting in arterial embolism.[63] Closure of a large PFO eliminated arterial bubbles in their study. At present, there is no justification for routinely closing a PFO in divers.

Fitness

Recreational diving is generally performed at a 3–4 METs exercise level.[64] However, because of unpredictable water conditions, exercise demand can quickly increase to 6–7 METs from currents, wind, and surface wave action. The study of Prendergast *et al.*[64] demonstrated a non-linear relationship between speed of swimming with scuba gear and energy demand (Figure 3). This can be theoretically derived from the hydraulics of fluid motion that describe the relationship between water resistance and velocity as a second order relationship (Figure 3). Most healthy individuals below age 50 with average conditioning can exercise comfortably at 6–7 METs.[65] Exercise demand greater that this level will usually exceed anaerobic and dyspnea thresholds, resulting in limits to exercise capacity, and often panic while diving. Recommended exercise capacity is 6–7 METs of steady-state exercise to manage contingencies. A peak capacity of twice the steady-state capacity would be a measure of safety for divers.

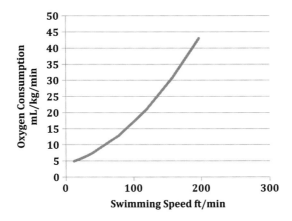

Figure 3.   Oxygen consumption vs. swimming speed for a diver with full scuba equipment. The curve shows a disproportionate increase in oxygen consumption as swimming speed increases. Data from Pendergast *et al.*[65]

Temperature

Diving and triathlon exposures occur primarily in water temperatures below usual skin temperature (85°F). In triathlons, a thermal protective dress is often used when water temperature is below 78°F, while in diving, thermal protection is usually needed even in water temperature of 80–82°F due to the lower exercise activity and longer duration of water exposure. Diving dress can be used for thermal protection in waters at 35–45°F, and often involves systems that supply constant hot water flow from the surface into a suit to maintain body temperature.[28] Commercial divers can be supported for multi-hour exposures with such systems. Thermal protection for SCUBA divers can consist of a neoprene wet suit that holds a fixed layer of water heated by body thermal energy. Once warmed, this warm water layer provides thermal insulation. Wet suits can be used for temperatures down to 60°F. At lower temperatures, full dress suits that are dry and provide thermal protection by an air layer are used. Hypothermia usually progresses slowly, and often is undetected until the diver develops mental changes, and motor incapacity. Rapid rewarming is essential for divers demonstrating clinical evidence of hypothermia. Concern has been expressed for the development of ventricular fibrillation in the heart of divers with profound hypothermia as rewarming occurs.

Medical Disorders and Diving

Because diving is a recreational sport, it often attracts candidates for the sport who have chronic medical disorders. Some disorders can be aggravated by diving and a knowledge of basic principles of diving exposure can aid in making decisions regarding fitness for diving.

ENT disorders

A chronically perforated tympanic membrane is considered to be a contraindication to diving because of the propensity of water to enter the middle ear and result in otitis media. There are specially designed diving masks that incorporate ear covers to prevent water from entering the ear canal. Using a dry diving system, with a full helmet, also prevents water from entering the middle ear. Chronic nasopharyngeal congestion due to allergies or infection prevents usual equalization of the middle ear and paranasal sinuses. Recurrent injury to the middle ear can impair hearing and cause a chronic otitis media that can extend into the mastoid cells. Chronic sinus infection can result from repeated sinus barotrauma. Unilateral neurologic hearing loss is considered a relative contraindication to diving because of the risk (although small) of neurologic injury to the functioning ear with permanent total hearing loss. Many ear surgeons consider surgical reconstruction of middle ear ossicles to be a contraindication because of the high likelihood of recurrent damage to the ossicles that would result from ear barotrauma.

Pulmonary disorders

Chronic obstructive lung disease is usually a contraindication to diving due to reduced exercise capacity, and chronically damaged lung parenchyma that makes the diver prone to pneumothorax. Asthma has been considered to be a contraindication to diving, but experience with asthmatic divers in the US and other countries suggests that most asthmatics can dive safely if their asthma is controlled with medication, and they are not experiencing an acute exacerbation at the time of diving.[66,67] A history of spontaneous pneumothorax due to congenital pleural blebs is considered a contraindication to diving as these often rupture due to the intrapulmonary pressures noted with diving, and result in a pneumothorax. Tetzlaff et al.[37] found an increased incidence of pulmonary lesions in divers who sustained unexplained lung barotrauma and arterial air embolism.

Cardiovascular disorders

Impaired exercise capacity due to cardiomyopathy, congenital heart disease, valvular, or ischemic heart disease is a relative contraindication to diving.[68] Limited exercise impairment with mild cardiac conditions often can be tolerated during recreational diving in low stress exposures (warm water, calm sea state, minimal current). Exercise testing to determine safe exercise capacity, presence of ischemia, and arrhythmias can guide decisions on fitness for diving in these patients. Patients with chronic right to left shunts due to congenital heart disease are at risk for para-doxical air embolism and should not dive. Most of these patients are cyanotic with reduced arterial oxygen saturation and limited exercise capacity. Elevated pulmo-nary pressure due to high pulmonary vascular resistance imposes significant limi-tations to exercise in these patients. Patients with right atrial to pulmonary artery conduits (Fontan, Glen shunts) are sensitive to volume shifts in the venous circula-tion and have limited exercise capacity. These patients might tolerate very low stress recreational diving, but would not manage increased exercise demands dur-ing diving.[69] Patients with NYHA Class I heart failure could participate safely in low stress recreational diving. Patients with significant impairment (NYHA Class III–IV) would experience limitations due to the demands of even minimal stress diving and should not dive.

Atrial Arrhythmias

Supraventricular tachycardia, paroxysmal atrial flutter, and fibrillation can be pro-voked by diving due to central blood shifts and atrial distention during water immersion. Divers who are prone to these arrhythmias can be advised to use PRN beta-blockers to reduce risk for these arrhythmias during diving. Patients with per-manent atrial fibrillation can undertake diving safely if they have adequate exercise tolerance, and are aware of bleeding risk from anticoagulants (see next section).

Pacers/ICDs

Patients with implanted pacemakers have been able to dive safely. Most manufac-turers provide specifications on pressure tolerance of pacemakers and many have been tested to pressures of 3–4 ATA (66–99 FSW[70]). Some patients with implant-able cardioverter defibrillators (ICD) report no problems while diving (personal communication). Like pacemakers, ICDs are usually designed to function in increased pressure environments. Review of the manufacturer specifications is essential for divers who wish to return to diving after having an ICD implanted. Lampert *et al.*[71] followed over 328 athletes with ICDs who returned to sports activ-ity. Many returned to competitive sports. Over a mean observation period of 31 months, there were 49 who experienced an ICD shock while participating in sports. There were no fatalities and most of the shocks were appropriate. No divers were included in her registry, however, comparable sport experience suggests that divers with implanted ICDs would be able to dive safely. The cardiac disorder requiring the ICD should also be considered. For patients with heart failure with reduced ejection fraction, the heart failure status is more likely to complicate diving than the presence of an ICD.

Long QT Syndrome

Ackerman *et al.*[72] reported a series of patients who had survived near drowning and were found to have the long QT syndrome. They ultimately identified patients with the LQT1 variant as being susceptible to ventricular tachycardia and fibrillation when swimming. Some portion of unexplained drowning is likely due to ventricular fibrillation developing in swimmers or divers with the LQT1 gene. Although risk of an arrhythmic event is low in these patients, and may be mitigated by an implanted ICD or medical therapy for LQT syndrome, divers should be cautioned about the risk.

Cardiac Transplantation

Diving is generally not recommended in patients with cardiac transplant due to immunosuppression and potential exposure to water borne pathogens that can be aspirated while breathing underwater. However, isolated reports describe heart transplant patients who have returned to limited diving.

Coronary Artery Disease

Most diving training organizations issue a certification for sport diving qualifications that is permanent, and can be used throughout a lifetime. Sport diving operations require a certification card to allow divers to participate, but in the absence of a time limit, many divers who were certified in their 3rd or 4th decade develop coronary disease later in life and still retain the initial certification that permits them to participate in diving. Most diving operations provide their divers with a medical questionnaire regarding history of important illnesses that might complicate diving, but the responses are personal and often not verified. Current experience indicates that the majority of sudden death events while diving are related to coronary disease.[73,74] Divers who develop coronary disease are at risk for cardiac events while diving and screening for safety should be done in any diver with coronary disease who wishes to participate.

Asymptomatic Coronary Disease

As with any other sport activity, an individual who seeks advice about safety during sports activity, needs to be screened for cardiovascular risk. For most individuals who wish to participate in recreational diving, an exercise capacity of 6–7 METs (see previous section) is needed to manage contingencies such as transporting heavy diving gear, swimming in currents or rough seas, assistance with a struggling diver, etc. Most exercise physiology texts[65] recommend a peak capacity of about twice the steady-state capacity, thus a peak capacity during exercise testing should be about 13 METs. The candidate should not demonstrate ischemic changes, arrhythmias, or severe hypertension at the 6–7 MET level. A standard CVD risk calculator can be used to assess CVD risk. If CVD risk exceeds 10% with the Framingham calculator[75] or 7.5% with the Pooled Cohort Equations,[76] further evaluation with stress testing should be recommended.

Known Coronary Disease

Patients with established coronary disease and stable angina should not undertake sport diving. The sport provides many opportunities for excess stress and unplanned high exercise demands that can provoke ischemia and an angina event. When diving, there is little opportunity to reduce activity or take sublingual nitroglycerin. Divers who develop angina while diving often need assistance or rescue, and can put other divers in jeopardy.

Coronary Revascularization

Many divers undergo either surgical or percutaneous coronary revascularization and wish to return to diving. Many sport divers have returned to sport diving after coronary revascularization. Of prime concern is the residual ischemia following the revascularization procedure. The coronary anatomy, and the arteries that were revascularized, residual coronary occlusive disease, and the status of left ventricular function all need to be considered after revascularization. If revascularization leaves no residual myocardial flow limitations, and the diver or diving candidate can exercise to 6–8 METs without evidence of ischemia or arrhythmias, low stress recreational diving can be permitted. Surgical bypass patients should wait 6 months to recover from surgery, regain exercise capacity, and undergo testing to evaluate exercise capacity and risk for ischemia. Percutaneous revascularization patients should wait at least 3 months post procedure and be tested for exercise capacity and ischemia before returning to diving.

Peripheral Arterial Disease

While risk of a sudden unexpected cardiac event while diving is likely to be lower than the risk associated with known coronary disease, many patients with peripheral arterial disease have generalized atherosclerosis that includes coronary disease that may be undiagnosed. These patients should undergo exercise testing before being approved for diving. If claudication limits swimming capacity, these divers should be instructed to avoid situations where high levels of exercise are anticipated.

Patients with thoracic aortic aneurysms may be at risk for aneurysm rupture due to the transient increase in stroke volume that follows a Valsalva maneuver.[77] Divers may be at risk for rupture of the ascending aorta if the diameter exceeds 4.5 cm. Guidance for managing thoracic aortic aneurysms can be found in current guidelines.[77]

Diabetes

While the apparent concern for diabetics is the risk of a hypoglycemic event while underwater, these have been rare. Of greater concern is the increased risk for occult coronary disease and an unexpected cardiac event while diving. Insulin dependent diabetics should not dive without special instructions on management of insulin during diving.[78] Insulin pumps must be removed before diving as they are susceptible to damage by increased pressure and water immersion. Non-insulin dependent diabetics are less likely to have difficulty with glucose management during diving, and should consider diving like any other physical activity and adjust their medication accordingly.

Medications

For recreational divers, diving exposure does not alter the effect or the metabolism of medications. Medications that induce sedation can exacerbate the narcotic effects of nitrogen, however, the nitrogen narcotic effects are not significant at usual sport diving depths. Divers who travel to tropical latitudes should be warned about sun sensitizing medications (e.g. amiodarone, tetracyline, etc.), and divers who are using diuretics should be cautioned about dehydration if they are in warm climates. Antihypertensive medications in usual doses are not a contraindication to diving, but divers should be cautioned about hypotension. One approach is to wait until diving is completed before taking daily antihypertensive medications. Usual doses of beta-blockers are well tolerated during diving. Anticoagulant medications are not a contraindication to diving, however, divers must be cautioned about ear and sinus barotrauma as there is likely to be excess bleeding into paranasal sinuses and the middle ear if a diver taking anticoagulants experiences a barotrauma event. Usual doses of antianxiety and antidepression medications are tolerated in recreational diving and are not a contraindication.

Summary

Diving underwater for military, commercial, and sport has been done for many years. At present, recreational diving exposes several million people to this environment. Changes in pressure and temperature, as well as exercise demands provide unique problems in this community. In addition, the number of athletes of all ages who compete in triathlons is increasing. The swimming component of this sport presents problems similar to problems related to immersion in divers. More detailed reviews of the topic can be found in Refs 79–81.

Personal Perspective

Alfred A. Bove

Dr. Bove was chief of Cardiology at Temple University Medical School for a total of 18 years between 1986 and 2009. He was president of the American College of Cardiology in 2009, and president of the Undersea and Hyperbaric Medical Society in 1984. He is trained as a Navy Undersea Medical Officer and served on active and reserve duty in the Navy for 33 years. He is board certified in Internal Medicine, Cardiology, and Undersea and Hyperbaric Medicine. He is the author of the text *Bove and Davis' Diving Medicine*, published by Elsevier in 2004, and Co-author of the text *Exercise Medicine* published by Academic Press in 1983. He is the director of the Temple University continuing education program in Diving Medicine, and continues to participate in sport diving for recreation. He has been a competitive runner since 1952, and has completed 23 marathons, 4–50 mi races, a Tin-Man triathlon, and 4 sprint triathlons, as well as numerous shorter distance races. Dr. Bove had been involved in clinical and basic research in heart failure, environmental medicine, telemedicine, exercise and sports medicine, and bioengineering.

References

1. http://en.wikipedia.org/wiki/Timeline_of_diving_technology. Accessed 1/23/2015.
2. Ferrigno M. Breath Hold Diving. In Bove AA (ed.), *Bove and Davis' Diving Medicine*. Philadelphia, Elsevier, 2004:77–94.
3. Hong SK, Cerretelli P, Cruz JC, *et al*. Mechanics of respiration during submersion in water. *J Appl Physiol* 1969;27:537–538.
4. http://wiki.answers.com/Q/How_many_recreational_scuba_divers_in_the_world. Accessed 3/14/2014.
5. Stefanko G, Lancashire B, Coombes JS, Fassett RG. Pulmonary oedema and hyponatraemia after an ironman triathlon. *BMJ Case Rep* 2009;pii:bcr04.2009.1764.

6. Boggio-Alarco JL, Jaume-Anselmi F, Ramirez-Rivera J. Acute pulmonary edema during a triathlon occurrence in a trained athlete. *Bol Asoc Med P R* 2006;98: 110–113.

7. Harris KM, Henry JT, Rohman E, Haas TS, Maron BJ. Sudden death during the triathlon. *J Am Med Assoc* 2010;303(13):1255–1257.

8. Boyle R. Defence of the Doctrine Touching the Spring and the Weight of the Air. In *New Experiments Physico-Mechanical. Touching the Air*. Oxford University Press, 1662.

9. Hunter SE, Farmer JC. Ear and Sinus Problems in Diving. *In* Bove AA (ed.), *Bove and Davis' Diving Medicine*. 4th (edn.), Philadelphia: WB Saunders, 2004:431–460.

10. Henry W. Experiments on the quantity of gases absorbed by water, at different temperatures, and under different pressures. *Philos T Roy Soc* 1803;93:29–274.

11. Fraser JA, Peacher DF, Freiberger JJ, Natoli MJ, Schinazi EA, Beck IV, Walker JR, Doar PO, Boso AE, Walker AJ, Kernagis DN, Moon RE. Risk factors for immersion pulmonary edema: Hyperoxia does not attenuate pulmonary hypertension associated with cold water immersed prone exercise at 4.7 ATA. *J Appl Physiol* 2011;110: 610–618.

12. Shupak A, Weiler-Ravell D, Adir Y, Daskalovic YI, Ramon Y, Kerem D. Pulmonary oedema induced by strenuous swimming: A field study. *Respir Physiol* 2000;121: 25–31.

13. Koehle MS, Lepawsky M, McKenzie DC. Pulmonary oedema of immersion. *Sports Med* 2005;35:183–190.

14. Pons M, Blickenstorfer D, Oechslin E, Hold G, Greminger P, Franzeck UK, Russi EW. Pulmonary oedema in healthy persons during scuba-diving and swimming. *Eur Respir J* 1995;8:762–767.

15. Adir Y, Shupak A, Gil A, Peled N, Keynan Y, Domachevsky L, Weiler-Ravell D. Swimming induced pulmonary edema: Clinical presentation and serial lung function. *Chest* 2004;126:394–399.

16. Zavorsky GS, Saul L, Decker A, Ruiz P. Radiographic evidence of pulmonary edema during high-intensity interval training in women. *Respir Physiol Neurobiol* 2006;153:181–190.

17. Zavorsky GS. Evidence of pulmonary oedema triggered by exercise in healthy humans and detected with various imaging techniques. *Acta Physiol* 2007;189: 305–317.

18. West JB, Mathieu-Costello O, Jones JH, Birks EK, Logemann RB, Pascoe IR, Tyler WS. Stress failure of pulmonary capillaries in racehorses with exercise-induced pulmonary hemorrhage. *J Appl Physiol* 1993;75:1097–1109.

19. Irving L, Solandt OM, Solandt DY, Fischer KC. The respiratory metabolism of the seal and its adjustment to diving. *J Cell Comp Physiol* 1935;7:137–151.

20. Irving L. Bradycardia in human divers. *J Appl Physiol* 1963;18:489–491.

21. Lindholm P, Lundgren C. The physiology and pathophysiology of human breath-hold diving. *J Appl Physiol* 2009;106:284–292.

22. Bove AA, Lynch PR, Connell JV, Harding JM. Diving reflex after physical training. *J Appl Physiol* 1968;25:70–72.

23. Whitman V, Sakeosian GM. The diving reflex in termination of supraventricular tachycardia in childhood. *J Pediatr* 1976;89:1032–1033.
24. Craig AB Jr. Causes of loss of consciousness during underwater swimming. *J Appl Physiol* 1961;16:583–586.
25. Craig AB Jr. Depth limits of breath hold diving (an example of Fennology). *Respir Physiol* 1968;5:14–22.
26. Muth CM, Radermacher P, Pittner A, *et al.* Arterial blood gases during diving in elite apnea divers. *Int J Sports Med* 2003;24:104–107.
27. Lindholm P, Lundgren CE. Alveolar gas composition before and after maximal breath-holds in competitive divers. *Undersea Hyperb Med* 2006;33:463–467.
28. Navy Department: U.S. Navy Diving Manual, Rev 6, Vol 5, Diagnosis and Treatment of Decompression Sickness and Arterial Gas Embolism. (Publication No. NAVSEA 0910-LP-106–0957). Washington, DC: U.S. Navy Department, 2008.
29. Bert P. Barometric Pressure: Researches in Experimental Physiology (Hitchcock MA, Hitchcock FA, transl). Columbus Book Co, 1943. Reprinted by the Undersea Medical Society, Bethesda, MD, 1878.
30. Butler FK, Bove AA. Infraorbital hypesthesia after maxillary sinus barotrauma. *Undersea Hyperb Med* 1999;26:257–260.
31. Butler F. Orbital hemorrhage following facemask barotrauma. *Undersea Hyperb Med* 2001;28:31–34.
32. Latham E, van Hoesen K, Grover I. Diplopia due to mask barotrauma. *J Emerg Med* 2011;41:486–488.
33. Hayden JD, Davies JB, Martin IG. Diaphragmatic rupture resulting from gastrointestinal barotrauma in a scuba diver. *Brit J Sports Med* 1998;32:75–76.
34. Behnke AR. Analysis of accidents occurring in training with the submarine "lung". *US Naval Med Bull* 1932;30:177–184.
35. Polak B, Adams H. Traumatic air embolism in submarine escape training. *US Naval Med Bull* 1932;30:165–177.
36. Schaefer KE, Nulty WP, Carey C, *et al.* Mechanisms in development of interstitial emphysema and air embolism on decompression from depth. *J Appl Physiol* 1958; 13:15–29.
37. Tetzlaff K, Reuter M, Leplow B, *et al.* Risk factors for pulmonary barotrauma in divers. *Chest* 1997;112:654–659.
38. Harker CP, Neuman TS, Olson LK, *et al.* The roentgenographic findings associated with air embolism in sport scuba divers. *J Emerg Med* 1993;11:443–449.
39. Massey EW, Greer HD. Neurologic Consequences of Diving. In Bove AA (ed.), *Bove and Davis' Diving Medicine* 4th (edn.), Philadelphia: WB Saunders, 2004;461–474.
40. Neuman TS, Spragg RG, Wagner PD, *et al.* Cardiopulmonary consequences of decompression sickness. *Respir Physiol* 1980;41:143–155.
41. Boycott AE, Damant GCC, Haldane J. The prevention of compressed air illness. *J Hyg* 1908;8:342–443.
42. Vann RD. Mechanisms and Risk of Decompression Sickness. In Bove AA (ed.), *Bove and Davis' Diving Medicine* 4th (edn.), Philadelphia: WB Saunders, 2004;127–164.

43. Golding FC, Griffiths P, Hempleman HV, *et al.* Decompression sickness during construction of the Dartford Tunnel. *Brit J Ind Med* 1960;17:167–180.

44. Francis TJR, Smith DH. Describing Decompression Illness (42nd UHMS Workshop). Kensington, Md, Undersea and Hyperbaric Medical Society, 1991.

45. Gempp E, Blatteau JE, Simon O, Stephant E. Musculoskeletal decompression sickness and risk of dysbaric osteonecrosis in recreational divers. *Diving Hyperb Med* 2009;39:200–204.

46. Gempp E, Louge P. Inner ear decompression sickness in scuba divers: A Review of 115 cases. *Eur Arch Otorhinolaryngology* 2013;270:1831–1837.

47. Farmer JC, Thomas WG, Youngblood DG, *et al.* Inner ear decompression sickness. *Laryngoscope* 1976;86:1315–1326.

48. Vann RD, Butler FK, Mitchell SJ, Moon RE. Decompression illness. *Lancet* 2011;377:153–164.

49. Ryles MT, Pilmanis AA. The initial signs and symptoms of altitude decompression sickness. *Aviat Space Environ Med* 1996;67:983–989.

50. Conkin J, Waligora JM, Foster PP, *et al.* Information about venous gas emboli improves prediction of hypobaric decompression sickness. *Aviat Space Environ Med* 1998;69:8–16.

51. McCallum RI, Walder DN. Bone lesions in compressed air workers. *J Bone Joint Surg* 1966;48:207–235.

52. Cimsit M, Ilgezdi S, Cimsit C, Uzun G. Dysbaric osteonecrosis in experienced dive masters and instructors. *Aviat Space Environ Med* 2007;78:1150–1154.

53. Carturan D, Boussuges A, Vanuxem P, *et al.* Ascent rate, age, maximal oxygen uptake, adiposity, and circulating venous bubbles after diving. *J Appl Physiol* 2002;93: 1349–1356.

54. Sulaiman ZM, Pilmanis AA, O'Conner RB. Relationship between age and susceptibility to altitude decompression sickness. *Aviat Space Environ Med* 1997;68: 695–698.

55. Gempp E, Blatteau JE. Influence of exercise on decompression sickness. *Appl Physiol Nutr Metab* 2008;33:666–670.

56. Leffler CT, White JC. Recompression treatments during the recovery of TWA Flight 800. *Undersea Hyperb Med* 1997;24:301–308.

57. Bove AA. Risk of decompression sickness with patent foramen ovale. *Undersea and Hyperba Med* 1998;25:175–178.

58. Torti SR, Billinger M, Schwerzmann M, *et al.* Risk of decompression illness among 230 divers in relation to the presence and size of patent foramen ovale. *Eur Heart J* 2004;25:1014–1020.

59. Germonpré P, Dendale P, Unger P, Balestra C. Patent foramen ovale and decompression sickness in sports divers. *J Appl Physiol* 1998;84:1622–1626.

60. Wilmshurst PT, Treacher DF, Crowther A, *et al.* Effects of a patent foramen ovale on arterial saturation during exercise and on cardiovascular responses to deep breathing, Valsalva manoeuvre, and passive tilt: Relation to history of decompression illness in divers. *Brit Heart J* 1994;71:229–231.

61. Kumar VK, Waligora JM, Billica RD. Utility of Doppler-detectable microbubbles in the diagnosis and treatment of decompression sickness. *Aviat Space Environ Med* 1997;68:151–158.
62. Eftedal OS, Lydersen S, Brubakk AO. The relationship between venous gas bubbles and adverse effects of decompression after air dives. *Undersea Hyperb Med* 2007;34:99–105.
63. Honek J, Sramek M, Sefc L, Januska J, Fiedler J, Horvath M, Tomek A, Novotny S, Honek T, Veselka J. Effect of catheter-based patent foramen ovale closure on the occurrence of arterial bubbles in scuba divers. *J Am Coll Cardiol Intv* 2014;7:403–408.
64. Pendergast DR, Tedesco M, Nawrocki DM, *et al*. Energetics of underwater swimming with SCUBA. *Med Sci Sports Exerc* 1996;28:573–580.
65. Levine BD. Exercise Physiology for the Clinician. In Thompson PD (ed.), *Exercise and Sports Cardiology*. New York: McGraw Hill, 2001:6–8.
66. Neuman TS, Bove AA, O'Connor RD, Kelsen SG. Asthma and diving. *Ann Allergy* 1994;73:344–350.
67. Elliott DH. Are Asthmatics Fit to Dive. *Kensington MD, Undersea Hyperb Med Society* 1996.
68. Bove AA. The cardiovascular system and diving risk. *Undersea Hyperb Med* 2011;38:261–269.
69. Goldberg DJ, Avitabile CM, McBride MG, Paridon SM. Exercise capacity in the Fontan circulation. *Cardiol Young* 2013;23:824–830.
70. Lafay V, Trigano JA, Gardette B, Micoli C, Carre F. Effects of hyperbaric exposures on cardiac pacemakers. *Brit J Sports Med* 2008;42(3):212–216.
71. Lampert R, Olshansky B, Heidbuchel H, Lawless C, Saarel E, Ackerman M, *et al*. Safety of sports for athletes with implantable cardioverter-defibrillators: Results of a prospective, multinational registry. *Circulation* 2013;127:2021–2030.
72. Ackerman MJ, Tester DJ, Porter CJ. Swimming, a gene-specific arrhythmogenic trigger for inherited long QT syndrome. *Mayo Clin Proc* 1999;74:1088–1094.
73. Denoble PJ, Caruso JL, Dear Gde L, Pieper CF, Vann RD. Common causes of open-circuit recreational diving fatalities. *Undersea Hyperb Med* 2008;35(6):393–406.
74. Mebane GY, Low N, Dovenbarger J. A review of autopsies on recreational scuba divers: 1989–1992. *Undersea Hyperb Med* 1993;20:70.
75. Wilson PW, D'Agostino RB, Levy D, Belanger AM, Silbershatz H, Kannel WB. Prediction of coronary heart disease using risk factor categories. *Circulation* 1998;97:1837–1847.
76. Goff DC, Lloyd-Jones DM, Bennett G, Coady S, D'Agostino RB, *et al*. 2013 ACC/AHA guideline on the assessment of cardiovascular risk: A report of the American College of Cardiology/American Heart Association Task Force on Practice Guidelines. *J Am Coll Cardiol* 2014 Jul 1;63(25 Pt B):2935–2959.
77. Hiratzka LF, Bakris GL, Beckman JA, Bersin RM, *et al*. ACCF/AHA/AATS/ACR/ASA/SCA/SCAI/SIR/STS/SVM guidelines for the diagnosis and management of patients with thoracic aortic disease. *J Am Coll Cardiol* 2010;55(14):1509–1544.

78. Scott DH, Marks AD. Diabetes and Diving. In Bove AA (ed.), *Bove and Davis' Diving Medicine*. WB Philadelphia: Saunders, 2004:507–518.
79. Bove AA. Diving Medicine. *Am J Respir Crit Care Med* 2014;189(12):1479–1486.
80. Bove AA. *Bove and Davis' Diving Medicine*. 4th (ed.), Philadelphia: Elsevier, 2004.
81. Adir Y, Bove AA. Lung injury related to extreme environments. *Eur Respir Rev* 2014;23:416–426.

Chapter 10

Heat Stress and Illnesses in Athletes

Luke N. Belval*, William M. Adams[†], and Douglas J. Casa*

*Korey Stringer Institute, Department of Kinesiology
University of Connecticut Storrs, CT, USA
[†]Department of Kinesiology, University of North Carolina
at Greensboro, Greensboro, NC, USA

Introduction

Three causes account for the majority of sudden death cases in sport: cardiac conditions, head injuries, and exertional heat stroke (EHS). In fact, 85% of fatalities in high school and college football are attributed to these three causes alone.[1] While cardiac conditions are likely the overall leading cause of sudden death in sport, in certain situations, EHS can be the chief concern for the clinician.[2] American football practices, military training, and warm-weather running road races are the three most common of these instances where heat-related illnesses occur on a more regular basis, regularly eclipsing other catastrophic illnesses and injuries.[3–5] However, even outside of these situations, heat-related illnesses are a large concern for the athlete, since the physiological strain of exercising in the heat can defeat even the strongest athlete.[6] In the U.S. Armed Forces, heat stress was a primary or contributory cause for 33% of cardiac deaths during basic training from 1997–2001.[6]

Exertional heat illnesses (EHI) primarily occur in athletes due to a failure of the homeostatic mechanisms responsible for thermoregulation during exercise. This chapter will begin with an overview of the physiological stresses imposed upon athletes exercising in the heat and how different situations can lead to the failure of the body's protective mechanisms. This is followed by an examination of the major EHI, including their prevention, recognition, and treatment. Finally, considerations for cardiologists treating EHI and prescribing medications to athletes exercising in the heat are presented.

Physiological Challenges of Exercise in the Heat

The physiological processes that regulate homeostatic functions during exercise are further stressed when that activity occurs in a warm environment. It is estimated that the body during exercise is approximately 20% efficient meaning roughly one quarter of the energy used is converted for movement.[7] Therefore, 80% of the energy consumed is released as metabolic heat. Even in colder conditions, this amount of heat would lead to dangerous hyperthermia without dissipation from the body. Therefore, the body relies on several physiological and physical processes to dissipate this massive amount of heat produced and prevent unsafe increases in body temperature.

Principles of thermoregulation

The basic thermoregulatory processes in the body are modeled by the heat balance equation.[8] In essence, this equation states that heat storage within the body is equal to the difference of heat production and heat loss. More specifically the equation can be represented as:

$$S = M - (W \pm C \pm R \pm K \pm \text{Resp}),$$

where S is the amount of heat storage in the body, M is the metabolic rate of heat production, W is the work rate, C is convection, R is radiation, K is conduction, and Resp is respiration.[9] Of note is that convection, conduction, and radiation can either contribute to heat gain or heat loss depending on environmental conditions. When there is an excess production or gain of heat in the body that cannot be overcome by the methods of dissipation, body temperature will rise leading to tissue stress and potentially exertional heat illness.

Methods of heat gain

Metabolism is the primary mode of heat gain for the exercising individual. The magnitude of difference in heat produced at the level of the muscle can be a factor of 15–20 during intense exercise.[8] The principle driver in this significant increase in metabolic heat production is the intensity of the activity. For example, while sitting, a human expends approximately 112 W, which can be contrasted to competitive rowing which can yield a metabolic rate of 1,800 W.[10] This helps to explain why individuals can become severely hyperthermic, even in milder climates.

Methods of heat dissipation

While the main driver to heat gain in the body comes from one source, there are multiple methods by which the body dissipates heat. In general, the body's circulatory system is used to move heat from the body's core and exercising muscles to the skin where it can be released into the environment. The primary method for this dissipation in hot environmental conditions and exercise is the evaporation of sweat from the skin surface.[10] However, this process becomes limited by a small water vapor pressure gradient. Consequently, when the humidity is high or when there is no air flow around the body, there is too small a gradient for additional water to evaporate off the skin into the environment, resulting in no net heat loss.[8,11] It can be postulated that this may be part of the reason exertional heat stroke is common in the Southeast of the US, wherein high ambient temperatures are often combined with high humidities.[4]

Radiation or the exchange of energy through radiative emission accounts for minimal heat loss during exercise in the heat. However, radiative heat gains from sun light exposure can significantly contribute to heat gain.[11] It is for this reason that the Wet-Bulb Globe temperature (WBGT), one of the most commonly used measures of environmental heat stress, uses a black globe thermometer as a component.[9]

Convection, the exchange of heat through a fluid medium, is the secondary method of heat dissipation during exercise in the heat. The ability of the body to cool convectively is limited by the size of the temperature gradient with the direct environment of the skin surface.[11] Therefore in conditions where the ambient temperature exceeds the skin temperature, convection is not an effective method of heat removal. Conversely, one of the body's natural accommodations to exercise in the heat is an increase in cutaneous blood flow that increases skin temperature and delays the failure of this system.

The body's methods for heat loss rely on a direct interface with the environment. One of the factors that influences some of this cooling is air flow around the skin surface. In order for the body to effectively use convective and evaporative cooling, a constant air flow is necessary to limit the creation of a small area around the body that is significantly warmer or more humid than the environment.[12] This is partially the reason why it is unusual to become hyperthermic while cycling compared to running; during cycling there is a much higher rate of air flow, allowing for greater evaporation of sweat and convective cooling. In contrast, if you limit the capacity of the surrounding environment around the body to cool, heat stress is significantly greater. One common way that individuals create these micro-environments is through the use of protective equipment, such as American football equipment or nuclear, biological, and chemical (NBC) gear. Individuals in this gear are known to fatigue quicker and reach higher rectal temperatures during exercise than their minimally clothed counterparts.[13]

Exercise and hydration

The human body is largely (50–70%) made up of water (total body water) with variation being attributed to body composition; lean mass contains ~73% water and fat mass contains ~10% water. Furthermore, total body water is distributed into both intracellular (65%) and extracellular (35%) compartments. The extracellular compartment is further divided into interstitial and plasma spaces. To put these values into perspective, a 70 kg male has a total body water volume of ~42 L. The intracellular and extracellular compartments contain ~28 L and ~14 L of water, respectively. When fluid losses exceed fluid gain, the body undergoes the process of dehydration resulting in a state of hypohydration. Rehydration is the process of returning to a state of euhydration and, conversely, when fluid gain exceeds fluid loss the body enters a state of hyperhydration.[15]

Fluid balance, defined as the balance between water intake (beverages, food, and metabolic production) and water output (sweat, urine and fecal losses, and insensible losses), is adequately maintained in free-living persons with *ad libitum* fluid intake that is controlled via neuroendocrine and renal responses within the body.[16,17] During exercise, especially in hot environmental conditions, *ad libitum* intake of fluid is often not sufficient to maintain fluid balance and it is not uncommon for a disruption of fluid balance (water output exceeds water intake) to occur due to the large volumes of sweat lost and the inability to replace fluid during exercise.[18–20]

Fluid deficits during exercise as a result of exercise-induced dehydration have been purported to cause performance deficits and increase the relative risk of exertional heat illness. Fluid losses of 2% body mass (~3% of total body water) from dehydration have been shown to increase cardiovascular[19,21,22] and thermoregulatory strain.[23–25] Evidence has shown that for every 1% body mass loss, body temperature increases ~0.22°C[24,26,27] and heart rate (HR) increases by 3 beats·min^{-1}.[28] With dehydration, there is a reduction in plasma volume, which results in a concurrent reduction in skin blood flow[29–31] and sweat rate,[32] limiting the body's effectiveness in dissipating metabolically produced heat, thus contributing to the rise in body temperature.[33–35] Furthermore, as environmental conditions become hotter, physiological strain becomes more pronounced, further exacerbating cardiovascular and thermoregulatory strain.[21,36,37]

The insult to the cardiovascular and thermoregulatory systems from exercise-induced dehydration is implicated as a factor impairing exercise performance.[24,27,38–40] During exercise in the heat, performance deficits become more

	Exercise in the Heat	Exercise in the Heat (Heat Acclimatized)	Exercise in the Heat (Hypohydrated)
Exercising Heart Rate	↑	↓	↑↑
Sweat Rate	↑	↑↑	↓
Rise of Core Temperature	↑	↓	↑↑
Skin Blood Flow	↑	↑	↓
Plasma Volume	↓	↑	↓↓
Cardiac Output	↓	↑	↓↓
Overall Exercise Performance	↓	↑	↓↓

←→: Negligible Change, ↑: Small Change ↑↑: Moderate Change, ↑↑↑: Large Change

Figure 1. Physiological responses during exercise in the heat.

pronounced as levels of dehydration increase.[25,36,41,42] The performance deficits observed with dehydration are declines in endurance performance,[34,38,40] anaerobic performance,[39,43] strength,[39,43] power,[39,43] and cognitive function.[44,45] Declines in endurance performance and cognitive function occur with as little as 2–3% body mass loss, whereas anaerobic performance, strength, and power deficits begin to manifest at fluid losses equating to 3–4% body mass loss. The former is postulated to occur at lower levels of dehydration due to the exacerbation of cardiovascular strain during prolonged exercise. Figure 1 describes the physiological responses during exercise in the heat and factors that can positively or adversely affect these responses. Heat acclimatization improves one's ability to perform in the heat,[46] but hypohydration drastically reduces physiological function, regardless of acclimatization status.[47]

Exertional Heat Illnesses

Heat illnesses represent a spectrum of conditions ranging from mild (heat syncope) to life-threatening (heat stroke). When these illnesses occur in exercise situations they are termed exertional heat illnesses. Failure of the thermoregulatory system affects a wide variety of exercising individuals, including athletes, laborers, and soldiers. A common misconception is that these conditions occur across continuum, with a less severe precipitating a more severe heat illness.[48] Rather, heat stroke can occur without an episode of heat syncope. Therefore, clinicians must use sound evidence-based reasoning and decision making when evaluating a potential exertional heat illness.

The three most common heat illnesses are heat syncope, heat exhaustion, and exertional heat stroke. It should be noted that other minor heat illnesses exist beyond the scope of this chapter.[7] In addition, "heat cramps" or exercise-associated muscle cramps have an etiology that extends beyond the environmental heat stress that they have been linked to in the past.[49]

Heat syncope

Heat syncope, a fainting episode occurring with exposure to environmental heat stress, has been most commonly correlated with unfit, unacclimatized individuals during the initial stages of heat exposure.[49–51] While the cause of syncope is multi-factorial, heat syncope results from hypotension, upright posture, and pooling of blood in the extremities.[49,50]

During the initial stages of heat exposure (within the first few days), the body's cardiovascular system lacks the ability to fully adapt to the elevated environmental temperatures. The pooling of blood caused by skin vasodilation during exercise in the heat reduces the ability of blood to return to the heart, causing a decline in cardiac filling, cardiac output, blood pressure, and insufficient oxygen delivery to the brain resulting in a syncope episode.[50,51]

Heat syncope may also present with individuals complaining of dizziness, tunnel vision, and may exhibit signs/symptoms of dehydration, a decreased pulse rate, and pale and/or sweaty skin.[49] Once heat syncope has been diagnosed, individuals should be removed from the source of heat stress and the medical provider should raise the individual's legs from the ground to restore blood pressure and monitor vital signs.[49] Individuals suffering from heat syncope respond quickly to treatment and will oftentimes recover within a short period of time.

Heat exhaustion

Heat exhaustion is defined as one's inability to continue exercise in the heat due to cardiovascular insufficiency, hypotension, energy depletion, and central fatigue.[50,52] Heat exhaustion is the most common heat-related illness, especially in unacclimatized and dehydrated individuals.[53] Heat syncope and heat exhaustion represent ~80% of all cases of exertional heat illnesses.[50]

The physiological causes of heat exhaustion are fluid–electrolyte imbalances in conjunction with exercising heat stress resulting in circulatory dysfunction and dehydration. Heat exhaustion causes a reduction in extracellular fluid volume, reducing cardiac output and limiting the body's ability to provide adequate blood flow to both the working muscles and the skin to dissipate metabolically produced heat.[50] Associated signs and symptoms of heat exhaustion include hypotension, orthostatic intolerance, dizziness, syncope, fatigue or weakness, nausea, tachycardia, muscle incoordination, and minor cognitive changes (i.e. dizziness, headache, confusion).[49,50]

Key criteria of heat exhaustion that can be used to differentiate it from exertional heat stroke are an elevated body temperature <40.5°C [105°F], the absence of significant altered mental status, and normal hematologic markers.[49] Clinicians suspecting heat exhaustion should monitor cognitive changes and assess body temperature (via rectal thermometry) to rule out exertional heat stroke, since the latter requires life-saving measures to prevent mortality and morbidity.[49,53] For heat exhaustion, the individual should be removed from the source of heat stress (physical activity) and allowed to rest in a shaded area with legs elevated to promote venous blood return to the heart.[49,53] Clothing should be loosened or removed to enhance body cooling. Cooling modalities such as iced towels may also be used. Fluids should be provided to help restore body water losses.[49,53] With appropriate treatment, recovery is often complete within 24–48 h without subsequent sequelae.[50]

Heat stroke

Exertional heat stroke (EHS) is a life-threatening condition and the most severe of the exertional heat illnesses. EHS occurs during intense or prolonged exercise, whereas classical heat stroke typically occurs in the elderly and infants during heat waves. Without rapid treatment, EHS can cause life-long sequelae or death.[54]

Epidemiology

Due to the highly situation-specific nature of EHS, establishing a global incidence remains difficult. However, there are three predominant situations in which EHS occurs in relatively high volume: road races, American football preseason practices, and military training. Beyond these scenarios, EHS can occur in a wide variety of exercise settings and environmental conditions. Epidemiological data from high school athletics show that boys' football has the greatest incidence of exertional heat illnesses, by a factor of 2.3 compared to the next highest group.[55] In the US Military, there are a recorded 0.23 heat stroke diagnoses per 1,000 person-years across active armed forces.[56] Finally, representing the extreme of EHS situations, the Falmouth Road Race has documented 2.13 EHS cases per 1,000 runners.[57] While identifying an exact incidence may be elusive, the commonality of these situations illustrates the factors that contribute to the highest occurrence of EHS: high environmental temperatures in conjunction with intense exercise.

The specific risk factors for EHS can be divided into two groups: (1) intrinsic and (2) extrinsic risk factors.[49] Intrinsic risk factors consist of individual items that increase the risk of exertional heat illness for a particular person. The most common intrinsic risk factors for EHS are underlying illness (especially febrile), dehydration, sleep loss, medications, lack of fitness, lack of heat acclimatization, and excess body mass.[49,54] All of the above factors either contribute to precipitous heat gain or impair heat loss, increasing the likelihood of dangerous increases in body temperature.

Extrinsic risk factors represent the factors outside the body that increase the risk of EHS. Environmental conditions (ambient temperature, humidity), exercise in excess of fitness, lack of water or lack of rest, and excess clothing or equipment are the most commonly noted extrinsic contributors to EHS.[49,58,59] Notably, most of these factors are controllable on an individual or institutional level.

Intense environmental conditions are a common situation that precipitate EHS.[5] However, ambient temperature alone does not fully account for the environmental stress. The WBGT is commonly used to assess heat stress from the environment.[49] This aggregate temperature accounts for humidity, dry temperature, and radiant heat and can be used to adjust workloads, work-to-rest ratios, and exercise timing.[60] Specific guidelines have been created for a variety of situations, including American football, the military, and laborers.[53,61]

Prevention

Prevention of EHS relies on mitigation of both intrinsic and extrinsic risk factors. The most successful strategies are multi-faceted and require advance planning and communication. In the athletic setting this typically entails cooperation between the medical staff, coaches, and administration. Heat acclimatization, hydration guidelines and practices, activity modifications, and body cooling are the largest components of a successful prevention plan.[62,63]

Heat acclimatization is a physiological process that allows the body to better accommodate to exercise in the heat.[64,65] This process traditionally occurs over the course of 10–14 days of exposure to exercise heat stress. Physiological changes include plasma volume expansion, decreased body temperature and heart rate at a given exercise intensity, and an increased sweat rate in conjunction with a decrease in sweat sodium losses.[65,66] Figure 2 shows an example of NCAA American football guidelines for heat acclimatization that allows for gradual increases in exercise intensity, duration, and equipment.[49] Similar guidelines exist for high school athletics.[67]

As previously mentioned, an individual's hydration status has the ability to profoundly impact their ability to exercise in the heat. Fluid needs are highly individualistic with typical sweat losses ranging from less than 1 L/h to >2 L/h.[68] What may be inadequate and leading to hypohydration for one athlete could create severe hyponatremia, due to serum sodium dilution for another. Therefore, it is recommended that athletes develop individualized hydration plans based on their sweat rates and the exercising conditions. The simplest technique often employed is measuring body weight changes over a typical exercise session.[64,69]

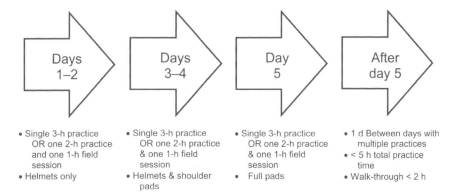

Figure 2.   NCAA heat-acclimatization guidelines. Taken from Ref. 49.

In many athletic situations, the environmental stressors can be easily modified through administrative controls. In even the most extreme environments, moving activities to either the early morning or evening can effectively decrease the risk of exertional heat illnesses.[49] In situations wherein activity cannot be delayed, increases in body temperature can be ameliorated by modifying work-to-rest ratio based on the WBGT to allow for hydration and body cooling interspersed with activity.[53,61]

The concept of body cooling before and during exercise is to lower the body temperature whenever possible to help offset rapid rises in body temperature that can occur during intense exercise.[70] It is common for elite athletes to cool right before competition or during organized breaks (e.g. half-time) in warm environmental conditions. There are a variety of techniques that can be used to varying success, including ice vests,[71] ice slurry,[72] and other more technical solutions.[64]

Policy changes to prevent heat illnesses

One of the key initiatives of the Korey Stringer Institute is to promote policy changes at the local, state, and national levels to prevent exertional heat illnesses. Heat acclimatization policies have been adopted in 8 states for high school athletics at the time this was written. Those states that have passed and followed these guidelines have had no deaths.[67] If previous trends had held true, approximately 20 athletes would have died in that time frame. This is an example of how policies can have a sweeping effect. Other policies that are recommended to minimize the risk of exertional heat illnesses are WBGT policies, coaching education, and emergency action plans. Details on the recommended policies can be found at ksi. uconn.edu.

Recognition

Recognition and diagnosis of EHS is dependent on two criteria: (1) deep body temperature >40.5°C and (2) central nervous system dysfunction.[49] There are a multitude of other signs and symptoms of EHS, (e.g. nausea, diarrhea, dehydration, tachycardia, hypotension, hyperventilation), however, definitive differentiation from other potential conditions can be determined by these two criteria.[73] In an exercising individual, rectal, esophageal, or gastrointestinal temperature are the only way to accurately assess deep body temperature.[74,75] However, due to the necessary patient compliance for esophageal temperature and the timing issues associated with gastrointestinal temperature, rectal temperature is the most widely accepted method to assess potential EHS.[47]

Figure 3 shows that the timing of this assessment can have profound impact on the outcome of an EHS. Animal models have demonstrated that survival from EHS is reliant on cooling the body within 30 min of the body temperature exceeding the threshold for critical cell damage (~40.5°C).[54] However, in many situations the time a patient initially becomes hyperthermic beyond this threshold and the time that they collapsed are not the same. Therefore, the time in which a clinician has to cool a patient may be much less than 30 min.[76]

Along with hyperthermia, CNS dysfunction is a hallmark of EHS. Presentations can range from minor mood changes to severe aggression.[77] It is not uncommon for a patient to become physically combative. In addition, a lucid interval may occur, wherein the patient is able to cognate fully only to deteriorate rapidly.[54] Due to the variation in CNS dysfunction, body temperature assessment can greatly assist clinical decision making.

Treatment

Survival of EHS is predicated upon rapid cooling. Prognosis from EHS is dependent on the total time the body is above the critical cell threshold, rather than the maximum temperature.[78] EHS is one of the few medical situations wherein transportation may be delayed if appropriate treatment (cooling) is available on site.[49] Figure 4 presents data from the Falmouth Road Race that demonstrates the effectiveness of rapid cooling on patient survival and disposition.[79] In this optimal situation, patients are triaged and immediately cooled upon confirmation of hyperthermia.[80] Based on this evidence, the overall goal of EHS care is to reduce body temperature to under 40.5°C within 30 min of collapse.[80,81]

Cold-water immersion has been coined the gold standard for EHS care. As demonstrated in Figure 5, the most superior cooling rates were associated with

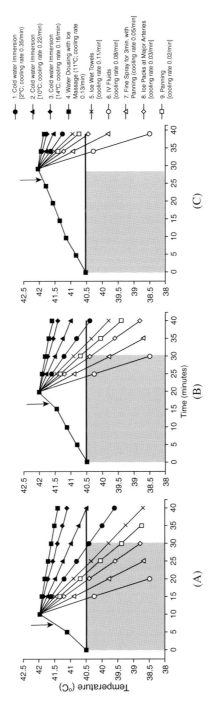

Figure 3. (A), (B), and (C). Three scenarios for EHS treatment where the shaded area indicates the 30-min window needed to cool the body to ensure survival and minimize long-term sequelae. The black line indicates a temperature measure just below the critical threshold. The arrows indicate the moment of recognition. (A) Optimal/immediate treatment, (B) Delayed treatment, (C) EHS recognition and treatment are absent.

Source: Taken from Ref. 78.

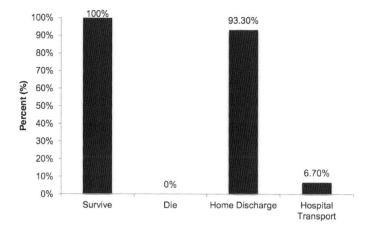

Figure 4.   Outcomes of 274 EHS with immediate rectal temperature assessment, on-site treatment using cold water immersion, and on-site physician clearance at the Falmouth Road Race. Adapted from Ref. 82.

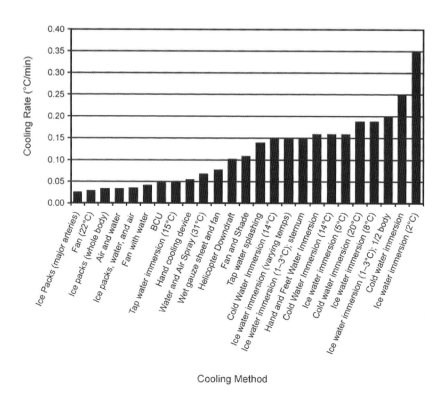

Figure 5.   Cooling rates associated with various modalities. Figure depicts experiments with healthy hyperthermic athletes and heatstroke victims. From Ref. 75.

either ice-water or cold-water immersion.[81] In situations where cold-water immersion is not readily available, water dousing, tarp-assisted cooling or rotating wet towels over the skin surface are the recommended treatments.[49,96,97]

Principally, heat stress alters the permeability of the intestinal wall, allowing for endotoxemia followed by systemic inflammatory response.[82,83] In cases where rapid cooling was not administered appropriately, liver and kidney damage are commonplace.[84,85]

Cardiac complications of heat stroke

Cardiac complications resulting from EHS are relatively rare and usually self-resolving for individuals cooled appropriately. However, several instances of cardiac related sequelae have been reported, primarily associated with direct thermal stress to the myocardium and a release of catecholamines during EHS.[86,87] This can present as S–T segment elevation, cardiac enzyme release, cardiogenic shock, and ventricular hypokinesis.[86,88] In one study, lactate dehydrogenase (LDH) elevation was present in 69% of EHS cases, with abnormal ECGs in 58% of cases, however, there is no mention of patient recovery.[88] A case study reported that an abnormal ECG indicating cardiomyopathy in an EHS patient was reversed by day 6.[88] Others observed cardiac hypokinesis that self-resolved in several days.[89] More research is needed to determine the exact cardiovascular complications of EHS, however, early evidence suggests that cardiac changes are reversible with appropriate treatment.

Rhabdomyolysis and exertional heat stroke

Rhabdomyolysis secondary to EHS is common due to both thermal and mechanical stress to the skeletal muscle.[90] The clinical course of non-complicated exertional rhabdomyolysis can aid in the understanding of the disease as a complication of heat stroke. Chemically, creatine kinase (CK) levels typically peak 48–96 h after injury with levels several 1,000-fold greater than normal. Normalization of CK levels is not an indication of recovery, but simply an indication that no further muscle damage is occurring.[91]

Return to play

Currently there are no evidence-based guidelines for return-to-activity following EHS so that return to activity guidelines are based primarily on anecdotes and case reports. Therefore, consensus recommendations are to await a complete resolution of clinical abnormalities followed by a return-to-play process that gradually introduces heat stress.[92,93] In addition, for individuals who have trouble returning to activity or who have had multiple EHS, heat tolerance testing may be indicated.[94]

Medications and heat illnesses

There are generally two types of medications that alter an individual's risk for EHI: (1) drugs that increase heat production or (2) drugs that inhibit heat loss.[94] Drugs, that raise metabolism or disturb skeletal muscle control either as an intended or side effect have the potential to precipitate dangerous rises in body temperature during exercise. In addition, illicit drugs like ecstasy or methamphetamine have been linked to dangerous rises in body temperature with minimal activity.[95]

There are two cardiac medications that clinicians should be aware of that may influence risk for exertional heat illnesses. Diuretics, due to the alterations in fluid balance, increase the risk of heat illness by producing dehydration.[82] In addition, beta-blockers alter skin blood flow which in turn may decrease the body's cooling capacity.[82]

Personal Perspective

Douglas J. Casa

Imagine this scene: We were driving on a rugged dirt road in the outback of Lackland Air Force Base outside of San Antonio, Texas, in late September. We kept driving, and driving, and driving. Eventually we made it to a remote training area where some of our most elite airmen train to protect our country. They are doing this for all of us, so we can have a safe country and the best opportunities.

The Air Force leadership had invited the Korey Stringer Institute (KSI) as a outside consultant to assess, educate, and train the members of the 559th Medical Group on managing exertional heat stroke (EHS) cases in remote settings that are common in military training. Previously, KSI had the privilege to provide this support for the US Army at Fort Benning, GA, and at Fort Bragg, NC, by interacting with an array of soldiers and special forces, including the Army Rangers. However, being in Lackland was different. This was not just an educational visit. They were seeking our expert opinions to revisit and update their policies that they implement at their training sites. Imagine a collapsed airman with EHS 9 mi from a medical station, with limited supplies and the clock ticking — and KSI is making the recommendation of what the best course of action would be to assure the airman's survival. This is not something that makes us nervous; in fact, we cherish this opportunity, and it is a chance to share our expertise to help protect the men and women who help protect us. It was the most professionally important moment of my life. As I (DJC) stood in this remote setting with my two colleagues from KSI, I realized that the tireless efforts since we created KSI are developing into an organization with great influence and opportunity.

Rewinding the time back to six weeks before the visit to Lackland, I was standing at the Falmouth Road Race medical tent in mid-August with a team of 35 people from KSI and 100 other volunteers who were working in the medical tent at the finish line. I know you are supposed to say that the day you get married or the birth of your first child should be the best day of your life, but for me it was this day. I am in charge of triage at the finish line medical tent and work under the direction of the two incredible medical directors (Drs. Robert Davis and John Jardine) and with the skilled direction of the medical coordinator (Chris Troyanos). Well, this was no average day at the office. We encountered 42 EHS (for real) and 55 heat exhaustion cases in the span of less than 2 h. We triaged at a rate of one case per minute, and the team worked in an impressive manner to assure rapid cooling for all patients. As a result, we saved every single EHS patient that was admitted to the medical tent. After the last patient was treated, I was truly exhausted but had never felt more useful in my life. It was a few hours later when I went for a swim in the ocean with two of my kids (who had also assisted in the medical tent) that I felt a satisfaction that I could never recapture. I was truly thankful to have made a difference, to be able to save the lives of runners who could have otherwise been in a critical condition after the race. It was in these two momentous events, in addition to many smaller ones leading to this point, I began to realize that I am beginning to pay back the 2nd chance I got at life when I survived my heat stroke 30 years ago. On August 8, 2015, I celebrated my 30th survival party at a beach in Montauk, NY, with my closest family and friends. The person who saved my life (Kent Scriber, ATC) was able to attend. As we stood on the beach talking that evening, I was smart enough to realize that the hand I had been dealt had been a royal straight flush (and playing poker is one of my favorite activities). From the amazing care for my EHS, loving parents, amazing colleagues at UCONN and KSI, and the family and friends that lift you toward a greater good, I am grateful for it all. I looked at my kids running on the beach and said, "Wow." I took a deep breath. Then I sat down, overwhelmed at what had transpired over the past 30 years (Pertinacity. Available at: http://opencommons. uconn.edu/pertinacity/4).

References

1. Boden BP, Breit I, Beachler JA, Williams A, Mueller FO. Fatalities in high school and college football players. *Am J Sports Med* 2013;41(5):1108–1116.
2. Yankelson L, Sadeh B, Gershovitz L, *et al.* Life-threatening events during endurance sports. *J Am Coll Cardiol* 2014;64(5):463–469.
3. Carter R III, Cheuvront SN, Williams JO, *et al.* Epidemiology of hospitalizations and deaths from heat illness in soldiers. *Med Sci Sport Exer* 2005;37(8):1338–1344.
4. Grundstein AJ, Ramseyer C, Zhao F, *et al.* A retrospective analysis of American football hyperthermia deaths in the United States. *Int J Biometeorol* 2012;56(1): 11–20.
5. Demartini JK, Casa DJ, Belval LN, *et al.* Environmental conditions and the occurrence of exertional heat illnesses and exertional heat stroke at the Falmouth Road Race. *J Athl Training* 2014;49(4):478–485.
6. Scoville SL, *et al.* Nontraumatic deaths during U.S. Armed Forces basic training, 1977–2001. *Am J Prev Med* 2004;26(3):205–212.
7. Armstrong, Lawrence E. Exertional Hearth Illnesses. Champaign, IL. Human Kinetics Publishers. Inc.; 2003.
8. Casa DJ. Exercise in the heat. I. Fundamentals of thermal physiology, performance implications, and dehydration. *J Athl Training* 1999;34(3):246.
9. Havenith, G. and Fiala, D. Thermal Indices and Thermophysiological Modeling for Heat Stress. *Comprehensative Physiology* 2015;6:255–302.
10. Höppe PR. Heat balance modelling. *Experientia* 1993;49(9):741–746.
11. Brotherhood JR. Heat stress and strain in exercise and sport. *J Sci Med Sport* 2008; 11(1):6–19.
12. Deren TM, Coris EE, Casa DJ, *et al.* Maximum heat loss potential is lower in football linemen during an NCAA summer training camp because of lower self-generated air flow. *J Strength Cond Res* 2014;28(6):1656–1663.
13. Armstrong LE, Johnson EC, Casa DJ, *et al.* The American football uniform: Uncompensable heat stress and hyperthermic exhaustion. *J Athl Training* 2010; 45(2):117–127.
14. Greenleaf J. Importance of fluid homeostasis for optimal adaptation to exercise and enviromental stess: Acceleration. *Perspecet Exer Sci Sports Med* 1990;3(9):309–346.
15. Armstrong LE, Epstein Y. Fluid-electrolyte balance during labor and exercise: Concepts and misconceptions. *Int J Sport Nutr* 1999;9(1):1–12.
16. Cheuvront SN, Kenefick RW. Dehydration: Physiology, assessment, and performance effects. *Compr Physiol* 2014;4(1):257–285.
17. Cheuvront SN, Kenefick RW, Charkoudian N, Sawka MN. Physiologic basis for understanding quantitative dehydration assessment. *Am J Clinical Nutrition* 2013; 97(3):455–462.
18. Noakes TD. Fluid replacement during exercise. *Exercise Sport Sci R* 1993; 21(1):297–330.

19. González-Alonso J, Mora Rodriguez R, Below PR, Coyle EF. Dehydration reduces cardiac output and increases systemic and cutaneous vascular resistance during exercise. *J Appl Physiol* 1995;79(5):1487–1496.

20. Cheuvront SN, Haymes EM. Ad libitum fluid intakes and thermoregulatory responses of female distance runners in three environments. *J Sport Sci* 2001;19(11):845–854.

21. González-Alonso J, Mora Rodriguez R, Coyle EF. Stroke volume during exercise: Interaction of environment and hydration. *Am J Physiol Heart C* 2000;278(2): H321–H330.

22. Montain SJ, Sawka MN, Latzka WA, Valeri CR. Thermal and cardiovascular strain from hypohydration: Influence of exercise intensity. *Int J Sports Med* 1998;19(2):87–91.

23. Sawka MN, Montain SJ, Latzka WA. Hydration effects on thermoregulation and performance in the heat. *Com Biochem Phys A* 2001;128(4):679–690.

24. Montain SJ, Coyle EF. Influence of graded dehydration on hyperthermia and cardiovascular drift during exercise. *J Appl Physiol* 1992;73(4):1340–1350.

25. Buono MJ, Wall AJ. Effect of hypohydration on core temperature during exercise in temperate and hot environments. *Pflüg Arch Eur J Physiol* 2000;440(3):476–480.

26. Sawka MN, Young AJ, Francesconi RP, Muza SR, Pandolf KB. Thermoregulatory and blood responses during exercise at graded hypohydration levels. *J Appl Physiol* 1985;59(5):1394–1401.

27. González-Alonso J, Mora Rodriguez R, Below PR, Coyle EF. Dehydration markedly impairs cardiovascular function in hyperthermic endurance athletes during exercise. *J Appl Physiol* 1997;82(4):1229–1236.

28. Adams WM, Ferraro EM, Huggins RA, Casa DJ. The influence of body mass loss on changes in heart rate during exercise in the heat: A systematic review. *J Strength Cond Res* 2014;28(8):2380–2389.

29. Nadel ER, Fortney SM, Wenger CB. Effect of hydration state of circulatory and thermal regulations. *J Appl Physiol* 1980;49(4):715–721.

30. Sawka MN, Cheuvront SN, Kenefick RW. High skin temperature and hypohydration impairs aerobic performance. *Exp Physiol* 2012;97(3):327–332.

31. Cheuvront SN, Kenefick RW, Montain SJ, Sawka MN. Mechanisms of aerobic performance impairment with heat stress and dehydration. *J Appl Physiol* 2010;109(6): 1989–1995.

32. Montain SJ, Latzka WA, Sawka MN. Control of thermoregulatory sweating is altered by hydration level and exercise intensity. *J Appl Physiol* 1995;79(5):1434–1439.

33. Coyle EF. Physiological determinants of endurance exercise performance. *J Sci Med Sport* 1999;2(3):181–189.

34. Armstrong LE, Costill DL, Fink WJ. Influence of diuretic-induced dehydration on competitive running performance. *Med Sci Sport Exer* 1985;17(4):456–461.

35. Coyle EF, Montain SJ. Thermal and cardiovascular responses to fluid replacement during exercise. *Perspect Exer Sci Sports Med* 1990;6:179–223.

36. Coyle EF, González-Alonso J. Cardiovascular drift during prolonged exercise: New perspectives. *Exercise Sport Sci R* 2001;29(2):88–92.

37. Ganio MS, Wingo JE, Carrolll CE, Thomas MK, Cureton KJ. Fluid ingestion attenuates the decline in VO$_2$ peak associated with cardiovascular drift. *Med Sci Sport Exerc* 2006;38(5):901–909.

38. Casa DJ, Stearns RL, Lopez RM, *et al*. Influence of hydration on physiological function and performance during trail running in the heat. *J Athl Training* 2010;45(2): 147–156.

39. Judelson DA, Maresh CM, Anderson JM, *et al*. Hydration and muscular performance: Does fluid balance affect strength, power and high-intensity endurance? *Sports Med* 2007;37(10):907–921.

40. Lopez RM, Casa DJ, Jensen KA, *et al*. Examining the influence of hydration status on physiological responses and running speed during trail running in the heat with controlled exercise intensity. *J Strength Cond Res* 2011;25(11):2944–2954.

41. Kenefick RW, Cheuvront SN, Palombo LJ, Ely BR, Sawka MN. Skin temperature modifies the impact of hypohydration on aerobic performance. *J Appl Physiol* 2010;109(1):79–86.

42. González-Alonso J, Teller C, Andersen SL, Jensen FB, Hyldig T, Nielsen B. Influence of body temperature on the development of fatigue during prolonged exercise in the heat. *J Appl Physiol* 1999;86(3):1032–1039.

43. Judelson DA, Maresh CM, Farrell MJ, *et al*. Effect of hydration state on strength, power, and resistance exercise performance. *Med Sci Sport Exer* 2007;39(10): 1817–1824.

44. Lieberman HR, Bathalon GP, Falco CM, Kramer FM, Morgan CA, Niro P. Severe decrements in cognition function and mood induced by sleep loss, heat, dehydration, and undernutrition during simulated combat. *Biol Psychiat* 2005;57(4): 422–429.

45. Benton D. Dehydration influences mood and cognition: A plausible hypothesis? *Nutrients* 2011;3(5):555–573.

46. Nielsen B, Hales JR, Strange S, Christensen NJ, Warberg J, Saltin B. Human circulatory and thermoregulatory adaptations with heat acclimation and exercise in a hot, dry environment. *J Physiol* 1993;460:467–485.

47. Sawka MN, Latzka WA, Matott RP, Montain SJ. Hydration effects on temperature regulation. *Int J Sports Med* 1998;19:S108–S110.

48. Lopez RM, lop. Do exertional heat illnesses occur in a continuum or can they occur independently of each other? *Quick Questions in Heat-Related Illness and Hydration*, Thorofare, NJ: SLACK Incorporated, 2015;(10).

49. Casa DJ, Demartini JK, Bergeron MF, *et al*. National athletic trainers' association position statement: Exertional heat illnesses. *J Athl Training* 2015;50(9):986–1000.

50. Armstrong LE, Johnson EC, Casa DJ, *et al*. The American football uniform: Uncompensable heat stress and hyperthermic exhaustion. *J Athl Training*, Champaign, IL: Human Kinetics Publishers. Inc., 2010;45(2):117–127.

51. Knochel JP. Environmental heat illness. An eclectic review. *Arch Intern Medi* 1974;133(5):841–864.

52. Nybo L, Rasmussen P, Sawka MN. Performance in the heat-physiological factors of importance for hyperthermia-induced fatigue. *Compr Physiol* 2014;4(2):657–689.

53. Armstrong LE, Casa DJ, Millard-Stafford ML, Moran DS, Pyne SW, Roberts WO. Exertional heat illness during training and competition. *Med Sci Sport Exer* 2007;39(3):556–572.

54. Casa DJ, Armstrong LE, Kenny GP, O'Connor FG, Huggins RA. Exertional heat stroke: New concepts regarding cause and care. *Curr Sports Med Rep* 2012;11(3): 115–123.

55. Kerr ZY, Casa DJ, Marshall SW, Comstock RD. Epidemiology of exertional heat illness among. *Am J Prev Med* 2013;44(1):8–14.

56. Armed Forces Health Surveillance Center (AFHSC). Update: Heat injuries, active component, U.S. Armed Forces, 2013. *Medical Surveillance Monthly Report* 2014; 21(3):10–13.

57. Demartini JK, Martschinske JL, Casa DJ, *et al.* Physical demands of National Collegiate Athletic Association Division I football players during preseason training in the heat. *J Strength Cond Res* 2011;25(11):2935–2943.

58. Goforth CW, Kazman JB. Exertional heat stroke in navy and marine personnel: A hot topic. *Crit Care Nurse* 2015;35(1):52–59.

59. Rav-Acha M, Hadad E, Epstein Y, Heled Y, Moran DS. Fatal exertional heat stroke: A case series. *Am J Med Sci* 2004;328(2):84–87.

60. Budd GM. Wet-bulb globe temperature (WBGT)—its history and its limitations. *J Sci Med Sport* 2008;11(1):20–32.

61. Grundstein A, Williams C, Phan M, Cooper E. Regional heat safety thresholds for athletics in the contiguous United States. *Appl Geogr* 2015;56:55–60.

62. Roberts WO. Determining a 'Do Not Start' Temperature for a marathon on the basis of adverse outcomes. *Med Sci Sport Exer* 2010;42(2):226–232.

63. Kerr ZY, Marshall SW, Comstock RD, Casa DJ. Exertional heat stroke management strategies in United States high school football. *Am J Sports Med* 2014;42(1): 70–77.

64. Pryor RR, Casa DJ, Adams WM, *et al.* Maximizing athletic performance in the heat. *Strength Condi J* 2013;35(6):24–33.

65. Armstrong LE, Maresh CM. The induction and decay of heat acclimatisation in trained athletes. *Sports Med* 1991;12(5):302–312.

66. Horowitz M. Heat acclimation, epigenetics, and cytoprotection memory. *Compr Physiol* 2014;4(1):199–230.

67. Casa DJ, Csillan D. Preseason heat-acclimatization guidelines for secondary school athletics. *J Athl Training* 2009;44(3):332.

68. Shirreffs SM, Armstrong LE, Cheuvront SN. Fluid and electrolyte needs for preparation and recovery from training and competition. *J Sports Sci* 2004;22(1):57–63.

69. Armstrong LE, Casa DJ. Methods to evaluate electrolyte and water turnover of athletes. *Athl Train Sports Health Care* 2009;1(4):169–179.

70. Bongers CCWG, Thijssen DHJ, Veltmeijer MTW, Hopman MTE, Eijsvogels TMH. Precooling and percooling (cooling during exercise) both improve performance in the heat: A meta-analytical review. *Brit J Sport Med* 2014;49(6):377–384.

71. Webster J, Holland EJ, Sleivert G, Laing RM, Niven BE. A light-weight cooling vest enhances performance of athletes in the heat. *Ergonomics* 2005;48(7):821–837.

72. Ihsan M, Landers G, Brearley MB, Peeling P. Beneficial effects of ice ingestion as a precooling strategy on 40-km cycling time-trial performance. *Int J Sports Physiol Perform* 2010;5(2):140–151.

73. Casa DJ. Preventing sudden death in sport and physical activity. 2011:367.

74. Ganio MS, Brown CM, Casa DJ, *et al*. Validity and reliability of devices that assess body temperature during indoor exercise in the heat. *J Athl Training* 2009;44(2): 124–135.

75. Casa DJ, Becker SM, Ganio MS, *et al*. Validity of devices that assess body temperature during outdoor exercise in the heat. *J Athl Training* 2007;42(3):333.

76. Adams WM, Hosokawa Y, Casa DJ. The timing of exertional heat stroke survival starts prior to collapse. *Curr Sports Med Rep* 2015;14(4):273–274.

77. Casa DJ, Armstrong LE, Ganio MS, Yeargin SW. Exertional heat stroke in competitive athletes. *Curr Sports Med Rep* 2005;4(6):309–317.

78. Hubbard RW, Bowers WD, Matthew WT, *et al*. Rat model of acute heatstroke mortality. *J Appl Physiol* 1977;42(6):809–816.

79. Hosokawa Y, Adams WM, Stearns RL. Heat stroke in physical activity and sports. *Pensar en Movimiento* 2014;12(2):1–21.

80. Demartini JK, Casa DJ, Stearns R, *et al*. Effectiveness of cold water immersion in the treatment of exertional heat stroke at the falmouth road race. *Med Sci Sports Exer* 2015;47(2):240–245.

81. Casa DJ, McDermott BP, Lee EC, Yeargin SW, Armstrong LE, Maresh CM. Cold water immersion: The gold standard for exertional heatstroke treatment. *Exer Sport Sci Rev* 2007;35(3):141–149.

82. Leon LR, Bouchama A. Heat stroke. *Compr Physiol* 2015;5(2):611–647.

83. Epstein Y, Roberts WO. The pathopysiology of heat stroke: An integrative view of the final common pathway. *Scand J Med Sci Spor* 2011;21(6):742–748.

84. Yudis M, Reid JW, Burd RM. Acute renal failure complicating heatstroke: Case report. *Mil Med* 1971;136(12):884–887.

85. Kew M, Bersohn I, Seftel H, Kent G. Liver damage in heatstroke. *Am J Med* 1970;49(2):192–202.

86. Wakino S, Hori S, Mimura T, Miyatake S, Fujishima S, Aikawa N. A case of severe heat stroke with abnormal cardiac findings. *Int Heart J* 2005;46(3):543–550.

87. Kew MC, Tucker RBK, Bersohn I, Seftel HC. The heart in heatstroke. *Am Heart J* 1969;77(3):324–335.

88. Chen W-T, Lin C-H, Hsieh M-H, Huang C-Y, Yeh J-S. Stress-induced cardiomyopathy caused by heat stroke. *Ann Emerg Med* 2012;60(1):63–66.

89. Atar S, Rozner E, Rosenfeld T. Transient cardiac dysfunction and pulmonary edema in exertional heat stroke. *Mil Med* 2003;168(8):671–673.

90. Capacchione JF, Muldoon SM. The relationship between exertional heat illness, exertional rhabdomyolysis, and malignant hyperthermia. *Anesth Analg* 2009;109(4): 1065–1069.

91. Szczepanik ME, Heled Y, Capacchione J, Campbell W, Deuster P, O'Connor FG. Exertional rhabdomyolysis: Identification and evaluation of the athlete at risk for recurrence. *Curr Sports Med Rep* 2014;13(2):113–119.

92. O'Connor FG, Casa DJ, Bergeron MF, *et al.* American college of sports medicine roundtable on exertional heat stroke — return to duty/return to play. Conf Proc. *Curr Sports Med Rep* 2010;9(5):314–321.

93. McDermott BP, Casa DJ, Yeargin SW, Ganio MS, Armstrong LE, Maresh CM. Recovery and return to activity following exertional heat stroke: Considerations for the sports medicine staff. *J Sport Rehabil* 2007;16(3):163–181.

94. Ben Kazman J, Heled Y, Lisman PJ, Druyan A, Deuster PA, O'Connor FG. Exertional heat illness: The role of heat tolerance testing. *Curr Sports Med Rep* 2013;12(2): 101–105.

95. Clark WG, Lipton JM. Drug-related heatstroke. *Pharmacol Therapeut* 1984;26(3): 345–388.

96. Hosokawa Y, Vandermark LW, Belval LN, Casa DJ. Tarp-assisted cooling as an alternative method of whole body cooling in hyperthermic individuals. *Annals Emerg Med* 2017;69(3):347–352.

97. Luhring KE, Butts CL, Smith CR, *et al.* Cooling effectiveness of a modified cold-water immersion method after exercise-induced hyperthermia. *J Athl Train* 2016;51(11):946–951. doi:10.4085/1062-6050-51.12.07.

Index